13

CURRENT CLINICAL TOPICS IN INFECTIOUS DISEASES

13

CURRENT CLINICAL TOPICS IN INFECTIOUS DISEASES

Edited by

JACK S. REMINGTON, MD

Professor of Medicine
Division of Infectious Diseases and Geographic Medicine
Stanford University School of Medicine

Marcus A. Krupp Research Chair and
Chairman, Department of Immunology
and Infectious Diseases, Research Institute
Palo Alto Medical Foundation

MORTON N. SWARTZ, MD

Professor of Medicine
Harvard Medical School

Chief, James Jackson Firm
Medical Services
Massachusetts General Hospital
Infectious Disease Unit
Massachusetts General Hospital

BLACKWELL SCIENTIFIC PUBLICATIONS
Boston   Oxford   London   Edinburgh   Melbourne   Berlin   Paris   Vienna

**Blackwell Scientific Publications
Editorial offices:**
238 Main Street, Cambridge, Massachusetts
02142, USA
Osney Mead, Oxford OX2 0EL, England
25 John Street, London WC1N 2BL, England
23 Ainslie Place, Edinburgh EH3 6AJ, Scotland
54 University Street, Carlton, Victoria 3053,
Australia
Arnette SA, 2 rue Casimir-Delavigne, 75006
Paris, France
Blackwell-Wissenschaft, Meinekestrasse 4, D-1000
Berlin 15, Germany
Blackwell MZV, Feldgasse 13, A-1238 Vienna,
Austria

Distributors:
USA
  Blackwell Scientific Publications
  238 Main Street
  Cambridge, Massachusetts 02142
  (Telephone orders: 800-759-6102 or
    617-876-7000)
Canada
  Times Mirror Professional Building
  130 Flaska Drive
  Markham, Ontario L6G 1B8
  (Telephone orders: 800-268-4178 or
    416-470-6739)
Australia
  Blackwell Scientific Publications
    (Australia) Pty Ltd
  54 University Street
  Carlton, Victoria 3053
  (Telephone orders: 03-347-5552 or
    03-347-0300)
Outside North America and Australia:
  Blackwell Scientific Publications, Ltd.
  c/o Marston Book Services, Ltd.
  P.O. Box 87
  Oxford OX2 0DT
  England
  (Telephone orders: 44-865-791155)

Typeset by Huron Valley Graphics, Inc.
Printed and bound by Braun-Brumfield, Inc.

**Library of Congress Cataloging in
  Publication Data**
The Library of Congress has catalogued this serial
publication as follows:
Current clinical topics in infectious diseases.
1-
  New York. McGraw-Hill Book Co.,
  © 1980–1988
  Boston, Blackwell Scientific Publications,
  © 1989–
  v. ill. 25 cm.
  Annual
  Key title: Current clinical topics in
  infectious diseases, ISSN 0195-3842.
  I. Communicative diseases—
  Periodicals.
  DNLM: 1. Communicable Diseases—
  Periodicals. W 1 CU786T
RC111.C87   616.9′05
  80-643590
ISBN 0-86542-278-8

To our fellows

Contents

Preface

As literature in the field of infectious diseases has increased in complexity and volume, a need has become evident for timely, concise summaries and critical commentaries on subjects pertinent to the student and practitioner of medicine, the specialist in infectious diseases, and those in allied fields. It is our intention that this series provide the reader with a true update of information in very specific areas of infectious diseases which require reevaluation.

Each author was requested to confine his/her chapter to a relatively narrow subject, to deal with only contemporary questions and problems, to gather and synthesize the information on recent advances which is often spread diffusely among numerous journals, to offer critical evaluation of this information, to place the information into perspective by defining its present status, and to point out deficiencies in the information and thereby indicate directions for further study. All of this was to be done within the most rigid deadlines to ensure that the chapters be written and published in less than a year. We are extremely grateful to the contributing authors, each of whom is a recognized authority in the particular field, for consenting to undertake such an admittingly difficult task.

Current Clinical Topics in Infectious Diseases: 13 is the thirteenth volume of a series which is published annually. Each text in the series consists of updates of a variety of subjects covering the wide scope of clinical infectious disease problems, including bacteriology, mycology, virology, parasitology, and epidemiology.

JACK S. REMINGTON
MORTON N. SWARTZ

Contributors

Gerald P. Bodey, MD
Professor of Medicine, Chairman, Department of Medical Specialties, Chief, Section of Infectious Diseases, The University of Texas M.D. Anderson Cancer Center, Houston, Texas

Samuel A. Bozzette, MD
Assistant Clinical Professor of Medicine, Division of Infectious Diseases, Department of Medicine, University of California, San Diego School of Medicine, The Health Sciences Program, Department of Social Policy, The Rand Corporation, San Diego, California

Laurence J. Cibley, MD
Assistant Clinical Professor of Obstetrics and Gynecology, Boston University School of Medicine; Co-Director, Colposcopy Clinic and Director, Vulvo-vaginitis Clinic, Boston City Hospital, Boston, Massachusetts

Dennis A. Clements, MD, PhD
Department of Pediatrics, Duke University Medical Center, Durham, North Carolina

Dieter R. Enzmann, MD
Professor, Department of Radiology, Stanford University School of Medicine, Stanford, California

Patricia M. Griffin, MD
Assistant Chief, Enteric Diseases Epidemiology Branch, Division of Bacterial and Mycotic Diseases, National Center for Infectious Diseases, Centers for Disease Control, Atlanta, Georgia

Dennis M. Israelski, MD
Clinical Assistant Professor, Department of Medicine, Division of Infectious Diseases, Stanford University School of Medicine; Chief of Infectious Diseases, San Mateo County General Hospital, San Mateo, California

Paul Kamitsuka, MD
Instructor of Medicine, Harvard Medical School; Chief, Infectious Diseases Unit, Brockton West Roxbury VA Medical Center, West Roxbury, Massachusetts

Samuel L. Katz, MD
Wilburt C. Davison Professor of Medicine, Department of Pediatrics, Duke University School of Medicine, Durham, North Carolina

Michael R. Keating, MD
Assistant Professor of Medicine, Mayo Medical School; Consultant, Division of Infectious Diseases, Department of Internal Medicine, Mayo Clinic, Rochester, Minnesota

Daniel R. Kuritzkes, MD
Assistant Professor of Medicine, Microbiology and Immunology, Division of Infectious Diseases, University of Colorado Health Sciences Center, Denver, Colorado

John M. Leedom, MD
Hastings Professor of Medicine; Chief, Division of Infectious Diseases, Department of Medicine, University of Southern California School of Medicine and Los Angeles County/USC Medical Center, Los Angeles, California

James M. Maguire, MD
Associate Professor of Medicine, Harvard Medical School; Associate Professor in Tropical Public Health, Harvard School of Public Health, Clinical Director, Division of Infectious Disease, Brigham & Women's Hospital, Boston, Massachusetts

Elizabeth J. McFarland, MD
Instructor in Pediatrics, Division of Pediatric Infectious Diseases, University of Colorado Health Sciences Center, Denver, Colorado

Charles N. Oster, MD
Associate Professor, Uniformed Services, University of the Health Sciences; Chief, Infectious Diseases Service, Walter Reed Army Medical Center, Washington

Julie Parsonnet, MD
Assistant Professor of Medicine, Division of Infectious Diseases and Geographic Medicine, Department of Medicine, Stanford University School of Medicine, Stanford, California

Kenneth V.I. Rolston, MD
Associate Professor of Medicine, Department of Medical Specialties, Section of Infectious Diseases, University of Texas M.D. Anderson Cancer Center, Houston, Texas

Jack S. Remington, MD
Professor of Medicine, Division of Infectious Diseases and Geographic Medicine, Stanford University School of Medicine; Marcus A. Krupp Research Chair, Chairman, Department of Immunology and Infectious Diseases, Research Institute, Palo Alto Medical Foundation, Palo Alto, California

Peter A. Rice, MD
Professor of Medicine, Boston University School of Medicine; Chief, Infectious Diseases, Director, The Maxwell Finland Laboratory for Infectious Diseases, Boston City Hospital, Boston, Massachusetts

Judith Steinberg, MD
Assistant Professor of Medicine, Boston University School of Medicine, Assistant Visiting Physician, Medical Co-Director, Sexually Transmitted Disease Clinic, Boston City Hospital, Boston, Massachusetts

Alan M. Sugar, MD
Associate Professor of Medicine, Boston University School of Medicine, Evans Memorial Department of Clincal Research and Department of Medicine, The University Hospital, Thorndike Memorial Laboratory, Department of Medicine, Boston City Hospital, Boston, Massachusetts

Edmund C. Tramont, MD
Professor, Director, Medical Biotechnology Center, University of Maryland Institute, Baltimore, Maryland

Arvid E. Underman, MD, FACP
Clinical Professor of Medicine and Microbiology, University of Southern California School of Medicine, Los Angeles, California; Assistant Director, Internal Medicine Residency, Huntington Memorial Hospital, Pasadena, California

Michael E. Weiss, MD
Assistant Clinical Professor of Medicine, Division of Allergy, University of Washington School of Medicine, Redmond Medical Center, Seattle, Washington

Mark P. Wilhelm, MD
Assistant Professor of Medicine, Mayo Medical School; Consultant, Division of Infectious Diseases, Department of Internal Medicine, Mayo Clinic, Rochester, Minnesota

Ray C. Williams, DMD
Associate Director and Head, Department of Periodontology, Associate Dean for Postdoctoral Education, Harvard School of Dental Medicine, Boston, Massachusetts

Drew J. Winston, MD
Associate Clinical Professor of Medicine, Division of Hematology and Oncology, UCLA Medical Center, Center for the Health Sciences, Department of Medicine, Los Angeles, California

Other Volumes in the Series

CURRENT CLINICAL TOPICS IN INFECTIOUS DISEASES 1

The Role of CT Scanning in Diagnosis of Infections of the Central Nervous System
Staphylococcus aureus Bacteremia
Cytomegalovirus Infection in Transplant and Cancer Patients
Diagnosis and Management of Meningitis Due to Gram-Negative Bacilli in Adults
Infection Prevention during Granulocytopenia
Infant Botulism
The Role of Surgery in Infective Endocarditis
Treatment of Bacterial Infections of the Eye
Giardiasis: The Rediscovery of an Ancient Pathogen
Legionnaires' Disease
Antibiotic-Associated Diarrhea
Antibiotic-Resistant Pneumococci
The Cancer Patient with Fever and Pulmonary Infiltrates: Etiology and Diagnostic Approach
Q Fever: An Update

CURRENT CLINICAL TOPICS IN INFECTIOUS DISEASES 2

Acute Epiglottitis, Laryngitis, and Croup
Urinary Tract Infections in the Female: A Perspective
Treatment of Cryptococcal, Candidal, and Coccidiodal Meningitis
Bacteriology, Clinical Spectrum of Disease, and Therapeutic Aspects in Coryneform Bacterial Infection
Rocky Mountain Spotted Fever: A Clinical Dilemma
The Doctor's Dilemma: Have I Chosen the Right Drug? An Adequate Dose Regimen? Can Laboratory
    Tests Help in My Decision?
Shock in Gram-Negative Bacteremia: Predisposing Factors, Pathophysiology, and Treatment
The Management of Patients with Mycotic Aneurysm
A Review of the "New" Bacterial Strains Causing Diarrhea
Endocarditis Complicating Parenteral Drug Abuse
The Cephalosporins and Cephamycins: A Perspective
The Diagnosis and Treatment of Gangrenous and Crepitant Cellulitis
Management of Acute and Chronic Otitis Media

CURRENT CLINICAL TOPICS IN INFECTIOUS DISEASES 3

Sexually Transmitted Enteric Disease
Nucleoside Derivatives and Interferons as Antiviral Agents

Prophylaxis and Treatment of Malaria
Guillain-Barré Syndrome
Newer Antifungal Agents and their Use, Including an Update on Amphotericin B and Flucytosine
Role of Ultrasound and Computed Tomography in the Diagnosis and Treatment of Intraabdominal
    Abscess
Treatment of Infections Due to Atypical Mycobacteria
Combination of Single Drug Therapy for Gram-Negative Sepsis
Deep Infections Following Total Hip Replacement
Treatment of the Child with Bacterial Meningitis
Diagnosis and Management of Meningitis Associated with Cerebrospinal Fluid Leaks
Prophylactic Antibiotics for Bowel Surgery
Infections Associated with Intravascular Lines
Diagnosis and Treatment of Cutaneous Leishmaniasis
Candida Endophthalmitis

CURRENT CLINICAL TOPICS IN INFECTIOUS DISEASES 4

Diagnosis and Management of Septic Arthritis
Kawasaki's Disease
A Critical Review of the Role of Oral Antibiotics in the Management of Hematogenous Osteomyelitis
When Can the Infected Hospital Employee Return to Work?
Endocardiography and Infectious Endocarditis
Orbital Infections
The Use of White Blood Cell Scanning Techniques in Infectious Disease
Antimicrobial Prophylaxis in the Immunosuppressed Cancer Patient
The Diagnosis of Fever Occurring in a Postpartum Patient
Management at Delivery of Mother and Infant When Herpes Simplex, Varicella-Zoster, Hepatitis, or
    Tuberculosis Have Occurred during Pregnancy
"Nonspecific Vaginitis," Vulvovaginal Candidiasis, and Trichomoniasis: Clinical Features, Diagnosis and
    Management
Radionuclide Imaging in the Management of Skeletal Infections
Comparison of Methods for Clinical Quantitation of Antibiotics
What is the Clinical Significance of Tolerance to β-lactam Antibiotics?
A Critical Comparison of the Newer Aminoglycosidic Aminocyclitol
The Third Generation Cephalosporins

CURRENT CLINICAL TOPICS IN INFECTIOUS DISEASES 5

Prostatitis Syndromes
Staphylococcus epidermidis: The Organism, Its Diseases, and Treatment
Management of Nocardia Infections
Current Issues in Toxic Shock Syndrome
Isolation and Management of Contagious, Highly Lethal Diseases
Nutrition and Infection
Infections Associated with Hemodialysis and Chronic Peritoneal Dialysis
New Perspectives on the Epstein-Barr Virus in the Pathogenesis of Lymphoproliferative Disorders
Staphyloccal Teichoic Acid Antibodies
Current Status of Granulocyte Transfusion Therapy
Infections Associated With Intrauterine Devices
Hospital Epidemiology: An Emerging Discipline
The Viridans Streptococci in Perspective
Current Status of Prophylaxis for Haemophilus influenzae Infections
Acute Rheumatic Fever: Current Concepts and Controversies

CURRENT CLINICAL TOPICS IN INFECTIOUS DISEASES 6

The Acquired Immunodeficiency Syndrome
Health Advice and Immunizations for Travelers

CURRENT CLINICAL TOPICS IN INFECTIOUS DISEASES 10

Genital Herpes and the Pregnant Woman
Home Management of Antibiotic Therapy
Serum Bactericidal Test: Past, Present and Future Use in the Management of Patients with Infections
Lyme Borreliosis
The Role of MR Imaging in the Diagnosis of Infections of the Central Nervous System
Imipenem and Aztreonam: Current Role in Antimicrobial Therapy
Progressive Multifocal Leukoencephalopathy
Campylobacter pylori: Its Role in Gastritis and Peptic Ulcer Disease
Nucleic Acid Probes in Infectious Diseases
Norfloxacin, Ciprofloxacin, and Ofloxacin: Current Clinical Roles
Liposomes in Infectious Disease: Present and Future
Antibiotic Prophylaxis: Non-abdominal Surgery
Prevention of *Haemophilus influenzae* type b Disease: Vaccines and Passive Prophylaxis

CURRENT CLINICAL TOPICS IN INFECTIOUS DISEASES 11

The Chlamydial Pneumonias
Human Immunodeficiency Virus (HIV)-Associated Pneumocystosis
Fever of Unknown Origin-Reexamined and Redefined
Echinococcal Disease
The Epidemiology of AIDS: A Decade of Experience
Antibiotic Resistance Among Enterococci: Current Problems and Management Strategies
Intraocular Infections: Current Therapeutic Approach
Bronchiectatis: A Current View
Infection of Burn Wounds: Evaluation and Management
Colonic Diverticulitis: Microbiologic, Diagnostic, and Therapeutic Considerations
Echocardiography in the Management of Patients with Suspected or Proven Endocarditis
The Clinical Spectrum of Human Parvovirus B19 Infections

CURRENT CLINICAL TOPICS IN INFECTIOUS DISEASES 12

Viral Aseptic Meningitis in the United States: Clinical Features, Viral Etiologies, and Differential
  Diagnosis
Aeromonas Species: Role as Human Pathogens
Neurologic Complications of Bacterial Meningitis in Children
Purulent Pericarditis
Diagnosis and Management of Infections of Implantable Devices Used for Prolonged Venous Access
Pancreatic Abscess and Infected Pseudocyst: Diagnosis and Treatment
Approach to the Febrile Traveler Returning from Southeast Asia and Oceania
Management of Septic Shock: New Approaches
The Increasing Prevalence of Resistance to Antituberculosis Chemotherapeutic Agents: Implications for
  Global Tuberculosis Control
Use of Immune Globulins in the Prevention and Treatment of Infections
Mycobacterium avium Complex in AIDS
Hepatitis B Immunization: Vaccine Types, Efficacy, and Indications for Immunization
Therapy of Cytomegalovirus Infections with Ganciclovir: A Critical Appraisal
Evaluation of Cryptic Fever in a Traveler to Africa

13

CURRENT CLINICAL TOPICS IN INFECTIOUS DISEASES

The pathogenesis, prevention, and management of urinary tract infection in patients with spinal cord injury

PAUL F. KAMITSUKA

INTRODUCTION

The impact of urinary tract infection on the survival of patients with spinal cord injury (SCI) has changed dramatically in the past few decades (1–3). In the preantibiotic era, approximately 80% of all deaths following SCI were due to pyelonephritis (1). Thirty to fifty percent of all deaths among patients sustaining SCI during World War II and the Korean War were from renal causes, including pyelonephritis, vesicoureteral reflux, hydronephrosis, and stones (4). With improvements in urologic management—in particular, the achievement of balanced bladder function and the avoidance where possible of indwelling catheters—and the advent of dialysis and improved antibiotics, many centers have reduced renal-related mortality to less than 5% of all deaths (5). The relative contribution of infection per se to renal failure in this population remains ill-defined. Unquestionably, however, urinary tract infection remains a major cause of morbidity among SCI patients and accounts for 47% to 72.4% of life-threatening bacteremias in this population (6,7).

NEUROGENIC VESICOURETHRAL DYSFUNCTION FOLLOWING SCI

The pathogenesis of neurogenic vesicourethral dysfunction following SCI has been reviewed recently (8,9). Briefly summarized, in the acute period following SCI, most patients present with a hypotonic, flaccid bladder ("shock bladder"), regardless of the level of injury. This self-limited phase usually lasts for several weeks, shorter in those with incomplete lesions. As spinal shock subsides, patients manifest neurogenic dysfunction which is determined by the level and completeness of injury. The upper motor neuron pattern of dysfunction is most common. Patients with upper motor neuron lesions (above T-11) have preserved reflex activity in the cord segments below the level of injury. These patients exhibit a hyperreflexic bladder with spasticity of the

1

pelvic floor. In addition, varying degrees of bladder-sphincter dyssynergia, i.e., the failure of the sphincter to relax during detrusor contractions, may contribute to a high-pressure system. A low-compliance bladder with detrusor hypertrophy may result, with impaired urinary drainage. On the other hand, patients with lower motor neuron lesions (involving the conus medullaris and cauda equina) have hyporeflexive or flaccid bladders, frequently with inadequate or absent opening of the bladder neck and large amounts of residual urine. Left untreated, such patients develop a large bladder with trabeculation and subsequently develop pseudodiverticuli and reflux into the upper urinary tract. Mixed bladder dysfunction occurs with lesions at T-12 and L-1.

With concerted effort and training, often in conjunction with pharmacotherapy instituted to modify either bladder or sphincter function (5,8–10), up to 70% of patients with myelopathy can develop reliable, timed bladder emptying to less than 100 mL (11). Patients with upper motor neuron dysfunction utilize stimuli such as light suprapubic stimulation to induce reflex detrusor contraction or anal stretch to relax the pelvic floor, with emptying facilitated by Valsalva's maneuver or an elastic abdominal binder. Patients with flaccid bladders may achieve emptying by using Valsalva's maneuver or by applying manual external force (Credé). In both cases, condom catheters may be worn by those with incontinence between voids. Several options are available for those unable to accomplish adequate emptying using these methods. Patients with preserved upper-extremity function are potential candidates for intermittent catheterization. Those with varying degrees of bladder-striated sphincter dyssynergia which is not ameliorated by pharmacotherapy may require external sphincterotomy, with or without bladder neck incision, and condom drainage. As a last resort, indwelling catheters are used. As will be reviewed below, indwelling catheters appear to be associated with an increased risk of urinary tract infections, although no prospective controlled trials have been performed to prove this point. Complications such as epididymitis, penoscrotal abscess, urethral fistula and strictures, and stones also appear more commonly with indwelling catheters (12,13). Finally, patients with chronic indwelling catheters are at risk for developing squamous cell carcinoma of the bladder (14,15).

The ultimate goal of urologic management of the SCI patient with neurogenic vesicourethral dysfunction is to maintain a so-called balanced bladder with low intravesical pressures and low residual volumes (5,8,9,16,17). Patients with high-pressure upper motor neuron dysfunction are at particular risk for vesicoureteral reflux and silent hydronephrosis, which may cause irreversible upper tract damage after only 1 to 2 years if left untreated (18). Intravesical pressures >40 cm water in patients with flaccid bladders can also lead to upper urinary tract deterioration (19). Moreover, a direct relationship has been demonstrated between increasing residual volumes between 100 to 250 mL and the incidence of bacteriuria (20). Thus, a thorough urologic evaluation, including urodynamic investigation, is mandatory for all patients with SCI, with pharmacological or surgical interventions made as needed to achieve a low-pressure, balanced system with low residual volumes. Also essential is the recognition that the urodynamic status of the SCI patient may change over time. Factors such as distal progression of lumbar injury due to a syrinx, anatomic/structural changes in the bladder, prostatic enlargement, obstruction secondary to stones, and urinary tract infection may all contribute to urodynamic dysfunction, resulting in upper tract damage if left unrecognized. This dynamic situation mandates a regular schedule of urologic follow-up to insure that a balanced system is maintained (5,21–26).

PATHOGENESIS OF URINARY TRACT INFECTION IN SCI PATIENTS

SCI patients are at increased risk for urinary tract infection due to a variety of factors, including (a) altered urinary defenses due to functional or mechanical abnormalities such as incomplete bladder emptying, vesicoureteral reflux, and the frequent presence of bladder or renal calculi which serve as indwelling foreign bodies and (b) frequent instrumentation. In addition, altered host defenses at a cellular level, such as an increase on uroepithelial cells of binding sites for bacteria, may play a role in the initiation of urinary tract infection in patients with indwelling catheters (27).

Several lines of data suggest that urinary tract infections in SCI patients result from the introduction into the bladder of bacteria colonizing the urethra and perineum, a process facilitated by instrumentation (28–30). The normal periurethral flora, consisting of diptheroids, *Streptococcus viridans*, and coagulase-negative staphylococci (plus lactobacilli in females) is replaced by gram-negative organisms (28). The perinea, groins, penile shafts, and urethras of SCI patients are heavily colonized by a range of gram-negative rods (GNR) (31,32). Serial cultures indicate that GNR may start to colonize the skin as early as 2 to 3 days following spinal cord injury. Some species such as *Citrobacter diversus* and *Escherichia coli* appear as transient colonizers, while others such as *Enterobacter aerogenes*, *Serratia marcescens* and *Klebsiella pneumoniae* become stable members of the flora (32). Giroux and Perkash found that, in 84% of those with predominantly condom catheter drainage, the infecting bladder organisms could simultaneously be cultured from their condom, drainage bag, perineum, or urethral swab (29). Likewise, among patients undergoing intermittent catheterization, Donovan and associates recently used plasmid profiling to demonstrate that identical strains of *K. pneumoniae* could be found in stool cultures obtained prior to or coincident with the onset of bacteriuria due to this organism, suggesting that the stool flora serves as a reservoir for subsequent urinary tract colonization, at least for this organism. Finally, in patients with indwelling catheters, organisms causing bacteriuria have been found to colonize the urethral meatus 2 to 5 days earlier. Along with contamination of the catheter-tubing junction and of the drainage bag, migration of bacteria extraluminally in the periurethral space constitutes a well-recognized pathway for entry of bacteria into the bladder (33–35).

In the recent literature a number of virulence factors relevant to the pathogenesis of urinary tract infection have been defined, including adhesins such as the pili-associated and afimbrial determinants of *E. coli* (36–38) or the mannose-resistant hemagglutinins of *Proteus* (39), bacterial exopolysaccharides or biofilms, and urease production. Bacterial virulence factors are less vital for the establishment of urinary tract infection in the SCI patient compared with the normal host because the presence of an abnormal urinary tract and frequent instrumentation enables microorganisms to bypass the usual host defense mechanisms and establish infection (37,40). The data of Johnson and associates illustrate this point (40). These investigators examined the relative incidence of P-fimbriated *E. coli* strains cultured from the blood and urine of uroseptic patients with and without urologic (abnormal urinary tract, instrumentation) or medical (diabetes mellitus, immunosuppressive therapy, etc.) abnormalities. While 100% of isolates from patients without any abnormalities were P-fimbriated, supporting the importance of P-fimbriae for upper tract infection with *E. coli* in normal hosts, a direct correlation was found between the number of host abnormalities and a decreased likelihood that the cultured isolate would be P-fimbriated. Most striking was the finding that none of the eight patients with an upper urinary tract abnormality had P-fimbriated *E. coli* ($p = 0.0002$).

The particular importance of bacterial virulence factors for the SCI patient is their role in maintaining *persistent* infections and in making eradication of infection difficult. Mobley and associates have presented data suggesting that expression of type I fimbriae may be required for the persistence of *E. coli* in patients with indwelling catheters (41). Biofilms, which are matrixes of polysaccharides secreted by bacteria, play a key role in protecting bacteria that are embedded within them from antibiotics and antiseptic agents (35,42–48). Such biofilms maintain bacterial populations on catheter surfaces as well as on the bladder wall. The establishment of bladder infection is facilitated by removal of the bladder's mucous coat, which normally provides a protective barrier against bacterial adherence to the transitional epithelium (27,49–51). A variety of urease-positive and urease-negative bacteria has been shown to directly damage the mucous coat (52). Moreover, increases in local ammonium concentration secondary to the activity of urease produced by organisms such as *Proteus* sp and *Providencia stuartii* may also damage the mucous coat, further facilitating the establishment of bacterial colonies adherent to the bladder wall (49,50). Bacterial biofilms, damage to the mucous coat, and bacterial urease production are also interrelated factors in the genesis of urinary tract stones, which are a further factor allowing persistent infections to occur. As adherent bacterial populations increase, protected by their biofilm matrix, other substances including mucoproteins, cellular debris, and crystals of struvite (magnesium, ammonium phosphate) and apatite (calcium phosphate) become entrapped within the matrix (53–55). Precipitation of struvite and apatite crystals is accelerated by the alkaline milieu of the urine caused by urease activity, giving rise to stones which provide stable sanctuaries for the imbedded microorganisms. Similar pathogenic mechanisms are also thought to be operative in the formation of renal stones and catheter-associated encrustations (45,46,56,57).

The incidence of bacteriuria among SCI patients with different modes of urinary drainage is difficult to define from the literature because authors have used different definitions of bacteriuria (ranging from 10^2 to 10^5 bacteria/mL), with patients maintained on varying regimens of antibiotic or antiseptic suppression. Indeed, there is no consensus as to what constitutes "significant" bacteriuria in this population. Gribble and associates found that among patients on intermittent catheterization, $>10^2$ cfu/mL provided optimal sensitivity and specificity, if one uses bacteriuria of any quantity cultured from a suprapubic aspirate as the "gold standard" (58). For voided samples obtained from those on condom drainage, particularly those with sphincterotomy, more stringent criteria (10^4 to 10^5) have been suggested because of contamination of such specimens with urethral flora (59,60).

PREVENTION OF BACTERIURIA IN THE SPINAL-CORD-INJURED PATIENT

Perhaps the single most important measure that can be taken to prevent bacteriuria in the spinal-cord-injured patient is to avoid an indwelling catheter. In addition, a number of different approaches have been tried in patients with the different modes of urinary drainage to prevent bacteriuria, including the topical application of antiseptic or antibiotic agents to the perineum and urethral meatus, addition of antiseptics to catheter drainage bags, bladder irrigation with antiseptic agents, the use of urinary catheters coated with antimicrobial agents, and the systemic administration of suppressive antiseptics or antibiotics.

Avoidance of indwelling catheters

Since Guttmann and Frankel presented their experience with the technique in a landmark paper published in 1966 (12), intermittent catheterization has become the preferred method of urinary drainage for those unable to reflex void. While Guttmann and Frankel stressed the importance of aseptic technique in performing intermittent catheterization, practical necessity has given way to the use of clean (but not sterile) intermittent catheterization in the outpatient setting (13,61–64), a practice first championed by Lapides, et al. (65,66). Well-controlled prospective trials have not been done comparing intermittent with indwelling catheterization, nor have sterile versus clean intermittent catheterizations been compared in this manner. However, the existing data suggest that bacteriuria rates are lower with intermittent catheterization. For example, Erickson and associates, using $>10^4$ cfu/mL to define bacteriuria (11), found that 29% of reflex voiders and 43% of those on intermittent catheterization were bacteriuric at their $>$15-month postrehabilitation follow-up visit, as compared to 100% of those with indwelling catheters. Others have estimated the incidence of bacteriuria among intermittently catheterized patients to be between 1.03 to 1.86/100 patient days (72,73).

Perineal/urethral antisepsis

Topical antiseptics have been used to wash the perineal area, and both antiseptic and antibiotic agents have been applied to the urethral meatus in an effort to suppress the flora which is considered to be the reservoir for urinary tract infection. Although variable results have been achieved, they have generally been poor. Sanderson and Weissler reported a marginal reduction (74% versus 60%, $p < 0.01$) in bacteriuria among male inpatients on intermittent catheterization who received daily baths using 4% chlorhexidine solution with the application of chlorhexidine cream to the urethral meatus after each catheterization, as compared to those washed with plain soap without meatal antisepsis (74). Among patients with indwelling catheters, meatal application of agents such as povidone-iodine or polyantibiotic cream has been found either to have no effect on the incidence of bacteriuria (75) or to actually increase bacteriuria rates (76). The increase has been attributed to urethral manipulation, which is thought to enhance the ingress of urethral organisms into the bladder (76).

Stickler and others have raised the concern that the use of certain antiseptic agents such as chlorhexidine may actually prove counterproductive, as they may select for perineal colonization with resistant gram-negative organisms (77–79). Although effective against both gram-positive and gram-negative organisms in vitro, chlorhexidine appears to have a negligible effect on gram-negative bacteria such as *Proteus mirabilis*, *Pseudomonas aeruginosa*, *P. stuartii*, and *K. pneumoniae* in vivo. Furthermore, Stickler et al. have presented data suggesting an association between chlorhexidine resistance and resistance to multiple antibiotics, an association not found with other antiseptics such as phenoxyethanol. The basis for this association is unclear.

Drainage bag antisepsis

A number of authors have examined the efficacy of adding antiseptics to catheter drainage bags in preventing urinary tract infections. Agents such as povidone-iodine (80,81) and hydrogen peroxide (82,83) have appeared in some studies to reduce the incidence of infection among those catheterized for brief periods (days) using closed catheter systems. However, others have been unable to show any benefit (84–86). With the possible exception of the acutely injured patient with a temporary indwelling catheter prior to the onset of intermittent catheterization, SCI patients would not benefit from this practice for at least two reasons. First, even if the antiseptic were fully effective in preventing bag contamination, the periurethral route of bacterial entry would remain (87,88) and eventually lead to bacteriuria. Secondly, the majority of catheterized (condom or indwelling) SCI outpatients switch daily from leg bags to bedside bags and thus maintain open catheter systems with far greater opportunities for contamination of the drainage bag as well as the proximal catheter. Giroux and Perkash have evaluated a variety of disinfectants for potential use in leg bags and found 0.06% sodium hypochlorite to be completely bactericidal against *Enterococcus* and a variety of gram-negative organisms with which the bags were inoculated (89). Whether the addition of disinfectants such as sodium hypochlorite to leg bags will lead to a significant reduction in bacteriuria is doubtful, although it has yet to be evaluated.

Bladder irrigation

Bladder irrigation with chlorhexidine has been shown to be of benefit in preventing urinary tract infections following instrumentation of previously uninfected bladders (90). However, neither chlorhexidine nor agents such as povidone-iodine and noxythiolin can be recommended for frequent or long-term bladder irrigation because of their tendency to produce erosive bladder reactions and hematuria (79).

Once infection is established, agents such as chlorhexidine are ineffective in reducing bacteriuria among catheterized patients (47,91). Stickler and associates performed bladder irrigation by introducing 100 cc of antiseptic into the bladder by injection through the catheter and clamping the drainage tube for 30 minutes, followed by serial quantitative urine cultures to assess the impact of this intervention on the urinary flora of chronically bacteriuric SCI patients. Irrigation with chlorhexidine produced only a minimal and transient reduction in bacterial titers, with restoration of initial concentrations within hours. These authors postulated that antiseptic-resistant, biofilm-imbedded bacteria, which are known to adhere to bladder walls, serve to repopulate bacterial populations in the urine following irrigation. In support of this hypothesis was their finding in the urinary sediment of bacterial microcolonies imbedded in a polysaccharide matrix, presumably shed from the bladder wall. The inability of other antiseptic agents such as povidone-iodine, trisdine, and noxythiolin to eradicate biofilm-associated bacteria was demonstrated in an in vitro bladder model system (92).

In an effort to overcome the protection from antimicrobials afforded biofilm-associated microorganisms, Stickler, et al. have recently examined the activity of antiseptic agents against that of bacteria growing as biofilms on silicone disks. Their studies demonstrate that mandelic acid (1% wt/vol), or a combination of mandelic and lactic acids (0.5% wt/vol each) significantly reduced the viability of individual microorganisms such as P. aeruginosa, P. mirabilis, K. pneumoniae, Citrobacter diversus, and E. coli (42,48). These agents also proved effective in a test system designed to mimic the multilayered polymicrobial biofilms found on urinary catheters (46). A 3- to 4-log reduction in the viability of the biofilm after 20 to 30 minutes of exposure and complete elimination of biofilm organisms after 2 hours was noted upon exposure of mixed community biofilms composed of P. aeruginosa, Citrobacter freundii, and Enterococcus faecalis at cell densities of $>10^9$ cfu/mL (93). Clinical trials of bladder irrigation using mandelic acid or the mandelic-lactic acid combination have yet to be performed.

Silver oxide-coated catheters

An ideal urinary catheter remains an elusive goal (94). Several groups have recently examined the influence of various coating materials on the incidence of catheter-associated bacteriuria. Ruggieri et al. noted a reduction in bacterial adherence to catheters coated with heparin (51). Likewise, Liedberg and Lundeberg demonstrated in an in vitro system that silver coating of latex prevents adherence and growth of P. aeruginosa (95). In recent clinical trials of the silver oxide catheter, however, the promise of short-term efficacy suggested by earlier studies (88,96) has not been confirmed, at least in male patients (97,98). In a large prospective trial involving 482 acutely hospitalized patients, Johnson et al. (98) noted similar rates (10%) of urinary tract infection among recipients of a silver oxide-coated catheter as compared to those with a control silicone catheter. A difference (0% silver versus 19% control, $p = 0.04$) was noted only for the subset of patients who were women not receiving antibiotics.

Methenamine salts

The efficacy of methenamine salts in preventing urinary tract infection is difficult to determine from the literature. Methenamine salts hydrolyze in acid urine (pH <6) to formaldehyde and ammonia, as well as to either mandelic or hippuric acid, depending on the form of salt administered. One to two hours are required for bacteriostatic concentrations (>25 μg/mL) of formaldehyde, the active moiety, to be achieved—a fact precluding the usefulness of these agents in chronically catheterized patients (99). Higher urinary levels of both methenamine and formaldehyde have been observed with the mandelate salt (100). Acidifying agents such as ascorbic acid or ammonium chloride are often administered along with these salts, although the benefit derived from this practice is uncertain (101). For example, Devenport et al. found that, while ascorbic acid caused a significant reduction in urine pH, no effect on formaldehyde concentration was observed (100). Others have found ascorbic to be a poor acidifying agent (102). Still others have found no statistical correlation between urinary pH and formaldehyde concentrations in patients receiving a combination of methenamine mandelate and ammonium chloride (103).

Conflicting results have been presented regarding the clinical efficacy of methenamine salts in preventing urinary tract infections among SCI patients. Vainrub and Musher (104) and Thorsteinsson and Keys (105) found these agents to be ineffective in patients treated with intermittent catheterization. In contrast, the findings of Stover and Fleming suggest some efficacy (71). These authors performed a prospective trial including 100 evaluable patients to determine the length of time that male SCI patients on either intermittent catheterization or reflex voiding with condom drainage maintained sterile urine (<1000 cfu/mL) during therapy with methenamine hippurate, as compared with a group on ascorbic acid. With methenamine hippurate, 41% of the patients maintained sterile urine for >4 weeks compared with only 4% of ascorbic acid recipients. No patient receiving ascorbic acid had sterile urine for >5 weeks, while 14% of methenamine hippurate recipients had sterile urine at 6 months.

The most carefully controlled evaluation of methenamine is the double-blind prospective evaluation performed by Kevorkian et al. in SCI patients treated with intermittent catheterization during initial bladder training following injury (103). Patients were randomized to receive either methenamine mandelate plus ammonium chloride or identical placebo tablets. Patients had sterile urine at the outset, and urologic procedures were performed to ensure that the urinary tract had no reflux, renal or bladder calculi, congenital abnormalities, chronic cystitis or diverticuli before the trial was begun. Both diet (acid ash) and fluid intake (1.6 to 2.0 liters per day) were controlled. Of the 39 who completed the trial, 19/22 (86%) on placebo developed bacteriuria ($\geq 10^4$ to 10^5 cfu/mL) as compared with 9/17 (53%) in the treatment group ($p < 0.02$). These data suggest that methenamine salts may be beneficial in selected SCI patients without indwelling catheters. The long-term benefit of methenamine in the outpatient setting, where factors such as diet, frequency of catheterization, residual urine volume, urine pH, etc. are much less controlled, remains uncertain. In addition, the risk of systemic acidosis precludes the use of either methenamine mandelate or ammonium chloride in patients with renal insufficiency.

In an effort to increase urinary formaldehyde levels and thereby enhance the efficacy of oral methenamine, Krebs and associates studied the adjunctive use of bladder irrigation with 5% hemiacidrin, a solution containing citric and gluconic acids with a pH of 3.9 (106). The incidence of bacteriuria ($>10^5$ cfu/mL) was significantly lower in the treatment group ($p < 0.001$). However, 25% of these patients experienced gross hematuria, which was attributed to high formaldehyde concentrations in the bladder.

Antibiotic prophylaxis

As in the case of methenamine, there are conflicting reports in the literature as to whether prophylactic antibiotic administration prevents bacteriuria in the SCI population (107–110). Kuhlemeier et al. (108) randomized patients with initially sterile urine undergoing intermittent catheterization to receive either single-strength cotrimoxazole b.i.d., 50 mg of nitrofurantoin macrocrystals t.i.d., or nalidixic acid 500 mg q.i.d. they were then compared with patients receiving either ascorbic acid alone or methenamine hippurate. Weekly urine cultures were obtained. After 15 days, all of the groups had 50% infection rates, suggesting that the antibiotics were ineffective. A similar lack of efficacy was noted by Thorsteinsson and Keys (105) in a comparison of cotrimoxazole with no therapy in intermittently catheterized patients and by Mohler et al. (109), who compared double-strength cotrimoxazole nightly with an identical placebo. In contrast, Maynard and Diokno (110) found a significant reduction in the incidence of asymptomatic bacteriuria among intermittently catheterized recipients of either cotrimoxazole or macrodantin prophylaxis as compared with no prophylaxis. Of note, however, the incidence of febrile and/or symptomatic urinary tract infections was *not* influenced by either antibiotic prophylaxis or by whether antibiotic treatment was provided for episodes of asymptomatic bacteriuria detected by serial urine culture, in agreement with the findings of Mohler et al. (109). However, both of these studies are difficult to interpret because of the multiplicity of therapeutic subgroups, the small numbers (≤50 total per study) of patients enrolled, uncertainty as to whether patients in each of the subgroups were in fact comparable, and the absence of blinding in the latter study.

ASYMPTOMATIC BACTERIURIA: TO TREAT OR NOT TO TREAT

In SCI patients with indwelling catheters, due to the inevitability of bacteriuria and the risk of selecting out resistant organisms, most would agree that treatment should be reserved for symptomatic or febrile episodes (35,111,112). For patients with reflex voiding, intermittent catheterization, or condom drainage, the issue of whether or not to treat asymptomatic bacteriuria remains controversial. The situation is rendered even more nebulous by the fact that, as noted below, the clinical signs and symptoms of urinary tract infection are blunted or altered in this population, blurring the margins of what one truly considers "asymptomatic" bacteriuria. The key problem is that definitive criteria for distinguishing between colonization and infection have not been defined for this population. Several authors have examined the utility of quantitative assessments of pyuria or of various localizing techniques as indicators of the need for treatment. Additional considerations relevant to this decision include assessments of (a) the impact of asymptomatic bacteriuria on renal function, (b) the risk of bacteriuria in terms of febrile morbidity and sepsis, (c) the impact of antibiotic use on the emergence of antimicrobial resistance, and (d) whether the cultured organism is urease-positive, increasing the risk of developing urinary tract calculi.

Pyuria

It has been suggested that the degree of pyuria might be useful to distinguish bacteriuric patients with asymptomatic colonization from those with invasive infection requiring antibiotic therapy (113–115). The relationship between bacteriuria and pyuria has been examined in both catheterized and catheter-free patients (113,114,116). Musher et al. (116) found that, in patients with indwelling catheters, 62/69 patients with $>10^5$ cfu/mL had >10 white blood cells (WBC) per mm^3 of urine, as compared with 40/149 patients with $<10^3$ cfu/mL. Peterson and Roth conducted a retrospective study of chronically catheterized SCI patients with bacteriuria ($\geq10^5$/mL) to assess the clinical course of patients with high-level pyuria (≥50 WBC per high-power field (HPF)) versus lower levels of pyuria (≤50 WBC/HPF) (117). Of those with high-level pyuria, 6 of 10 (60%) developed febrile episodes, as compared with 3 of 22 (13.6%) of those with lesser degrees of pyuria ($P < 0.01$). Among a group of 48 spinal-cord-injured patients on intermittent catheterization with bacteriuria of $\geq10^5$, Hooton et al. found that 45 (94%) had ≥10 WBC/mm^3 (118).

However, interpretation of these data is difficult for several reasons. The commonly used method of counting the number of WBC per high-power field in spun sediments, as used by Peterson and Roth (117), has been shown to be an inaccurate measure of pyuria that does not correlate with the leukocyte excretion rate (113). The major source of inaccuracy is accounted for by the wide variations in the volume of fluid used to resuspend the centrifuged pellet. A far more accurate method is to quantitate WBC in unspun urine using a counting chamber. Moreover, urinary concentrations of WBC vary significantly, depending upon the method of sampling. Terminal catheter urine contains significantly higher concentrations of WBC than either midstream catheter specimens or suprapubic aspirates ($p < 0.0001$) (119). Also, the degree of pyuria found appears to vary with the type of microorganism cultured from the urine. Anderson and Hsieh-Ma (120) noted that bacteriuria due to gram-negative bacteria is associated with a significantly higher level of pyuria as compared with bacteriuria due to gram-positive organisms (445 ± 145 WBC/mm^3 versus 31 ± 10 WBC/mm^3, respectively). While the absence of pyuria reasonably predicts the absence of significant gram-negative bacillary bacteriuria, sterile pyuria is common in the SCI population, perhaps due to factors such as irritation of the bladder wall by catheters (119–121).

Thus, the key study assessing the utility of quantitative assessments of pyuria has yet to be done. Among other things, such a study would need to employ the counting chamber method of quantitation, control for factors such as the method of urinary drainage and the method of urinary sampling, and include data regarding the microorganisms cultured from the patient.

Localizing procedures

Short of performing quantitative cultures of urine collected by ureteric catheterization, which is not only too invasive for routine use but also technically difficult in patients who may have thickened and trabeculated bladder walls, there unfortunately is no reliable method for localizing the site of urinary tract infection in spinal-cord-injured patients. The Fairley bladder washout technique (122) is difficult to perform due to a number of factors, including the inability to achieve initial sterilization of either the urethra and/or bladder, the presence of bladder diverticuli, or the presence of vesicoureteral reflux (118,123–126). Likewise, the experience with the antibody-coated bacteria (ACB) test has been poor. Some investigators have noted a high incidence of false negatives in the face of clinical evidence strongly suggesting upper tract involvement, such as the presence of fever, rigors, and bacteremia (127) or positive cultures by ureteral catheterization (126). Others have noted false-positive ACB test results due to prostatitis or chronic/recurrent cystitis (128). Finally, localization of infection to the prostate is both cumbersome and difficult to achieve in this population, and the methods used have not been fully validated (126,128). Collection of prostatic secretions for quantitative culture involves the insertion of a catheter into the bladder, with traction applied throughout the procedure to prevent reflux from the urethra into the bladder; subsequent bladder irrigation is followed by prostatic massage and the collection of expressed secretions. Because abnormal bladders (e.g., large atonic bladders, trabeculated bladders, bladders with diverticuli) are difficult to sterilize, a difference in colony count between the samples obtained is often not achieved (126).

Effect of chronic bacteriuria on renal function

The impact of urinary tract infection on renal function among patients with spinal cord injury has been incompletely evaluated. It is likely, though unproven, that uncomplicated infection in the absence of anatomic or functional urinary tract dysfunction contributes little to a decline in renal function (129). Over a period of five years Sotolongo and Koleilat (70) prospectively studied 56 SCI patients on condom catheter drainage, all of whom were bacteriuric with greater than 10^5 cfu/mL. Careful attention was paid to maintaining a balanced, low-pressure system with regular urologic follow-up and urologic interventions as needed. During this period, none of the patients sustained evidence of urinary tract deterioration as assessed by upper tract imaging as well as serum creatinine levels.

A progressive decline in renal function has been documented, however, in chronically bacteriuric SCI patients with indwelling catheters. Using more sensitive indices of renal function, including inulin and para-aminohippurate (PAH) clearances to measure glomerular filtration rate (GFR) and renal plasma flow, respectively, Falls and Stacy prospectively followed the renal function of 18 such patients for a period of more than five years (130). At the outset, renal function was found to be normal in all patients. Over the follow-up period, only three of the patients remained free of complications, including vesicoureteral reflux, calculi, sepsis, or hypertension. However, even these patients demonstrated several of the alterations in renal function that were noted among all of the patients followed: stable inulin clearances, but a steady decrease in PAH clearance with associated increase in filtration fraction. The authors speculated that their findings were caused by the development of small foci of scarring and atrophy leading to loss of nephron units, with associated hyperfiltration in the remaining units. The degree to which chronic bacteriuria contributed to these changes is unclear. Also, whether similar changes in renal function would be found in patients managed without indwelling catheters and whether eradicating bacteriuria would lead to different results are issues that require clarification by prospective studies, carefully controlling for variables of urologic dysfunction.

Risk of febrile morbidity

Several investigators have attempted to quantitate the incidence of febrile or symptomatic urinary tract infections in patients with spinal cord injury. Lewis and co-workers
prospectively followed 52 SCI patients with uncomplicated neurogenic bladders (stable
upper tracts, no vesicoureteral reflux, and small vesical residuals) (131). All but two of
the patients were catheter-free, with 39 on intermittent catheterization and 11 on reflex
voiding. Over the course of 6 months, only 7 of 52 (13%) developed a febrile urinary
infection requiring antibiotic therapy. Even among patients with chronic indwelling
catheters, the incidence of febrile urinary tract infections is reasonably low. Estimates
among non-SCI patients with chronic indwelling catheters are 0.21 episode/patient-
month at risk for males (132), and 1.1 episode/100 patient-days at risk for females (133),
respectively. Ruutu et al. noted that 40% of SCI patients with abnormal upper tracts
developed ≥ 1 febrile urinary tract infection per year, as compared with 10% of those
with normal anatomy by urogram (22).

Antimicrobial resistance and urease-producing organisms

Although the risk of selecting for resistant organisms with repeated antibiotic courses is
well-recognized in a general sense, there are no prospective controlled studies addressing this issue among SCI patients without indwelling catheters. Moreover, while some
have adopted the policy of treating asymptomatic bacteriuria when the cultured organism is a urea splitter such as *Proteus* (123), the merits of this policy, while seemingly
reasonable, also have not been prospectively evaluated.

In summary, the issue of whether or not to treat asymptomatic bacteriuria in the
spinal-cord-injured patient without an indwelling catheter remains unsettled. Some
authors, such as Zhanel et al., contend that all such patients should be treated (112).
Others, such as Stickler and Chawla (134), argue for witholding antibiotic treatment on
the ground that the benefit of preserving antimicrobial susceptibility outweighs that of
initiating therapy in the absence of symptoms. As noted above, the precise risk of
emerging resistance has not been defined. However, in support of the latter policy are
data suggesting a relatively low risk of febrile morbidity associated with asymptomatic
bacteriuria in patients free of urologic complications such as upper tract abnormalities,
vesicoureteral reflux, or high residual volumes (131). Also, the data of Mohler et al.
(109) and Maynard and Diokno (110) suggest that the incidence of febrile or symptomatic urinary tract infection is not reduced by the practice of treating asymptomatic
bacteriuria in this population. However, if bacteriuria is to be left untreated, it is
crucial that close urologic follow-up be maintained, since the urologic status of SCI
patients may silently deteriorate over time. In the setting of occult obstruction with
hydronephrosis, for example, untreated bacteriuria may well contribute to a loss of
renal function and will certainly predispose to the development of overt sepsis. Yet
another consideration is the finding, reviewed below, that an increased risk of both
bladder and renal calculi occurs during the first year following spinal cord injury, and
during the initial three months in particular (135,136). A policy of treating bacteriuria
due to urease-producing organisms, especially during this stone-prone period, may

therefore make sense. Clearly, there is an urgent need for prospective trials to evaluate these issues in order to develop a rational therapeutic policy.

CLINICAL PRESENTATION OF URINARY TRACT INFECTION IN SCI PATIENTS

The spinal-cord-injured patient who presents with fever, systemic toxicity, and the recent development of foul, cloudy urine presents little diagnostic challenge. However, in the absence of such signs, the presentation of urinary tract infection in the SCI patient may be exceedingly subtle. Symptoms such as dysuria, frequency, and urgency are absent in most patients and may be unreliable when present. Deprived of sensation below the level of injury, patients may complain only of an ill-defined sense of malaise or of unexplained diaphoresis, suggesting associated autonomic dysreflexia (137).

Febrile episodes are often blamed on the urinary tract because of the frequency with which pyuria and bacteriuria are encountered in this population. However, a complete search for other febrile sources is obligatory before concluding that the urinary tract is the culprit. Just as the absence of sensation may alter the clinical presentation of urinary tract infection, a lack of symptoms may lead the unwary clinician to overlook other sites of infection as well.

Among febrile patients in whom the urinary tract is deemed to be the most likely source, an assessment of the upper tracts should be carried out to look for evidence of calculi, hydronephrosis, and purulent collections requiring drainage. An initial assessment is most easily accomplished by ultrasound, which should be performed without delay (138). All too often, clinicians inexperienced in treating SCI patients are surprised to find upper tract obstruction with extensive renal and/or perinephric collections of pus in patients who have exhibited few symptoms other than low-grade fever and malaise.

TREATMENT OF URINARY TRACT INFECTIONS

In treating SCI patients with urinary tract infections, several considerations apply. First, in contrast to populations such as young women in whom *E. coli* predominates, a variety of gram-negative organisms and *Enterococci* are recovered from the urine of SCI patients, including the finding of polymicrobial infection in almost half of cases (70). In the nosocomial setting, multiply-resistant microorganisms are frequently encountered. Second, preliminary studies have suggested that the pharmacokinetics of aminoglycosides differ in patients with spinal cord injury. Among other findings, an increase in the volume of distribution has been noted for both para- and quadriplegics compared with a literature-derived mean for normal subjects (139–141). In addition, some studies have suggested that aminoglycosides as monotherapy may be less effective than certain beta-lactams in treating urinary tract infections in this population, although these data require confirmation by a formal study (142,143). Inhibition of the antimicrobial activity of gentamicin by human urine has been demonstrated in vitro

(144). Whether diminished urinary concentrations due to a combination of under-dosing and renal insufficiency, along with the inhibitory effect of urine, may account for diminished efficacy of aminoglycosides in some patients remains to be determined.

Thus, for the febrile SCI patient with suspected urinary tract infection who is in the nosocomial setting or is known to harbor antibiotic-resistant organisms, empiric institution of therapy with a ureidopenicillin plus an aminoglycoside while awaiting culture and susceptibility results would seem reasonable. The ureidopenicillin would provide coverage for *Enterococci*, as well as additional coverage for gram-negative bacilli pending susceptibility data. For febrile outpatients presenting to the hospital without a recent history of antibiotic exposure, the combination of ampicillin and gentamicin would be appropriate. Unfortunately, there are no prospective controlled trials to clearly define the optimum duration of antibiotic therapy in this population. For febrile patients without demonstrable upper tract complications, it has been our practice to treat for a total duration of 14 days, with an oral antibiotic substituted for intravenous therapy at 24 to 72 hours following defervescence and once antimicrobial susceptibilities are known. For afebrile, nontoxic patients with otherwise symptomatic infection, a seven-day course of oral antibiotics is provided. Again, prospective trials are needed to validate these or other approaches.

INFECTION STONES IN PATIENTS WITH SPINAL CORD INJURY

The incidence of urolithiasis (bladder, renal, ureteral calculi) among patients with spinal cord injury is estimated at from 8% to 30% (23,53,145,146). The vast majority (98%) of these stones are composed of a combination of magnesium-ammonium-phosphate (struvite) and calcium phosphate (147,148). The pathogenesis of stone formation was discussed above. While urease activity is not a prerequisite for struvite stone formation (149,150), there is extensive evidence to suggest that urease-positive bacteria play a key role in the genesis of these calculi in humans. A wide variety of bacteria are capable of producing urease (54), but *P. mirabilis* plays the most prominent role, perhaps due to the fact that the enzyme of this organism acts some 6 to 25 times faster than ureases produced by other organisms (151,152). Indeed, this organism was isolated from 87% of the infection stones recovered by Silverman and Stamey (153). That non-urease-producing organisms may play an adjunctive role in struvite stone formation is suggested by the finding of these, in the absence of urease-positive organisms, in a minority of such stones (154). Urease nonproducers, such as *E. coli*, become imbedded in the biofilm matrix as mineralization occurs and appear, in fact, to serve as nuclei for the deposition of struvite/apatite crystals (155).

DeVivo et al. utilized logistic regression analysis to identify risk factors for bladder and renal calculi among SCI patients in Alabama (135,136). The risk of stones at both sites is greatest during the first year following injury, and during the first three months in particular. One may speculate that a factor contributing to this early occurrence is the immobility-associated hypercalciuria that occurs during the initial months following spinal cord injury (156,157). The presence of a neurologically complete lesion is another risk factor common to both bladder and renal stones. Risk factors specific for bladder calculi developing prior to discharge from the initial admission include *Klebsiella* infections at admission and white race. Patients developing bladder stones within two years of hospital discharge were most likely to be young and white, have indwelling urethral catheters, and have either *Proteus* or polymicrobial infections at discharge. According to DeVivo's analysis, the presence of a bladder stone(s) was itself a risk factor for renal calculi, while the method of urinary drainage did not appear significant. Conversely, Hall et al. (145) did not find bladder stones to be a risk factor for renal stones and suggested that a Foley catheter was a risk for stones at both sites. These authors also determined vesicoureteral reflux to be a risk factor for the ipsilateral development of renal calculi.

As in the case of urinary tract infection, the signs and symptoms of urolithiasis may be subtle or misleading in this population. Patients with acute renal colic may present with nothing more than nausea or vomiting, leading the clinician to consider gastrointestinal disease. Other patients may present either with bacteriuria refractory to multiple antibiotic courses or with fever and sepsis (23).

Several authors have emphasized that struvite stones in the kidney, particularly large staghorn calculi, pose a major threat to renal function (23,54,158–163). Left untreated, patients with infected staghorn calculi stand a 50% chance of losing the affected kidney, while untreated bilateral staghorns are reported to result in a 25% mortality within 5 years and a 40% mortality within 10 years (164). Neglected struvite stones may lead to hydronephrosis with loss of renal function and to other problems including intra- or perinephric abscess and xanthogranulomatous pyelonephritis.

As with renal stones in general, the therapeutic approach to infection stones in patients with spinal cord injury has been revolutionized by the development of endourologic techniques and the advent of both percutaneous and extracorporeal shock wave lithotripsy (ESWL) (165–170). Struvite calculi are quite amenable to dissolution by lithotripsy. However, the success of lithotripsy depends directly on the stone burden (171). A large body of collected experience suggests that struvite calculi with a diameter greater than 2 cm will require a combination of percutaneous and extracorporeal lithotripsy for successful dissolution; ESWL alone is associated with a high incidence of residual calculi in these instances (146,166,167,169,171–179). Percutaneous lithotripsy via a nephrostomy tract is often performed initially to break up the stone into smaller fragments, followed by ESWL. A ureteral stent is placed in most cases to facilitate clearance of stone fragments from the upper tracts (180–182). In some cases, irrigation of the upper tracts with acidic solutions such as hemiacidrin may be employed as an adjunct to these procedures (50,153,168,183,184). Surgical intervention is reserved for very large stones (175). However, even with surgical nephrolithotomy, residual stone fragments are left in between 17% and 45% of cases (153,178,185,186).

Struvite calculi are occasionally incompletely radioopaque and thus may be inapparent on plain radiographs. Tomograms performed at low kilovoltage (60 to 80 kV) and 0.5-cm cuts through the kidneys are useful to demonstrate the location and extent of such calculi (183).

Residual stone fragments serve as a nidus for persistent infection (153,161,163,173, 186,187), as well as for recurrent stone growth, which may occur quite rapidly in some patients (188). Beck and Riehle analyzed the fate of stone fragments left following

ESWL monotherapy in 53 patients with infection stones (158). Of 9 kidneys with fragments of more than 5 mm after the final treatment, 7 (78%) had residual fragments at 3 months, with evidence of stone progression. In contrast, of 9 kidneys with sand remaining, 6 (66%), and all three kidneys that appeared to be free of stones after ESWL, were without stones at follow-up. For patients with residual stones ≥5 mm diameter on a radiograph taken after the last sequential ESWL, these authors advocate a repeat radiograph within 2 to 3 weeks and early retreatment or endourological intervention if the stone is still present.

An adjunctive approach to the treatment of patients with struvite stones has been to administer inhibitors of the enzyme urease. Urease inhibitors have been employed in attempts to eradicate medically stones not removed by surgery or ESWL or to prevent the growth (or regrowth) of stones in patients chronically infected with urease-positive organisms. A variety of inhibitors have been examined, but only one, acetohydroxamic acid (AHA), has been evaluated in prospective controlled trials (189,190). Williams et al. (187) randomized subjects with struvite nephrolithiasis and infection with a urea-splitting organism to receive either AHA ($n = 18$) or placebo ($n = 19$) over mean follow-up periods of 15 to 19 months; changes in stone sizes between the two groups were then assessed. All patients were maintained on suppressive antibiotics throughout the study. AHA effectively prevented stone growth, but at a cost of adverse reactions in half of the recipients, including tremulousness in 5 of 18 and deep venous thrombosis in 3 of 18, with one of these patients experiencing a pulmonary embolus. Since that study, an association between AHA use and a hypercoagulable state, as reflected by elevated fibrinopeptide A levels and an associated drop in platelet count, has been confirmed (191). More recently, Griffith et al. (190) reported a much larger study comparing AHA ($n = 121$) with placebo ($n = 89$) among SCI patients with stones and chronic infection with a urease-producing organism. No attempt was made to control antibiotic use in this study. Only 35 AHA recipients and 58 placebo controls completed two years of therapy. Although a significant reduction in the extent of stone growth was noted at 12 months for those taking AHA ($P = 0.017$), no significant difference was noted at 24 months ($p = 0.26$). The occurrence rate for adverse reactions was significantly higher for those receiving AHA ($p \leq 0.0001$), with nausea, headache, tremulousness, skin rashes, and anemia most commonly noted. Of note, however, the AHA group did not experience a significantly higher incidence of phlebitis, with four cases noted in the drug group and two in the placebo. Thus, in summary, although some evidence for the efficacy of AHA exists, its utility is clearly limited by a high incidence of side effects. In addition, this compound is both mutagenic and teratogenic in animals (50).

Other urease inhibitors that have been subjected to limited evaluation include flurofamide (192–194) and propionhydroxamic acid (PHA) (195–203). Although perhaps less toxic than AHA, a number of side effects including hair loss has been noted with regularity in trials employing higher doses of this drug (198,199). At doses that are better tolerated, antiurease activity has been confirmed in some (197,200,203) but not other (196,199) studies. Significant reduction in stone size has not been noted in uncontrolled clinical trials (201,202). Preclinical data regarding other urease inhibitors have recently been presented by Satoh et al. (202). The search for an effective, yet nontoxic, inhibitor of urease activity continues.

Precise guidelines regarding the use of antibiotics around the time of surgical intervention for infection stones have not been established, and the practice varies among authors. Pode et al. (173) administered antibiotics for 12 hours before and 24 hours after lithotripsy, with ten days of antibiotics given post-ESWL to the 23% of their patients who developed fever or sepsis following the procedure. Michaels et al. (205) treated their patients with 3 to 8 days (mean 4.7 days) of parenteral antibiotics before and after ESWL, with oral antibiotics administered for 14 to 34 days (mean 25 days) thereafter.

In the absence of prospective controlled data, three observations are relevant to the issue of how long patients should receive antibiotics perioperatively. Charton et al. (206) found that fever always developed in their patients treated with less than four days of antibiotics prior to ESWL, with septicemia occurring in 4.5% of cases. Pode (173) observed that the incidence of fever was directly proportional to the size of the stone in their series. Finally, Michaels et al. (205) found that, in contrast to patients left with large fragments, sterilization of the urine of patients left with minute fragments (sand) was possible in the majority of their patients with antibiotics alone for two weeks. Based on this information, a rational approach would be to treat for at least seven days pre-ESWL for those with large stone burdens and positive cultures and for at least two weeks post-ESWL, during which upper tract irrigation may be performed in selected cases. Since sterilization of large (≥ 5 mm) residual fragments is unlikely with antibiotics alone (158,189), patients with such fragments whose infection relapses after completion of postoperative antibiotics should receive further intervention to eradicate the remaining stone fragments. In choosing antibiotics appropriate for the patient, a careful review of the susceptibility profiles of organisms previously isolated from the patient should be performed, recognizing that urine cultures may correlate with the bacteriology of infection stones in as little as 13% of cases (207).

In summary, the management of infection stones in patients with spinal cord injury has been in a state of evolution since the advent of ESWL. Although most would agree that staghorn calculi associated with chronic infection in patients with preserved renal function should be pursued aggressively, the optimal clinical approach to stable stones without infection remains undefined (23). Percutaneous lithotripsy is not without risks, with major complications such as respiratory arrest, perinephric abscess, and hydrothorax noted in 8.5% of patients and bleeding requiring transfusion occurring in 17% (176). The long-term effects of repeated ESWL on renal function and the development of hypertension are also unknown (172,208). The potential promise of urease inhibitors as adjunctive therapy has been dampened by the high incidence of side effects noted with existing agents, although safer and more effective drugs may be forthcoming. Finally, the precise role of antibiotics in patients with infection stones remains to be clarified.

CONCLUSIONS

Many questions remain unanswered with regard to urinary tract infections in the spinal-cord-injured population. From the clinical standpoint, particularly vexing issues include: (a) the continued search for better methods to prevent bacteriuria; (b) the development of criteria for distinguishing bladder colonization from true infection; (c) clarification of whether efforts to prevent or treat asymptomatic bacteriuria are warranted in patients in whom properly balanced vesicourethral function is maintained, particularly in regard to whether treating asymptomatic bacteriuria leads to significant decreases in febrile morbidity, deterioration of renal function, and the emergence of urinary tract calculi; (d) distinction between upper and lower urinary tract infection and determination of the optimal duration of antibiotic therapy for each; (e) determination of the optimal approach to urinary tract calculi, with particular reference to a risk/benefit analysis, defining the extent to which the eradication of such stones should be vigorously pursued and to the development of precise guidelines regarding the appropriate duration of pre- and postintervention antibiotic therapy; and (f) the continued search for more effective and less toxic urease inhibitors. The observation has been made that the management of the neurogenic bladder has historically been "by response to trends rather than objective measurement of outcomes" (13). There is indeed an urgent need for well-controlled prospective trials to address these challenging and important issues.

REFERENCES

1 DeVivo MJ, Kartus PL, Stover SL, Rutt RD, Fine PR. Cause of death for patients with spinal cord injuries. *Arch Intern Med* 1989; 149:1761.

2 Geisler WO, Jousse AT, Wynne-Jones M, Breithaupt D. Survival in traumatic spinal cord injury. *Paraplegia* 1983;21:364.

3 Borges PM, Hackler RH. The urologic status of the Vietnam war paraplegic: a 15-year prospective follow-up. *J Urol* 1982;127:710.

4 Hackler RH. A 25-year prospective mortality study in the spinal cord injured patient: Comparison with the long-term living paraplegic. *J Urol* 1977;117:486.

5 O'Donnell WF. Urological management in the patient with acute spinal cord injury. *Crit Care Clin* 1987;3:599.

6 Bhatt K, Cid E, Maiman D. Bacteremia in the spinal cord injury population. *J Am Paraplegia Soc* 1987;10:11.

7 Montgomerie JZ, Chan E, Gilmore DS, Canawati HN, Sapico FL. Low mortality among patients with spinal cord injury and bacteremia. *Rev Infect Dis* 1991;12:867.

8 Fam BA, Sarkarati M, Yalla SV. Spinal cord injury. In: Yalla SV, McGuire EJ, Elbadawi A, Blaivas JG, eds. *Neurourology and Urodynamics*. New York: Macmillan Publishing Co., 1988;291–302.

9 Thomas DG, Lucas MG. The urinary tract following spinal cord injury. In: Chisolm GD, Fair WR, ed. *Scientific Foundations of Urology, 3rd ed*. St Louis, MO: Mosby Year Book Inc., 1990;286–290.

10 Barkin M, Dolfin D, Herschorn S, Bharatwal N, Comisarow R. The urologic care of the spinal cord injury patient. *J Urol* 1983;129:335.

11 Erickson RP, Merritt JL, Opitz JL, Ilstrup DM. Bacteriuria during follow-up in patients with spinal cord injury. I. Rates of bacteriuria in various bladder emptying methods. *Arch Phys Med Rehabil* 1982;63:409.

12 Guttmann L, Frankel H. The value of intermittent catheterization in the early management of traumatic paraplegia and tetraplegia. *Paraplegia* 1966;4:63.

13 Cardenas DD, Mayo ME. Bacteriuria with fever after spinal cord injury. *Arch Phys Med Rehabil* 1987;68:291.

14 Broecker BH, Klein FA, Hackler RH. Cancer of the bladder in spinal cord injury patients. *J Urol* 1981;125:196.

15 Kaufman JM, Fam B, Jacobs SC, et al. Bladder cancer and squamous metaplasia in spinal cord injury patients. *J Urol* 1977; 118:967.

16 Gardner BP, Parsons KF, Machin DG, Galloway A, Krishnan KR. The urological manage-

ment of spinal cord damaged patients: a clinical algorithm. *Paraplegia* 1986;24:138.

17   Lloyd LK. New trends in urologic management of spinal cord injured patients. *Central Nervous System Trauma* 1986;3:3.

18   Storer M. Alterations in the urinary tract after spinal cord injury—diagnosis, prevention and therapy of late sequelae. *World J Urol* 1990; 7:205.

19   McGuire EJ, Savastano JA. Long-term follow-up of spinal cord injury patients managed by intermittent catheterization. *J Urol* 1983;129:775.

20   Merritt JL. Residual urine volume: correlate of urinary tract infection in patients with spinal cord injury. *Arch Phys Med Rehabil* 1981; 62:558.

21   Wyndaele JJ, Maes D. Clean intermittent self-catheterization: a 12-year follow-up. *J Urol* 1990;142:906.

22   Ruutu M, Kivisaari A, Lehtonen T. Upper urinary tract changes in patients with spinal cord injury. *Clin Radiol* 1984;35:491.

23   Culkin DJ, Wheeler JS. Current management of urolithiasis in the spinal cord injured patient. *J Am Paraplegia Soc* 1987;10:23.

24   Gardner BP, Parsons KF, Galloway A, Krishnan KR. The urological management of spinal cord damaged patients: a clinical algorithm. *Paraplegia* 1986;24:138.

25   Lloyd LK. New trends in the urologic management of spinal cord injured patients. *Cent Nerv Syst Trauma* 1986;3:3.

26   Sher AT. Changes in the upper urinary tract as demonstrated on intravenous pyelography and micturating cystourethrography in patients with spinal cord injury. *Paraplegia* 1975;13:157.

27   Daifuku R, Stamm WE. Bacterial adherence to bladder uroepithelial cells in catheter-associated urinary tract infection. *N Engl J Med* 1986; 314:1208.

28   Moloney PJ, Doyle AA, Robinson BL, Fenster H, McLoughlin MG. Pathogenesis of urinary tract infection in patients with acute spinal cord injury on intermittent catheterization. *J Urol* 1981;125:672.

29   Giroux J, Perkash I. Limited value of the Fairley test in urologic infections in patients with neuropathic bladders. *J Am Paraplegia Soc* 1985;8:10.

30   Donovan WH, Hull R, Cifu CX, Brown HD, Smith NJ. Use of plasmid analysis to determine the source of bacterial invasion of the urinary tract. *Paraplegia* 1990;28:573.

31   Montgomerie JZ, Morrow JW. Pseudomonas colonization in patients with spinal cord injury. *J Epidemiol* 1978;108:328.

32   Fawcett C, Chawla JC, Quoraishi A, Stickler DJ. A study of the skin flora of spinal cord injured patients. *J Hosp Infect* 1986;8:149.

33   Schaeffer AJ, Chmiel J. Urethral meatal colonization in the pathogenesis of catheter-associated bacteriuria. *J Urol* 1983;130:1096.

34   Classen DC, Larsen RA, Burke JP, Stevens LE. Prevention of catheter-associated bacteriuria: Clinical trial of methods to block three known pathways of infection. *Am J Infect Control* 1991;19:136.

35   Stamm WE. Catheter-associated urinary tract infections: epidemiology, pathogenesis, and prevention. *Am J Med* 1991;91(suppl 3B):65S.

36   MacKenzie WR, O'Hanley P. Recent advances related to virulence and host factors in urinary tract infections. *Curr Opin Infect Dis* 1991; 4:31.

37   Reid G, Sobel JD. Bacterial adherence in the pathogenesis of urinary tract infection: a review. *Rev Infect Dis* 1987;9:470.

38   Stamm WE, Hooton TM, Johnson JR, et al. Urinary tract infections: from pathogenesis to treatment. *J Infect Dis* 1989;159:400.

39   Mobley HLT, Chippendale GR. Hemagglutinin, urease, and hemolysin production by *Proteus mirabilis* from clinical sources. *J Infect Dis* 1990;161:525.

40   Johnson JR, Roberts PL, Stamm WE. P fimbriae and other virulence factors in *Escherichia coli* urosepsis: association with patients' characteristics. *J Infect Dis* 1987;156:225.

41   Mobley HLT, Chippendale GR, Tenney JH, Hull RA, Warren JW. Expression of type 1 fimbriae may be required for persistence of *Escherichia coli* in the catheterized urinary tract. *J Clin Microbiol* 1987;25:2253.

42   Stickler D, Dolman J, Rolfe S, Chawla J. Activity of antiseptics against *Escherichia coli* growing as biofilms on silicone surfaces. *Eur J Clin Microbiol Infect Dis* 1989;8:974.

43   Ladd TI, Schmiel D, Nickel JC, Costerton JW. The use of a radiorespirometric assay for testing the antibiotic sensitivity of catheter-associated bacteria. *J Urol* 1987;138:1451.

44   Nickel JC, Reid G, Bruce AW, Costerton JW. Ultrastructural microbiology of infected urinary stones. *Urology* 1986;28:512.

45   Cox AJ, Hukins DWL, Sutton TM. Infection of catheterized patients: bacterial colonization of encrusted foley catheters shown by scanning electron microscopy. *Urol Res* 1989;17:349.

46   Nickel JC, Downey JA, Costerton JW. Ultrastructural study of microbiologic colonization of urinary catheters. *Urology* 1989;34:284.

47 Stickler DJ, Clayton CL, Chawla JC. The resistance of urinary tract pathogens to chlorhexidine bladder washouts. *J Hosp Infect* 1987;10:28.

48 Stickler DJ, Dolman J, Rolfe S, Chawla J. Activity of some antiseptics against urinary tract pathogens growing as biofilms on silicone surfaces. *Eur J Clin Microbiol Infect Dis* 1991;10:410.

49 Hess B. Prophylaxis of infection-induced kidney stone formation. *Urol Res* 1990;18(Suppl 1):S45.

50 Lerner SP, Gleeson MJ, Griffith DP. Infection stones. *J Urol* 1989;141:753.

51 Ruggieri MR, Hanno PM, Levin RM. Reduction of bacterial adherence to catheter surface with heparin. *J Urol* 1987;138:423.

52 Grenabo L, Hedelin H, Hugosson J, Pettersson S. Adherence of urease-induced crystals to rat bladder epithelium following acute infection with different uropathogenic microorganisms. *J Urol* 1988;140:428.

53 Griffith DP, Osborne CA. Infection (urease) stones. *Mineral Electrolyte Metab* 1987;13:278.

54 McLean RJC, Nickel JC, Cheng KJ, Costerton JW. The ecology and pathogenicity of ureaseproducing bacteria in the urinary tract. *CRC Crit Rev Microbiol* 1988;16:37.

55 Nickel JC, Olson M, McLean RJC, Grant SK, Costerton JW. An ecological study of infected stone genesis in an animal model. *Br J Urol* 1987;59:21.

56 Kunin CM, Chin QF, Chambers S. Indwelling urinary catheters in the elderly. *Am J Med* 1987;82:405.

57 Kunin CM. Blockage of urinary catheters: role of microorganisms and constituents of the urine on formation of encrustations. *J Clin Epidemiol* 1989;42:835.

58 Gribble MJ, McCallum NM, Schecter MT. Evaluation of diagnostic criteria for bacteriuria in acutely spinal cord injured patients undergoing intermittent catheterization. *Diagn Microbiol Infect Dis* 1988;9:197.

59 Deresinski SC, Perkash I. Urinary tract infections in male spinal cord injured patients. *J Am Paraplegia Soc* 1985;8:4.

60 Nicolle LE, Harding GEM, Kennedy J, McIntyre M, Aoki F, Murray D. Urine specimen collection with external devices for the diagnosis of bacteriuria in elderly incontinent men. *J Clin Microbiol* 1988;26:1115.

61 Hill VB, Davies WE. A swing to intermittent clean self-catheterization as a preferred mode of management of the neuropathic bladder for the dextrous spinal cord patient. *Paraplegia* 1988;26:405.

62 Maynard FM, Diokno AC. Clean intermittent catheterization for spinal cord injury patients. *J Urol* 1982;128:477.

63 Maynard FM, Glass J. Management of the neuropathic bladder by clean intermittent catheterization: 5 year outcomes. *Paraplegia* 1987;25:106.

64 McGuire EJ, Savastano JA. Long-term followup of spinal cord patients managed by intermittent catheterization. *J Urol* 1983;129:775.

65 Lapides J, Diokno AC, Silber SJ, Lowe BS. Clean, intermittent self-catheterization in the treatment of urinary tract disease. *J Urol* 1972;107:458.

66 Lapides J, Diokno AC, Lowe BS, Kalish MD. Follow up on unsterile, intermittent self-catheterization. *J Urol* 1974;111:184.

67 Breitenbucher RB. Bacterial changes in the urine samples of patients with long-term indwelling catheters. *Arch Intern Med* 1984;144:1585.

68 Grahn D, Norman DC, White ML, et al. Validity of urinary catheter specimen for diagnosis of urinary tract infection in the elderly. *Arch Intern Med* 1985;145:1858.

69 Warren JW, Tenney JH, Hoopes JM, et al. A prospective microbiologic study of bacteriuria in patients with chronic indwelling catheters. *J Infect Dis* 1982;146:719.

70 Sotolongo JR, Koleilat N. Significance of asymptomatic bacteriuria in spinal cord injury patients on condom catheter. *J Urol* 1990;143:979.

71 Stover SL, Fleming WC. Recurrent bacteriuria in complete spinal cord injury patients on external condom drainage. *Arch Phys Med Rehabil* 1980;61:178.

72 Rhame FS, Perkash I. Urinary tract infections occurring in recent spinal cord injury patients on intermittent catheterization. *J Urol* 1979;122:669.

73 Mohler JL, Cowen DL, Flanigan RC. Suppression and treatment of urinary tract infection in patients with an intermittently catheterized neurogenic bladder. *J Urol* 1987;138:336.

74 Sanderson PJ, Seissler S. A comparison of the effect of chlorhexidine antisepsis, soap and antibiotics on bacteriuria, perineal colonization and environmental contamination in spinally injured patients. *J Hosp Infect* 1990;15:235.

75 Classen DC, Larsen RA, Burke JP, Alling DW, Stevens LE. Daily meatal care for prevention of

catheter-associated bacteriuria: results using frequent applications of polyantibiotic cream. *Infect Control Hosp Epidemiol* 1991;12:157.

76 Burke JP, Garibaldi RA, Britt MR, Jacobson JA, Conti M, Alling DW. Prevention of catheter-associated urinary tract infections. *Am J Med* 1980;70:655.

77 Stickler DJ, Thomas B, Chawla JC. Antiseptic and antibody resistance in gram-negative bacteria causing urinary tract infection in spinal cord injured patients. *Paraplegia* 1981;19:50.

78 Fawcett C, Chawla JC, Quoraishi A, Stickler DJ. A study of the skin flora of spinal cord injured patients. *J Hosp Infect* 1986;8:149.

79 Chawla JC, Clayton CL, Stickler DJ. Antiseptics in the long-term urological management of patients by intermittent catheterization. *Brit J Urol* 1988;62:289.

80 Al-Juburi AZ, Cicmanec J. New apparatus to reduce urinary drainage associated with urinary tract infections. *Urology* 1989;33:97.

81 Sujka SK, Petrelli NJ, Herrera L. Incidence of urinary tract infections in patients requiring long-term catheterization after abdominoperineal resection of rectal carcinoma: does Betadine in the foley drainage bag make a difference? *Europ J Surg Oncol* 1987;13:341.

82 Holliman R, Seal DV, Archer H, Doman S. Controlled trial of chemical disinfection of urinary drainage bags. *Brit J Urol* 1987;60:419.

83 Maizels M, Schaffer AJ. Decreased incidence of bacteriuria associated with periodic instillations of hydrogen peroxide into the urethral catheter drainage bag. *J Urol* 1980;123:841.

84 Gillespie WA, Jones JE, Teasdale C, et al. Does the addition of disinfectants to urine drainage bags prevent infection in catheterized patients? *Lancet* 1983;1:1037.

85 Thompson RL, Haley CE, Searcy MA, et al. Catheter-associated bacteriuria. *JAMA* 1984; 251:747.

86 Sweet DE, Goodpasture HC, Holl K, et al. Evaluation of H_2O_2 prophylaxis of bacteriuria in patients with long term indwelling Foley catheters. *Infection Control* 1985;6:263.

87 Daifuku R, Stamm WE. Association of rectal and urethral colonization with urinary tract infection in patients with indwelling catheters. *JAMA* 1984;252:2028.

88 Schaeffer AJ, Story KO, Johnson SM. Effect of silver oxide trichloroisocyanuric acid antimicrobial urinary drainage system on catheter-associated bacteriuria. *J Urol* 1988;139:69.

89 Giroux J, Perkash I. In vitro evaluation of current disinfectants for leg bags. *J Am Paraplegia Soc* 1985;8:13.

90 Ball AJ, Carr TW, Gillespie WA, Kelly M, Simpson RA, Smith PJB. Bladder irrigation with chlorhexidine for the prevention of urinary infection after transurethral operations: a prospective controlled study. *J Urol* 1987;138:491.

91 Davies AJ, Desai HN, Turton S, Dyas A. Does instillation of chlorhexidine into the bladder of catheterized geriatric patients help reduce bacteriuria? *J Hosp Infect* 1987;9:71.

92 Stickler DJ, Clayton CL, Chawla JC. Assessment of antiseptic bladder washout procedures using a physical model of the catheterized bladder. *Brit J Urol* 1987;60:413.

93 Stickler D, Hewett P. Activity of antiseptics against biofilms of mixed bacterial species growing on silicone surfaces. *Eur J Clin Microbiol Infect Dis* 1991;10:416.

94 Kunin CM. Can we build a better catheter? *N Engl J Med* 1988;319:365.

95 Liedberg H, Lundeberg T. Silver coating of urinary catheters prevents adherence and growth of Pseudomonas aeruginosa. *Urol Res* 1989;17:357.

96 Liedberg H, Lundeberg T. Silver alloy coated catheters reduce catheter-associated bacteriuria. *Brit J Urol* 1990;65:379.

97 Liedberg H, Lundeberg T, Ekman P. Refinements in the coating of urethral catheters reduces the incidence of catheter-associated bacteriuria. *Eur Urol* 1990;17:236.

98 Johnson JR, Roberts PL, Olsen RJ, Moyer KA, Stamm WE. Prevention of catheter-associated urinary tract infection with a silver oxide-coated urinary catheter: clinical and microbiologic correlates. *J Infect Dis* 1990; 162: 1145.

99 Musher DM, Griffith DP. Generation of formaldehyde from methenamine: effect of pH and concentration, and antibacterial effect. *Antimicrob Agents Chemother* 1974;6:708.

100 Devenport JK, Swenson JR, Dukes GE, Sonsalla PK. Formaldehyde generation from methenamine salts in spinal cord injury. *Arch Phys Med Rehabil* 1984;65:257.

101 Gleckman R, Alvarez S, Joubert DW, Matthews SJ. Drug therapy reviews: methenamine mandelate and methenamine hippurate. *Am J Hosp Pharm* 1979;36:1509.

102 Hetey SK, Kleinberg ML, Parker WD, Johnson EW. Effect of ascorbic acid on urine pH in patients with injured spinal cords. *Am J Hosp Pharm* 1980;37:235.

103 Kevorkian CG, Merritt JL, Ilstrup DM. Methenamine mandelate with acidification: an ef-

fective urinary antiseptic in patients with neurogenic bladder. *Mayo Clin Proc* 1984;59:523.

104 **Vainrub B, Musher DM.** Lack of effect of methenamine in suppression of, or prophylaxis against, chronic urinary infection. *Antimicrob Agents Chemother* 1977;12:625.

105 **Thorsteinsson G, Keys T.** The frequency and type of urinary tract infections in patients on intermittent catheterization by self and by catheterization team. *Arch Phys Med Rehabil* 1983;64:519.

106 **Krebs M, Halvorsen RB, Fishman IJ, Santos-Mendoza N.** Prevention of urinary tract infection during intermittent catheterization. *J Urol* 1984;131:82.

107 **Merritt JL, Erickson RP, Opitz JL.** Bacteriuria during follow-up in patients with spinal cord injury: II. Efficacy of antimicrobial suppressants. *Arch Phys Med Rehabil* 1982; 63:413.

108 **Kuhlemeier KV, Stover SL, Lloyd LK.** Prophylactic antibacterial therapy for preventing urinary tract infections in spinal cord injury patients. *J Urol* 1985;134:514.

109 **Mohler JL, Cowen DL, Flanigan RC.** Suppression and treatment of urinary tract infection in patients with an intermittently catheterized neurogenic bladder. *J Urol* 1987;138:336.

110 **Maynard FM, Diokno AC.** Urinary infection and complications during clean intermittent catheterization following spinal cord injury. *J Urol* 1984;132:943.

111 **Woods DR, Bender BS.** Long-term urinary tract catheterization. *Med Clin NA* 1989; 73:1441.

112 **Zhanel GG, Harding GEM, Guay DRP.** Asymptomatic bacteriuria. *Arch Intern Med* 1990;150:1389.

113 **Stamm WE.** Measurement of pyuria and its relation to bacteriuria. *Am J Med* 1983; 75(suppl 1B):53.

114 **Deresinski SC, Perkash I.** Urinary tract infections in male spinal cord injured patients. *J Am Paraplegia Soc* 1985;8:7.

115 **Menon EB, Tan ES.** Pyuria: index of infection in patients with spinal cord injuries. *Brit J Urol* 1992;69:144.

116 **Musher DM, Thorsteinsson SB, Airola VM.** Quantitative urinalysis. Diagnosing urinary tract infection in men. *JAMA* 1976;236:2069.

117 **Peterson JR, Roth EJ.** Fever, bacteriuria, and pyuria in spinal cord injured patients with indwelling urethral catheters. *Arch Phys Med Rehabil* 1989;70:839.

118 **Hooton TM, O'Shaughnessy EJ, Clowers D, Mack L, Cardenas DD, Stamm WE.** Localiza-

tion of urinary tract infection in patients with spinal cord injury. *J Infect Dis* 1984;150:85.

119 **Gribble MJ, Puterman ML, McCallum NM.** Pyuria: its relationship to bacteriuria in spinal cord injured patients on intermittent catheterization. *Arch Phys Med Rehabil* 1989;70:376.

120 **Anderson RU, Hsieh-Ma ST.** Association of bacteriuria and pyuria during intermittent catheterization after spinal cord injury. *J Urol* 1983;130:299.

121 **Steward DK, Wood GL, Cohen RL, et al.** Failure of urinalysis and quantitative urine culture in diagnosing symptomatic urinary tract infections in patients with long-term urinary catheters. *Am J Infect Control* 1985; 13:154.

122 **Fairley KF, Bond AG, Brown RB, Habersberger P.** Simple test to determine the site of urinary tract infection. *Lancet* 1967;2:427.

123 **Perkash I, Giroux J.** Prevention, treatment, and management of urinary tract infections in neuropathic bladders. *J Am Paraplegia Soc* 1985;8:15.

124 **Giroux J, Perkash I.** Limited value of the Fairley test in urologic infections in patients with neuropathic bladders. *J Am Paraplegia Soc* 1985;8:10.

125 **Wyndaele JJ, Oosterlinck W, DeSy WA, Claessens H.** The use of the bladder wash-out test in patients with spinal cord lesions who have urinary tract infection. *Paraplegia* 1983; 21:294.

126 **Kuhlemeier KV, Lloyd LK, Stover SL.** Failure of antibody-coated bacteria and bladder washout tests to localize infection in spinal cord injury patients. *J Urol* 1983;130:729.

127 **Galloway A, Green HT, Menon KK, Gardner BP, Pemberton S, Krishnan KR.** Antibody coated bacteria in urine of patients with recent spinal injury. *J Clin Pathol* 1990;43:953.

128 **Merritt JL, Keys TF.** Limitations of the antibody-coated bacteria test in patients with neurogenic bladders. *JAMA* 1982;247:1723.

129 **Ronald AR, Pattullo ALS.** The natural history of urinary infection in adults. *Med Clin NA* 1991;75:299.

130 **Falls WF, Stacy WK.** A prospective analysis of renal function in patients with spinal cord injuries and persistent bacilluria. *Milit Med* 1986;151:116.

131 **Lewis RI, Carrion HM, Lockhart JL, Politano VA.** Significance of asymptomatic bacteriuria in neurogenic bladder disease. *Urology* 1984; 23:3437.

132 **Ouslander JG, Greengold B, Chen S.** Complications of chronic indwelling urinary cathe-

ters among male nursing home patients: a prospective study. *J Urol* 1987;138:1191.

133 Warren JW, Damron D, Tenney JH, Hoopes JM, Deforge B, Muncie HL. Fever, bacteremia, and death as complications of bacteriuria in women with long-term urethral catheters. *J Infect Dis* 1987;155:1151.

134 Stickler DJ, Chawla JC. An appraisal of antibiotic policies for urinary tract infections in patients with spinal injuries undergoing long-term intermittent catheterization. *Paraplegia* 1988;26:215.

135 DeVivo MJ, Fine PR, Cutter GR, Maetz HM. The risk of bladder calculi in patients with spinal cord injuries. *Arch Intern Med.* 1985;145:428.

136 DeVivo MJ, Fine PR, Cutter GR, Maetz HM. The risk of renal calculi in spinal cord injury patients. *J Urol* 1984;131:857.

137 Erickson RP. Autonomic hyperreflexia: Pathophysiology and medical management. *Arch Phys Med Rehabil* 1980;61:431.

138 Hammond MC, Britell CW, Little JW, DeLisa JA. Diagnostic ultrasound: its value in acute urinary tract infection in spinal cord injury. *Arch Phys Med Rehabil* 1987;68:743.

139 Segal JL, Gray DR, Gordon SK, Eltorai IM, Konsari F. Gentamicin disposition kinetics in humans with spinal cord injury: a preliminary report. *J Am Paraplegia Soc* 1983:6:41.

140 Segal JL, Brunnemann SR, Gray DR. Gentamicin bioavailability and single-dose pharmacokinetics in spinal cord injury. *Drug Intell Clin Pharm* 1988;22:461.

141 Segal JL, Brunnemann SR, Gordon SK, Eltorai IM. Amikacin pharmacokinetics in patients with spinal cord injury. *Pharmacotherapy* 1988;8:79.

142 Montgomerie JA, Morrow JW, Canawati HN, et al. Ceftizoxime in the treatment of urinary tract infection in spinal cord injury patients: comparison with tobramycin. *J Antimicrob Chemother* 1982;10(Suppl C):247.

143 Sapico FL, Lindquist LB, Montgomerie JZ, Jiminez EM, Morrow JW. Short-course aminoglycoside therapy in patients with spinal cord injury. *Urology* 1980;15:457.

144 Minuth JN, Musher DM, Thorsteinsson SB. Inhibition of the antibacterial activity of gentamicin by urine. *J Infect Dis* 1976; 133:14.

145 Hall MK, Hackler RH, Zampieri TA, Zampieri JB. Renal calculi in spinal cord-injured patient: association with reflux, bladder stones, and foley catheter drainage. *Urology* 1989; 34:126.

146 Wahle S, Kramolowsky E, Loening S. Extracorporeal shock wave lithotripsy in paraplegic and quadriplegic patients. *J Am Paraplegia Soc* 1988;11:6.

147 Burr RG. Urinary calculi composition in patients with spinal cord lesions. *Arch Phys Med Rehabil* 1978;59:84–88.

148 Nikakhtar B, Vaziri ND, Khonsari F, Gordon S, Mirahmadi MD. Urolithiasis in patients with spinal cord injury. *Paraplegia* 1981; 19:363.

149 Wexler BC, McMurtry JP. Kidney and bladder calculi in spontaneously hypertensive rats. *Brit J Exp Path* 1981;62:369.

150 Boistelle R, Abbona F, Berland Y, Grandvuillemin M, Olmer M. The crystalization of magnesium ammonium phosphate (struvite) in acidic sterile urine. In: Schwille PO, Smith LH, Robertson WG, Vahlensieck W, eds. *Urolithiasis and Related Clinical Research.* New York: Plenum Press, 1985;793.

151 Michaels EK, Fowler JE. Extracorporeal shock wave lithotripsy for struvite renal calculi: prospective study with extended follow-up. *J Urol* 1991;146:728.

152 Mobley HLT, Warren JW. Urease-positive bacteriuria and obstruction of long-term catheters. *J Clin Microbiol* 1987;25:2216.

153 Silverman DE, Stamey TA. Management of infection stones: the Stanford experience. *Medicine* 1983;62:44.

154 Bratell S, Brorson JE, Gernabo L, Hedelin H, Pettersson S. The bacteriology of operated renal stones. *Euro Urol* 1990;17:58.

155 Hugosson J, Grenabo L, Hedelin H, Pettersson S, Seeberg S. Bacteriology of upper urinary tract stones. *J Urol* 1990;143:965.

156 Claus-Walker J, Campos RJ, Carter RE, Vallbona C, Lipscomb HS. Calcium excretion in quadriplegia. *Arch Phys Med Rehabil* 1972;53:14.

157 Claus-Walker J, Carter RE, Campos RJ, Spencer WA. Hypercalcemia in early traumatic quadriplegia. *J Chron Dis* 1975;28:81.

158 Beck EM, Riehle RA. The fate of residual fragments after extracorporeal shock wave lithotripsy monotherapy of infection stones. *J Urol* 1991;145:6.

159 Koga S, Arakaki Y, Matsuoka M, Ohyama C. Staghorn calculi—long-term results of management. *Br J Urol* 1991;68:122.

160 Motola JA, Smith AD. Therapeutic options for the management of upper tract calculi. *Urol Clin NA* 1990;17:191.

161 Blandy JP, Singh M. The case for a more aggressive approach to staghorn stones. *J Urol* 1976;115:505.

162 Kracht H, Buscher H-K. Formation of staghorn calculi and their surgical implications in paraplegics and tetraplegics. *Paraplegia* 1974; 12:98.

163 Rous SN, Turner WR. Retrospective study of 95 patients with staghorn calculus disease. *J Urol* 1977;118:902.

164 Wojewski A, Zajaczkowski T. The treatment of bilateral staghorn calculi of the kidneys. *Int Urol Nephrol* 1974;5:249.

165 Atala A, Steinbock GS. Extracorporeal shock-wave lithotripsy of renal calculi. *Am J Surg* 1989;157:350.

166 Brown RD, Preminger GM. Changing surgical aspects of urinary stone disease. *Surg Clin NA* 1988;68:1085.

167 Chaussy CG, Fuchs GJ. Current state and future developments of noninvasive treatment of human urinary stones with extracorporeal shock wave lithotripsy. *J Urol* 1989;141:782.

168 Dretler SP. Ureteral stone disease. *Urol Clin NA* 1990;17:217.

169 Holmes SAV, Whitfield HN. The current status of lithotripsy. *Br J Urol* 1991;68:337.

170 Liong ML, Clayman RV, Gittes RF, Lingeman JE, Huffman JL, Lyon ES. Treatment options for proximal ureteral urolithiasis: review and recommendations. *J Urol* 1989; 141:504.

171 Lazare JN, Saltzman B, Sotolongo J. Extracorporeal shock wave lithotripsy treatment of spinal cord injury patients. *J Urol* 1988; 140:266.

172 Lingeman JE, Woods J, Toth PD, Evan AP, McAteer JA. The role of lithotripsy and its side effects. *J Urol* 1989;141:793.

173 Pode D, Lenkovsky, Shapiro A, Pfau A. Can extracorporeal shock wave lithotripsy eradicate persistent urinary infection associated with infection stones? *J Urol* 1988;140:257.

174 Segura JW. Role of percutaneous procedures in the management of renal calculi. *Urol Clin NA* 1990;17:207.

175 Spirnak JP, Resnick MI. Retrograde percutaneous nephrostomy. *Urol Clin NA* 1988; 15:393.

176 Culkin DJ, Wheeler JS, Nemchausky BA, Fruin RC, Canning JR. Percutaneous nephrolithotomy in the spinal cord injury population. *J Urol* 1986;136:1181.

177 Kahnoski RJ, Lingeman JE, Coury TA, Steele RE, Mosbaugh PG. Combined percutaneous and extracorporeal shock wave lithotripsy for staghorn calculi: an alternative to anatrophic nephrolithotomy. *J Urol* 1986;135:679.

178 Niedrach WL, Davis RS, Tonetti FW, Cockett ATK. Extracorporeal shock-wave lithotripsy in patients with spinal cord dysfunction. *Urology* 1991;38:152.

179 Schulze H, Hertle L, Graff J, Funke P-J, Senge T. Combined treatment of branched calculi by percutaneous nephrolithotomy and extracorporeal shock wave lithotripsy. *J Urol* 1986;135:1138.

180 Riehle RA. Selective use of ureteral stents before extracorporeal shock-wave lithotripsy. *Urol Clin NA* 1988;15:499.

181 Saltzman B. Ureteral stents. *Urol Clin NA* 1988;15:481.

182 Shabsigh R, Gleeson MJ, Griffith DP. The benefits of stenting on a more-or-less routine basis prior to extracorporeal shock-wave lithotripsy. *Urol Clin NA* 1988;15:493.

183 Shortliffe LMD, Spigelman SS. Infection stones. *Urol Clin NA* 1986;13:717.

184 Nemoy NJ, Stamey TA. Surgical, bacteriological, and biochemical management of "infection stones". *JAMA* 1971;215:1470.

185 Comarr AE, Kawaichi GH, Bors E. Renal calculosis of patients with traumatic cord lesions. *J Urol* 1962;87:647.

186 Sleight MW, Wickham JEA. Long term follow-up in 100 cases of renal calculi. *Br J Urol* 1977;49:601.

187 Hugosson J, Grenabo L, Hedelin H, Lincoln K, Pettersson S. Chronic urinary infection and renal stones. *Scand J Urol Nephrol* 1988;23:61–66.

188 Griffith DP, Moskowitz PA, Carlton CE. Adjunctive chemotherapy of infection-induced staghorn calculi. *J Urol* 1979;121:711.

189 Williams JJ, Rodman JS, Peterson CM. A randomized double-blind study of acetohydroxamic acid in struvite nephrolithiasis. *N Engl J Med* 1984;311:760.

190 Griffith DP, Khonsari F, Skurnick JH, et al. A randomized trial of acetohydroxamic acid for the treatment and prevention of infection-induced urinary stones in spinal cord injured patients. *J Urol* 1988;140:318.

191 Rodman JS, Williams JJ, Jones RL. Hypercoagulability produced by treatment with acetohydroxamic acid. *Clin Pharmacol Ther* 1987; 42:346.

192 Bagley DH. Pharmacologic treatment of infection stones. *Urol Clin NA* 1987;14:347.

193 Millner OE, Anderson JA, Appler ME, et al. Flurofamide: a potent inhibitor of bacterial urease with potential clinical utility in the

treatment of infection induced urinary stones. *J Urol* 1982;127:346.

194   Texier-Maugein J, Clerc M, Vekris A, Bebear C. Ureaplasma urealyticum-induced bladder stones in rats and their prevention by flurofamide and doxycycline. *Israel J Med Sci* 1987;23:565.

195   Bruno M, Marangella M, Tricerri A, Martini C, Linari F. Physicochemical changes of urine environment on propionhydroxamic acid therapy. *Contr Nephrol* 1987;58:207–211.

196   Colussi G, Surian M, De Ferrari ME, Rombola G, Rolando P, Minetti L. Low-dose propionhydroxamic acid therapy in infection-induced stones. *Contr Nephrol* 1987;58: 230–232.

197   Di Silverio F, Gallucci M, Alpi G, Ricciutti GP, Fini D, Molinari C. Tolerance and side effects of propionhydroxamic acid. *Contr Nephrol* 1987;58:215–218.

198   Fini M, Romagnoli P, Mannini D, et al. The value of propionhydroxamic acid in the prevention and therapy of infection-induced stones. *Contr Nephrol* 1987;58:226–229.

199   Mandressi A, Dormia G, Montanari E, et al. Propionhydroxamic acid for the prophylaxis of recurrences of infection-induced renal stones. *Contr Nephrol* 1987;58:222–225.

200   Martelli A, Buil P, Spatafora S. Clinical experience with low dosage of propionohydroxamic acid (PHA) in infected renal stones. *Urology* 1986;28:373–375.

201   Martelli A, Buli P, Cortecchia V, Spatafora S, Fiore F, Tiozzi E. Urease inhibition in the treatment of infected renal stones: propionhydroxamic acid. *Contr Nephrol* 1987; 58:196–200.

202   Puppo P, Germinale F, Bottino P, Ricciotti G, Giuliani L. Propionhydroxamic acid in the management of struvite urinary stones. *Contr Nephrol* 1987;58:201–206.

203   Tizzani A, Carone R, Casetta G, Piana P, Vercelli D. Low dosage treatment with propiono-hydroxamic acid in paraplegic patients. *Eur Urol* 1989;16:36–40.

204   Satoh M, Munakata K, Takeuchi H, Yoshida O, Takebe S, Kobashi K. Effects of a novel urease inhibitor, N-(diaminophosphinyl)isopentenoylamide on the infection stone in rats. *Chem Pharm Bull* 1991;39: 897–899.

205   Michaels EK, Fowler JE, Mariano M. Bacteriuria following extracorporeal shock wave lithotripsy of infection stones. *J Urol* 1988; 140:254.

206   Charton M, Vallancien G, Veillon B, et al. Use of antibiotics in conjunction with extracorporeal lithotripsy. *Eur Urol* 1990;17:134.

207   Fowler JE, Jr. Bacteriology of branched renal calculi and accompanying urinary tract infection. *J Urol* 1984;131:213.

208   Wilson WT, Preminger GM. Extracorporeal shock wave lithotripsy. *Urol Clin NA* 1990; 17:231.

Epidemiologic considerations in the evaluation of undifferentiated fever in a traveler returning from Latin America or the Caribbean

JAMES H. MAGUIRE

INTRODUCTION

Each year, increasing numbers of persons travel between the United States and the countries that lie south of its borders. The most recent statistics are from 1989, when nearly six million U.S. residents visited Latin America, and a greater number of travelers from Latin America and the Caribbean region visited this country (1). During the same year, 60% of the one million legal immigrants and most of the unnumbered illegal immigrants arrived from Latin America or the Caribbean basin (1).

The incidence of fever following recent travel in this region is unknown. Certainly, fever is a less common health problem than either traveler's diarrhea and sunburn in tourists or intestinal parasites and positive tuberculin skin tests in immigrants. More-over, serious fever-producing infections of high prevalence in Latin America and the Caribbean occur relatively infrequently in travelers. For instance, in 1990, the U.S. Centers for Disease Control (CDC) registered fewer than 100 cases of dengue among travelers to the region despite an ongoing epidemic affecting 76,000 persons in Peru and the occurrence of tens of thousands of cases in other countries (2–4). In the 1980s, when reported cases of malaria in Latin America and the Caribbean increased to over one million per year, cases originating in the region and diagnosed in the United States numbered only several hundred each year (5,6).

Whatever its frequency, fever following travel in the Americas presents a challenge. Unusual and life-threatening infections must be distinguished from common and benign processes. The intent of this chapter is to present a perspective on the relative frequency of the various causes of fever and to highlight epidemiologic features that may assist in the diagnosis of an unfamiliar or exotic disease. The focus is on those infections that may present with undifferentiated fever within three to six months of travel.

RISK OF INFECTION BY REGION

The differential diagnosis of fever following travel in Latin America or the Caribbean is extensive, even after causes of fever unrelated to travel have been excluded. The risk of infection differs according to locale, and wide variation is expected for a region that covers over eight million square miles and includes several of the largest cities in the world, as well as vast expanses of rain forest, desert, and snow-covered mountains (Figure 2.1). Risk of infection also depends on individual factors such as the reason for travel, duration of residence, types of exposures, level of prior immunity, and use of prophylactic medications (7–11).

In general, fevers in tourists or other short-term travelers to developing countries are due to acute infectious diseases (8,9). Diarrheal diseases, acute respiratory tract infections, acute hepatitis, and sexually transmitted diseases are the most frequent infections associated with short visits, while malaria, dengue, typhoid fever, and amebiasis occur less commonly (12–16).

In the absence of a dengue epidemic, tourists visiting resorts in the Caribbean islands experience little exposure to endemic diseases (17). There have been relatively few outbreaks of diarrheal illnesses such as shigellosis in Caribbean tourist hotels or on cruise ships, although food eaten during onshore visits to Haiti or Mexico may pose a special risk (17–20). An outbreak of legionnaires' disease in tourists visiting the U.S. Virgin Islands was traced to contaminated potable water in a single hotel (21). Recreational activities may present unique hazards: soft-tissue infections with *Vibrio alginolyticus* and other halophilic *Vibrio* species have followed coral injuries and contact with saltwater, and human immunodeficiency virus (HIV) infection and other sexually transmitted diseases are prevalent throughout the Caribbean (22).

A greater risk of infection may be encountered during short-term travel to Haiti, Mexico, and Central America, where rates of enterically transmitted diseases such as travelers' diarrhea, typhoid fever, and amebiasis are high, and there is a risk of malaria (23). Short visits to major South American cities are usually uneventful unless there is an outbreak of dengue or typhoid, or a blood transfusion or shared needle exposes the traveler to acute Chagas' disease, hepatitis, or HIV infection. The hazards of venereal diseases in Latin American cities is well illustrated by the experience of a U.S. Navy ship on a five-month goodwill tour to 22 port cities (24). Among approximately 400 crew members, there were 115 culture-confirmed acute cases of gonorrhea, 23 of which were due to penicillin-resistant strains of *Neisseria gonorrhoeae*. Chancroid, donovanosis, and lymphogranuloma venereum are also prevalent in certain areas (25). Short expeditions to forests or rural areas of South America may lead to malaria, arboviral infections, leishmaniasis, rickettsioses, leptospirosis, and enteric infections.

Immigrants and long-term residents of developing countries may be less susceptible to certain acute infections because of prior exposure, but are more likely than short-term travelers to import chronic and exotic infections (8,9). For instance, the differential diagnosis of fever in a recent arrival from Haiti includes malaria, typhoid fever, active tuberculosis, filarial lymphadenitis, and reactivation toxoplasmosis or histoplasmosis complicating acquired immunodeficiency syndrome (AIDS) (9). Amebiasis, brucellosis, malaria, and typhoid fever are diagnostic considerations in immigrants

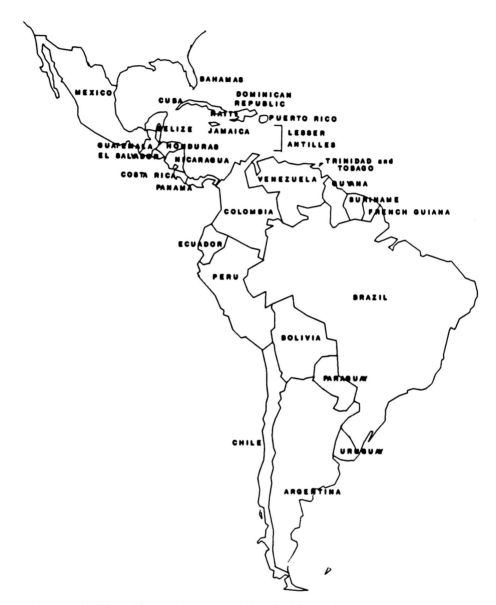

Figure 2.1 Map of Latin America and the Caribbean. The Lesser Antilles include Anguilla, Antigua and Barbuda, British Virgin Islands, Dominica, Grenada, Guadeloupe, Martinique, Montserrat, Netherlands Antilles (Aruba, Bonaire, Curaçao, Saba, Saint Eustatius, Saint Maarten), Saint Kitts and Nevis, Saint Lucia, Saint Martin (French), Saint Vincent and the Grenadines, Virgin Islands (U.S.). Also not shown: Cayman Islands, Turks and Caicos Islands.

Table 2.1   Endemic diseases associated with fever: partial listing by area

Widely distributed throughout Latin America and the Caribbean		
Commonly a cause of fever in travelers	*Occasionally a cause of fever in travelers*	*Uncommonly a cause of fever in travelers*
Bacterial diarrhea Respiratory tract infections	Enterovirus infections Hepatitis Influenza Sexually transmitted diseases Typhoid fever Tuberculosis	Acute HIV infection Acute rheumatic fever Leptospirosis Measles Meningococcal infection Murine typhus Q fever Toxocariasis Toxoplasmosis Trichinosis Tropical pyomyositis

		Present in:		
Frequency as a cause of fever in travelers:	*Caribbean*	*Mexico and Central America*	*Tropical South America*	*Temperate South America and the Andes*
Occasional	Malaria Dengue	Amebiasis Arboviral fevers (?) Brucellosis Coccidioidomycosis Dengue Malaria	Amebiasis Arboviral fevers (?) Brucellosis Dengue Malaria	
Uncommon or rare	Anthrax Cysticercosis Filariasis Histoplasmosis Relapsing fever Schistosomiasis	Angiostrongylosis (abdominal) Arboviral fevers (?) Chagas' disease Cysticercosis Filariasis Histoplasmosis Paracoccidioidomycosis Rabies Relapsing fever Spotted fever Typhus Visceral leishmaniasis	Arboviral fevers (?) Brazilian purpuric fever Chagas' disease Coccidioidomycosis Cysticercosis Filariasis Histoplasmosis Paracoccidioidomycosis Plague Rabies Relapsing fever Spotted fever Schistosomiasis Visceral leishmaniasis Yellow fever	Bartonellosis Bolivian and Argentine hemorrhagic fevers Chagas' disease Plague Rabies Relapsing fever Typhus

Note: Most diseases are not evenly distributed within a given area. Some diseases are more likely to be encountered among immigrants or long-term residents than among short-term visitors. Some diseases have never been encountered in travelers or are extremely unlikely to cause fever in travelers.
SOURCE From References 9, 15, 16, 27. See references and text for details.

from Mexico (9,26). Reactivation of paracoccidioidomycosis, Chagas' disease, or visceral leishmaniasis would be unusual and exotic causes of fever in South American immigrants.

Table 2.1 is an abbreviated summary of diseases that may cause fever according to geographic area. In the following sections, further information about the occurrence of individual diseases is presented. The references should be consulted for details about clinical features, diagnosis, and treatment.

MALARIA

Occurrence and risks

The incidence of malaria in many countries in Latin America and the Caribbean has increased dramatically during the past decade, largely because of deteriorating socioeconomic conditions (5). Nevertheless, rates of malaria in travelers to the region are five to 20 times lower than rates among travelers to parts of Africa and Asia (28,29). The risk of developing malaria for U.S. travelers returning from Haiti has been estimated to be 1:4,800. For European travelers who did not use chemoprophylaxis, the incidence of malaria was less than 10 cases and 50 cases per 100,000 travelers per month for travel to Central and South America, respectively (28,29). This relatively low risk reflects the absence of transmission in frequently visited cities and tourist resorts and the patchy distribution of malaria in rural areas (29,30).

In 1984, 70% of malaria cases imported into the United States from Latin America and the Caribbean occurred among foreign nationals (6). Immigrants from malarious regions often fail to take prophylaxis when visiting their country of origin because they do not realize that acquired immunity can be lost (29,31). A survey by the CDC in 1984 showed that only 27% of 1,445 travelers to Haiti took recommended chemoprophylaxis without interruption, and none of 58 reported patients with *Plasmodium falciparum* infections acquired in Haiti between 1980 and 1984 had used any prophylaxis (32). However, malaria has occurred in persons taking chloroquine and even mefloquine while traveling in areas with chloroquine-resistant *P. falciparum* (33,34).

Between 1959 and 1987, only six of 68 reported deaths due to falciparum malaria among U.S. travelers occurred in persons who had visited Haiti or South America (33). This relatively low number of deaths reflects the fact that less than 10% of malaria cases imported from the Americas are due to *P. falciparum* (6).

Since 1986, several outbreaks of *P. vivax* malaria involved migrant agricultural workers from Mexico who were infected shortly after arriving in the United States (35,36). Apparently, local anopheline mosquitoes had taken blood meals from other migrant workers who had untreated and often asymptomatic malaria. These outbreaks have occurred mainly in San Diego County, California, but other rural areas in the Southwest and along the Gulf of Mexico that have large populations of migrant workers living near mosquito breeding sites are also at risk for "introduced malaria" (35,36).

In 1990, imported *P. vivax* malaria was reported in two U.S. citizens who had received intramuscular injections of infected human blood in Mexico (37). They had been referred to practitioners in Mexico for malariotherapy of late-stage Lyme disease, based on the unproven practice of malariotherapy for neurosyphilis.

Geographic distribution and occurrence of drug resistance

Table 2.2 lists countries where malaria is endemic; transmission tends to be focal in each country and restricted to rural areas (27,38). In the Caribbean, malaria is found only in the island of Hispaniola. All cases in Haiti and all but a few in the Dominican Republic are due to *P. falciparum*, because *P. vivax* is unable to infect black persons whose erythrocytes lack the Duffy blood group determinants (39). In the other Caribbean islands, malaria has disappeared or been eradicated, but anopheline mosquitoes persist, and there is a risk of transmission from imported or recrudescent cases (40,41).

In Mexico and Central America west of the Canal Zone, more than 90% of cases are due to *P. vivax* (38). Major resort areas along the Pacific and Gulf coasts of Mexico are considered free of malaria, although, in 1985, 12 U.S. tourists to Puerto Vallarta and Acapulco contracted *P vivax* (42).

Both *P. vivax* and *P. falciparum* occur in varying proportions in most endemic areas of South America and Panama east of the Canal Zone; *P. malariae* and *P. ovale* are unusual. During the past decade transmission has increased dramatically in the Amazon basin following massive human migration into the region for purposes of agriculture and

Table 2.2   Distribution of malaria in the Americas

Area	Countries with malaria	Species	Chloroquine-resistant P falciparum confirmed
Caribbean	Haiti, Dominican Republic	*P. falciparum*	No
Mexico and Central America (including Panama west of Canal Zone)	All	*P. vivax* > 90%; rest *P. falciparum*	No
Andean area (Colombia, Venezuela, Ecuador, Peru) and Panama east of Canal Zone	All	*P. vivax* predominates; *P. falciparum* 5% to 30%; occasional *P. malariae*; rare *P. ovale*	Yes
Guayanas	All	>65% *P. falciparum*; rest *P. vivax*	Yes
Brazil	Mostly Amazon basin	*P. falciparum* and *P. vivax* in about equal portions	Yes
Southern Cone (Argentina, Chile, Paraguay, Uruguay)	Paraguay, northern provinces of Argentina	Mostly *P. vivax*	No

SOURCE From References 4, 5, 27, 38. For more detailed information about geographic distribution, see References 27 and 38.

mining (43). Induced malaria has become a problem in Brazil among intravenous drug users who share needles (44).

There is no confirmed chloroquine-resistant *P. falciparum* in the Caribbean, Mexico, or Central America (27). Chloroquine resistance is widespread in South America and Panama east of the Canal Zone. In western parts of the Amazon region, resistance to chloroquine and pyrimethamine-sulfadoxine has been detected in over 80% of *P. falciparum* isolates studied (45). There is a single reported clinical case of mefloquine-resistant *P. falciparum* infection acquired from the Amazon region; the patient developed bloodsmear-confirmed falciparum malaria while receiving 250 mg weekly of mefloquine and experienced a clinical relapse with negative smears after a treatment dose of 1,500 mg of mefloquine (34). Treatment of falciparum malaria from areas of Latin America where chloroquine-resistant *P. falciparum* is known to occur should include quinine or quinidine and a tetracycline (46). In the Amazon region of Brazil, clindamycin and quinine have been used extensively for treatment of chloroquine-resistant falciparum malaria. However, the use of clindamycin alone has been associated with a slow response to therapy (47). Halofantrine, the most recently introduced antimalarial agent, is available in Brazil for treatment of chloroquine-resistant falciparum malaria.

To date, there are no reports of chloroquine-resistant *P. vivax* in the Americas as described recently in New Guinea and the Solomon islands (48). However, relapses of vivax malaria after standard doses of chloroquine and primaquine have been reported in Latin America (49). These have not recurred after repeated doses of primaquine have been given, suggesting that relative primaquine resistance rather than chloroquine resistance was responsible.

TYPHOID FEVER

More than two-thirds of the approximately 500 cases of typhoid fever diagnosed in the United States each year occur in international travelers, and, of these, approximately 40% originate in Mexico and 20% originate elsewhere in the Caribbean or Latin America (50). During the last decade, the highest attack rates occurred among travelers returning from Haiti, Chile, and Peru and were two to five times higher than the rate of 20 cases per million among travelers to Mexico (50). U.S. citizens, particularly students, accounted for more than half the cases, and only 5% had been vaccinated within two years of travel (50,51). Of note, the inactivated parenteral vaccine and the new live, attenuated oral Ty21a vaccine are both only 50% to 80% effective in preventing the disease (50,51). The mortality of typhoid acquired during travel was 0.5% during the period 1975–1984 (50).

Typhoid fever is widely endemic in the region and occasionally occurs in epidemics (52,53). Endemic typhoid has been problematic along the western coast of South America, especially in Lima, Peru and Santiago, Chile. The remarkable incidence of 170 cases per 100,000 per year in Santiago has been attributed to a large number of chronic carriers with gallstones and the use of untreated waste water for irrigation of crops in the summer (54,55).

There is some suggestion that typhoid in the Western Hemisphere is a less severe illness than the highly lethal disease that occurs in parts of Asia (55,56). Typhoid fever in infants in Santiago may present as a mild, self-limited illness with low-grade fever and none of the features of classic enteric fever (55). An epidemic of typhoid fever in San Antonio, Texas in 1981 was remarkable for the frequent occurrence of mild and nonspecific symptoms and a uniformly benign outcome (57). An atypical clinical picture has been reported in AIDS patients with *Salmonella typhi* or *paratyphi* B bacteremia in Lima who presented with severe diarrhea, ulcerative lesions on proctoscopy, and a high rate of relapse after completing therapy (58). Persons with HIV infection appear to be at high risk for typhoid in endemic areas: The incidence in a cohort of HIV-infected patients in Lima was estimated to be approximately 60 times that in the general population (58).

Plasmid-mediated antibiotic resistance in *S. typhi* in general has not been a persistent problem in Latin America and the Caribbean. During a nationwide outbreak of multiply-resistant *S. typhi* in Mexico in 1972 and 1973, 80 cases of chloramphenicol-resistant *S. typhi* were reported in the United States (59). The epidemic subsided in 1973, and no further cases were seen in the United States. In Santiago, only 0.23% of isolates studied between 1975 and 1983 were resistant to chloramphenicol (60). However, following an endemic of multiply-resistant *S. typhi* in Peru in 1979–1980, strains resistant to chloramphenicol and, in some cases, ampicillin and trimethoprim remained endemic (52). Between 1975 and 1984, only 3.6% of strains of *S. typhi* acquired during foreign travel and reported to the CDC showed resistance to chloramphenicol, ampicillin, or trimethoprim-sulfamethoxazole (50). Third-generation cephalosporins and new quinolones are active against resistant isolates (52). Norfloxacin and ciprofloxacin have been used in Peru and Chile for the treatment of chronic typhoid carriers, with success rates of 78% to 92% in small groups of patients followed for one year (61,62).

BACTERIAL DIARRHEAL DISEASES

Fever, often with chills and other constitutional symptoms, may precede the onset of diarrhea and frequently accompanies the diarrhea caused by invasive bacteria such as *Shigella*, *Campylobacter*, and *Salmonella*. Fever is not seen as a rule with infections due to enterotoxigenic *Escherichia coli*, the most common cause of traveler's diarrhea in persons visiting the region, or *Vibrio cholerae*, which continues to spread rapidly through South and Central America and Mexico (63). The risk of developing traveler's diarrhea varies according to countries visited, with rates of 20% to 50% or higher in Mexico and other parts of Latin America and rates less than 10% to 20% in many Caribbean Islands except for Haiti (23). Rates of infection with individual invasive organisms usually are less than 10%, although *Shigella* has been isolated in as many as 20% of persons traveling to Mexico in several studies (64,65).

In 1988, a fivefold increase in the number of *Shigella dysenteriae* type 1 infections reported in the United States was traced to tourists visiting the Yucatan peninsula in Mexico (66). Illness among these travelers was severe: More than half of the persons interviewed had been hospitalized and two individuals developed a hemolytic uremic syndrome. Isolates from Mexico and from an outbreak in Guatemala in 1991 were resistent to ampicillin, chloramphenicol, and trimethoprim-sulfamethoxazole (67). Genetic analysis of isolates suggests that these outbreaks were due to the same strain that caused the disastrous pandemic in Central America from 1969 to 1972 (66–68).

Nontyphoidal salmonella infections account for up to 5% of cases of diarrhea in travelers to the region (65). Multiresistant strains of *Salmonella typhimurium* are becoming serious problems in urban centers of Brazil and Mexico (69). Cases of *S. arizonae* infection in the United States have been caused by ingestion of capsules of dried rattlesnake meat (70). The capsules were obtained in Mexico, or illegally in the United States, for treatment of a variety of illnesses, including cancer and AIDS. Pet iguanas, which are lizards native to the tropical Americas, have been the source of *S. marina* infections in infants (71). Systemic salmonellosis may cause undifferentiated and prolonged fever in persons with HIV infection, schistosomiasis, bartonellosis, falciparum malaria, disseminated histoplasmosis, louse- and tick-borne relapsing fever, and sickle cell anemia, all of which occur in the region (58,72–77).

AMEBIASIS

Fever is common in invasive amebiasis and may be the only symptom in persons with amebic liver abscesses. In several recent case series of amebic liver abscesses, the majority of patients were persons who had recently traveled in or emigrated from Mexico and South America (78–80). The risk of acquiring *Entamoeba histolytica* infection during short-term travel in endemic areas varies from none to a few percent (81–83). In a study of patients with amebic liver abscesses seen in Germany, a third had spent less than six weeks in an endemic area, and 95% developed amebic liver abscesses within eight to 20 weeks following return (84). Rarely, liver abscess or amebic colitis develops 10 or more years after leaving an endemic area (84,85).

Stool and serologic surveys for *Entamoeba histolytica* indicate a high prevalence of infection in many urban and rural areas throughout Latin America and the Caribbean (86). However, invasive amebiasis is not found uniformly throughout the region. The incidence of invasive amebiasis is extremely high in Mexico and may account for as many as five to six million clinical cases and 10,000 to 30,000 deaths a year (86,87). Invasive amebiasis is common in Colombia, Venezuela, and parts of Central America, but the incidence appears to be lower elsewhere in the region (86,87). For instance, in Jamaica, where the prevalence of infection is 5% to 30% by stool examination, only one case of liver abscess and two cases of colitis were seen in 20 years (88).

It has been shown that invasive amebiasis, including hepatic amebiasis, is produced by strains of amebas that can be differentiated from nonpathogenic amebas by DNA probes, monoclonal antibodies, or characterization of isoenzymes (89–91). In a group of 2,700 German travelers returning from the tropics, 106 had *E. histolytica* infection, but only eight had symptoms of invasive disease, and, of these, all five whose isolates were tested had pathogenic zymodemes (isoenzyme patterns); none of the asymptomatic persons were infected with a pathogenic zymodeme (92). Pathogenic amebas have been isolated from patients with invasive amebiasis in Mexico, and limited data are available on the zymodemes of South American strains (93). In the northeast of Brazil, where the prevalence of amebic infection is high but symptomatic amebiasis is unusual, virtually all strains of amebas studied were nonpathogenic (93,94). However, pathogenic zymodemes of E. *histolytica* have been identified in a few instances in the Amazon region of Brazil and in Ecuador, and, in fact, sporadic cases of invasive amebiasis occur in most countries in the Caribbean and Latin America (93,95). Nonpathogenic strains of E. *histolytica* do not appear to cause morbidity in patients with AIDS (96).

VIRAL HEPATITIS

Acute viral hepatitis is an occasional cause of undifferentiated fever in a traveler from the Caribbean or Latin America. In a study of Swiss travelers to developing countries, the incidence of hepatitis was four per 1,000 travelers per month, a rate higher than that of gonorrhea and malaria (12). All five hepatitis viruses (A–E) are endemic in the region; rates of infection vary according to the area visited and types of exposures.

Hepatitis A is the most commonly recognized cause of acute hepatitis among travelers, and, in the United States, approximately 7% of cases occur in international travelers (12,97). Acute hepatitis A is more often an illness of U.S. travelers, of whom only 10% to 20% have antibodies by age 20 years, than of immigrants or visitors arriving from developing countries, most of whom have acquired immunity earlier in life (98). Over 90% of children in areas such as Mexico City and Peru experience acute infection by age five years (99,100). Children shedding massive quantities of virus into the environment account for the high risk to nonimmune travelers. Appropriate use of pooled immune serum globulin by travelers has an efficacy of greater than 85% in preventing hepatitis A (98).

The prevalence of hepatitis B surface antigenemia varies from 1% or less in Mexico, temperate South America, and many Caribbean islands to 4% to 8% in the Amazon basin, Haiti, the Dominican Republic, St. Kitts, and Nevis (4). Travelers at risk typically spend prolonged periods of time with local populations and have sexual contact with chronic carriers or other intimate exposure to blood or body fluids. Unusually high numbers of cases of fulminant hepatitis and of chronic liver disease have occurred among inhabitants of areas in South America where hepatitis B is highly endemic, such as the Amazon region ("Labrea hepatitis"), northern Colombia ("hepatitis of the Sierra Nevada of Santa Marta"), and remote Amerindian settlements in Venezuela (101–104). The origin of these cases has been shown to be due to delta virus superinfection following direct person-to-person contact rather than percutaneous needle exposures.

Hepatitis C poses a risk to recipients of blood transfusions throughout the region (4,105). Hepatitis E, an enterically transmitted virus, has been responsible for documented outbreaks of acute hepatitis in Mexico and probably numerous other epidemics and sporadic cases in the region (4,105,106). The disease is usually self-limiting except for women in the third trimester of pregnancy, who have a fatality rate of 10% to 20%. Hepatitis E was confirmed serologically in a U.S. traveler following a day trip to Mexico (107). A newly described fluorescent-antibody blocking assay that detects antibodies to a recombinant structural protein of the hepatitis E virus should identify more cases of travel-associated hepatitis E in the future (107).

DENGUE, YELLOW FEVER, AND OTHER ARBOVIRUSES

Various arthropod-borne viruses are endemic in the Caribbean and Latin America (Table 2.3). After an incubation period of less than two weeks, most produce nonspecific febrile illnesses that are mild and self-limited. Because most arboviral fevers go undiagnosed, the frequency among travelers is unknown. The same virus may produce encephalitis or a hemorrhagic syndrome in addition to fever (108). Diagnosis is made by viral isolation from blood or demonstration of a specific antibody response. No antiviral drugs are known to be effective.

Dengue

Many of the cases of dengue diagnosed in the United States in recent years were acquired in the Caribbean and Latin America, where the number of cases has risen abruptly since 1981 following the resurgence of *Aedes aegypti* in the region (2,4,113–115). *A. aegypti* is a day-biting mosquito that breeds in water containers inside and around human dwellings in all countries in the region except Bermuda, the Cayman Islands, Costa Rica, Uruguay, and Chile (115). Dengue is now endemic in most areas where the vector is found, and massive and prolonged epidemics have become frequent, including suburban areas and coastal resorts in Mexico, major cities such as Rio de Janeiro, and Aruba, Barbados, Puerto Rico, and other Caribbean islands that

Table 2.3   Arboviruses and hemorrhagic fever viruses of the Americas

Arboviruses that cause undifferentiated fevers		Arboviruses that cause encephalitis
Dengue	Bussuquara	Venezuelan equine encephalitis
Oropouche	Catu	Rocio
Mayaro	Changuinola	Ilheus
Sand fly fever viruses	Cotia	St. Louis encephalitis
(Chagres, Punta Toro,	Guama	Western equine encephalitis
Candiru, Alenquer)	Guaroa	Eastern equine encephalitis
Group C viruses (Apeu,	Ilheus	**Viruses that cause hemorrhagic fever**
Caraparu, Tiaqui,	Taciuma	
Madrid, Marituba,	Vesicular	
Murutucu, Nepuyo,	Stomatitis	Yellow fever
Oriboca, Ossa,	Wyeomyia	Dengue (dengue hemorrhagic fever)
Restan)		Junin (Argentine hemorrhagic fever)*
		Machupo (Bolivian hemorrhagic fever)*
		Guanarito (Venezuelan hemorrhagic fever)*

*Arenaviruses transmitted via infected rodent excreta.
SOURCE: From References 108–112.

depend heavily on the tourist industry (4,116–118). The risk of dengue for most tourists seems to be small, except when an epidemic is in progress (116).

Dengue in travelers is usually of the "classic" variety, with sudden onset, high fever, severe headache, muscle and joint pain, and rash (116). Classic dengue may be confused with other viral illnesses, as, for instance, during an outbreak in Mexico when 10% of persons with a clinical diagnosis of dengue were later shown to have had acute rubella infection by serologic testing (119). Dengue hemorrhagic fever and shock syndrome are uncommon in U.S. travelers because their pathogenesis requires a second infection with a different serotype of the virus (120). Three serotypes (DEN-1, DEN-2, DEN-4) now circulate in the Americas, and sporadic cases and epidemics of dengue hemorrhagic fever and dengue shock syndrome have become common (4,116). A previously infected immigrant who returns to an endemic country is at risk for these potentially fatal illnesses.

Suspected cases of imported dengue should be reported to public health authorities because of the potential for indigenous transmission, as occurred in Texas in 1986 (121). Both *Aedes aegypti* and *Aedes albopictus* infest the southern United States (122,123). Since its importation from Asia in 1985, *A. albopictus*, an exceptionally aggressive vector of dengue, has spread throughout the southern, eastern, and midwestern states as far north as downtown Chicago.

Yellow fever

Undifferentiated fever occurs in the early stage of yellow fever before jaundice and bleeding develop and may be one of the only symptoms in mild cases, which are five to 10 times more common than classic cases (124). The last reported case of imported yellow fever in the United States was in 1924, and the last case of urban yellow fever in the Americas occurred in 1942 (125,126). Jungle yellow fever remains enzootic in monkeys in South America, Panama, and Trinidad and causes several hundred human cases in South America a year, usually among unvaccinated young men working in forested areas of Brazil, Colombia, Ecuador, Peru, and Bolivia (4,126,127). At present, only travelers who visit enzootic forested areas and have not received a highly effective yellow fever 17D vaccine are at risk. However, the recent invasion of *Aedes aegypti* into areas adjacent to forests may allow yellow fever to spread to more densely populated coastal regions (127,128).

Undifferentiated arboviral fevers

Many arboviruses cause self-limited febrile illnesses, which may or may not be associated with rash, conjunctival infection, myalgia, arthralgia, or arthritis (108–110). The vectors include various species of mosquitoes, phlebotomine sand flies, and *Culicoides* midges that inhabit forested regions of northern and eastern South America, Panama, and Trinidad (109). Sporadic cases and outbreaks typically occur when nonimmune settlers or soldiers enter the forest, although there have been outbreaks of Oropouche virus infection in urban centers in Brazil (109,110,129). Mayaro virus infection has been frequently encountered among settlers along the Trans-Amazon Highway in

Brazil (130). Ilheus virus occurs in Central America as well as South America and may cause mild encephalitis (109). Vesicular stomatitis virus (VSV), which may produce vesicles in the mouth and skin, is transmitted widely throughout the Americas by arthropods and other mechanisms (109,131).

Arbovirus encephalitis

A febrile illness may precede neurologic disease or may be the only manifestation of infection with arboviruses that cause encephalitis. Venezuelan equine encephalitis (VEE) virus is enzootic throughout tropical and subtropical regions from Florida to Argentina and has caused large epidemics with human fatalities in Trinidad, northern South America, Central America, Mexico, and Texas (111). Human infections have been most common during the rainy season in tropical coastal regions. Another mosquito-borne agent, Rocio virus, is found only in coastal plains of São Paulo state in Brazil, where it has produced epidemics of encephalitis (132). Although no clinical cases have been detected since 1980, there is serologic evidence of ongoing transmission. The viruses of St. Louis, eastern equine, and western equine encephalitis are present in tropical America and have caused sporadic cases in association with forest exposures in the Caribbean, South America, and Panama (112).

VIRAL HEMORRHAGIC FEVERS

In addition to dengue hemorrhagic fever and yellow fever, there are three viruses in South America that cause hemorrhagic disease: Junin virus, the agent of Argentine hemorrhagic fever; Machupo virus, the agent of Bolivian hemorrhagic fever; and the newly described Guanarito virus that causes Venezuelan hemorrhagic fever (133–135). All are arenaviruses and, like the closely related Lassa fever virus in Africa, appear to be transmitted by aerosolized rat excreta. The fatality rate without treatment is high. Transmission occurs peridomestically or in agricultural fields in well-defined rural areas of northwestern Argentina, eastern Bolivia, and central Venezuela. Travel-associated cases have not been reported, but there is a risk of person-to-person and nosocomial spread of infection (133,134).

In all three diseases, nonspecific illness with high fever, headache, conjunctivitis, and cervical lymphadenopathy precedes the hemorrhagic complications or may occur in the absence of hemorrhage (133,134). Diagnosis by detection of specific antibodies or by isolation of the highly contagious viruses from serum should be carried out in a containment facility (135). Administration of immune plasma is beneficial in Argentine hemorrhagic fever, and ribavirin has increased survival in rodents (135).

HIV AND HTLV-I INFECTIONS

Fever is common during acute HIV infection, "AIDS-related complex," and full-blown AIDS. The rapid spread of HIV has led to reports of AIDS from all countries and territories in the Americas (4,136,137). Brazil, Mexico, and Haiti account for more than one-half of the cases of AIDS reported from Latin America and the Carribean. Most HIV isolates have been identified as HIV-1, although HIV-2 has been demonstrated in Brazil and the Caribbean (136–138). In many parts of the region, heterosexual contact has become the predominant mode of transmission, and bisexual men, who account for 15% to 25% of AIDS cases, may act as the primary bridge for infection between the homosexual and heterosexual communities (4,137). High rates of transfusion-induced infection in the area are due to the use of paid donors and inadequate serologic screening of blood and blood products.

Fever in an immigrant from the region who has AIDS may be due to different opportunistic pathogens than are commonly seen in U.S. citizens with AIDS. Latin American and Haitian AIDS patients have a higher incidence of tuberculosis, toxoplasmosis, and salmonellosis than U.S.-born AIDS patients (139). Latent paracoccidioidomycosis, histoplasmosis, Chagas' disease, and visceral leishmaniasis may reactivate in patients with AIDS (140).

Human T-cell lymphotropic virus type I (HTLV-I), the retrovirus associated with adult T-cell leukemia and lymphoma (ATL), tropical spastic paraparesis, and HTLV-1-associated myelopathy, is endemic in the Caribbean and parts of Central and South America (4,137). Fever with lymphadenopathy and skin lesions or opportunistic infections may be the initial presentation of ATL.

OTHER VIRAL INFECTIONS: MEASLES, POLIOMYELITIS, AND RABIES

Although the fever of measles is usually accompanied by classic findings of cough, coryza, conjunctivitis, and rash, misdiagnoses are not uncommon. Failure to recognize measles and institute precautions among a group of persons who had acquired infection in Mexico resulted in 41 secondary cases during an outbreak in Washington state in 1990 (141). More than three-quarters of persons infected in the outbreak had never received the measles vaccine, and nearly half of these were immigrants or visitors from Latin America. Imported measles accounts for up to 7% of cases reported each year in the United States, and travel by U.S. citizens to Latin America accounts for about 35% of imported cases (141,142). Despite great progress made during the last decade by the World Health Organization's Expanded Programme on Immunization, measles are still transmitted throughout the Americas, and prospects for eradication are poor (143,144).

On the other hand, poliomyelitis as a cause of fever in a traveler from Latin America or the Caribbean is now extremely unlikely because of the success of the Pan American Health Organization's vaccination campaign (145). Only 11 new cases of wild-type polio virus infections were reported in the Americas in 1990, and no new cases have been reported since 1991 (145).

Fever of 105°F to 106°F may occur in rabies, and the diagnosis may not be obvious if there is no history of animal exposure. In the last decade, nine of the 16 reported cases in the United States were imported (146). Canine rabies is endemic along the U.S.-Mexican border and in cities and towns in other parts of Mexico, Central and South America, and several Caribbean islands (26,147). Mongoose rabies is found in the

Caribbean, and vampire bat bites have caused human cases, including an outbreak affecting 5% of two rural communities in the Amazon region of Peru in 1990 (148,149). In a recent investigation of rabies among immigrants without a known source of infection, DNA analysis after amplification of viral DNA by the polymerase chain reaction showed that one of the infections had originated in Mexico (150).

TUBERCULOSIS

Active tuberculosis is more likely to follow prolonged residence in Latin America and the Caribbean than a short trip. The rate of active infection among foreign-born persons arriving in the United States is 13 times that of the general population (151). Compared to 20,000 cases per year in the United States, over 200,000 cases of active tuberculosis are reported in the region, and the actual number may be as high as 800,000 (4,152). The infection rate in Cuba is as low as the U.S. rate, while rates are slightly higher in the English-speaking Caribbean, Costa Rica, and Uruguay; the rate is 10 to 20 times higher in Haiti and Bolivia, and between these aforementioned extremes for Mexico, Brazil, and other countries (4).

Vaccination with Bacille Calmette-Guérin (BCG) is practiced widely throughout the region and is encouraged by the Pan American Health Organization as a measure of control (4). In the interpretation of the tuberculin reaction of an immigrant with suspected tuberculosis, a history of BCG vaccination should be disregarded because the efficacy of the vaccine in the prevention of tuberculosis is unproven, vaccination may not result in a reactive skin test, and a positive reaction may wane with time (151,153).

Surveys have demonstrated isoniazid resistance in 22% of isolates from central Haiti. Resistance to one or more antituberculous drugs has been found in 34% of strains isolated from Haitian immigrants in Florida and in 38% of strains from Mexican immigrants in Los Angeles (154–156). Drug-resistant tuberculosis is being recognized increasingly among HIV-infected patients from Haiti and Latin America (157). Treatment of immigrants with four-drug regimens until susceptibilities return is advisable; and, if susceptible organisms are isolated, this combination allows for short courses of therapy and improved compliance (158).

BRUCELLOSIS

Fever in brucellosis can be acute or insidious, and the diagnosis is often elusive until appropriate serologic tests are requested or the fastidious organism is isolated from blood, tissues, or other body fluids (159). Despite active control programs, brucellosis remains an important health problem in Mexico and several Central and South American countries, and sporadic cases continue to occur in the Caribbean (160). While bovine brucellosis due to *Brucella abortus* remains prevalent in many Latin American countries, recent travel-associated cases diagnosed in the United States have more often been due to *B. melitensis* in unpasteurized goat's milk cheese (161–163). Sporadic cases have been associated with travel to Mexico, and epidemics related to ingestion of Mexican goat cheese have occurred in Texas and Colorado (162,163). In Texas, between 1982 and 1986, 67% of human cases of brucellosis were associated with ingestion of goat's cheese, and rates are especially high along the U.S.-Mexican border (162,163).

SPIROCHETAL INFECTIONS

Fever occurs in early Lyme disease and in the secondary stage of syphilis and yaws, often in association with skin lesions. Although potential tick vectors of *Borrelia burgdorferi* have been detected in South America, and both serological evidence and compatible clinical cases have been reported from Central and South America and the Caribbean, the occurrence and distribution of Lyme disease in the region requires confirmation (164–166). Before 1950, yaws was found in all countries of the Americas between the tropics of Cancer and Capricorn but, as a result of eradication programs, is now transmitted only sporadically in a few foci in the region (167).

Fever, chills, and headache of abrupt onset with intercurrent afebrile intervals is characteristic of relapsing fever. Louse-borne recurrent fever due to *Borrelia recurrentis* is endemic in high mountains of South America, especially Bolivia and Peru (168,169). Tick-borne relapsing fever due to several different species of *Borrelia* has been reported from Puerto Rico, Mexico, Central America, and the northern and western parts of South America (168). A recent imported case occurred in a U.S. citizen who had been working as a park ranger in the U.S. Virgin Islands (169).

Leptospirosis is widespread in the Americas and is particularly common in tropical regions during the rainy season when flooded fields, swamps, and city streets facilitate transmission. Among U.S. soldiers undergoing jungle training in Panama who did not use doxycycline prophylaxis, the attack rates ranged from 2% to 8%; most persons presented with fever, myalgia, and headache without signs of Weil's syndrome (170). Documented imported leptospirosis in travelers returning from the region has otherwise been unusual (171).

BARTONELLOSIS

The clinical picture of severe bartonellosis or Oroya fever was illustrated by an epidemic in a Peruvian village in 1987 in which 30 persons developed fever, chills, headache, pallor, and severe hemolysis, and 88% of untreated persons died (172). Phlebotomine sand flies transmit this rare disease in remote mountainous regions of Colombia, Ecuador, Peru, Bolivia, Chile, and probably Guatemala. Disease due to *Bartonella bacilliformis* also has a chronic benign phase characterized by verrucous skin lesions, *verruga peruana*. According to analysis of 16s rRNA, *B. bacilliformis* belongs to the purple bacteria (class Proteobacteria) and is closely related to *Rochalimaea quintana* and *Brucella abortus* (173). A common and life-threatening complication of Oroya fever is salmonella bacteremia, perhaps due to reticuloendothelial blockade from phagocytosed hemolyzed erythrocytes (73). Chloramphenicol is effective against *B. bacilliformis* and most local strains of salmonella.

BRAZILIAN PURPURIC FEVER

Brazilian purpuric fever, due to a pathogenic clone of *Hemophilus influenzae* biogroup aegyptius, was first recognized in 1984 when 10 children in a town of 20,000 persons in Brazil died of an acute febrile illness associated with shock and hemorrhagic skin lesions (174–176). Symptoms typically begin several days to weeks after a purulent conjunctivitis has resolved. Skin lesions may not be present even at the time the organism is isolated from the blood (177). Epidemics and sporadic cases have been reported from the states of São Paulo, Parana, and Mato Grosso, and the disease may occur elsewhere in central and southern Brazil (175). Oral rifampin appears to be effective for conjunctival eradication of the pathogen, and intravenous ampicillin or chloramphenicol, but not trimethoprim-sulfamethoxazole, early in the systemic illness reduce mortality (175,177).

OTHER BACTERIAL INFECTIONS

Meningococcal disease occurs sporadically throughout the region and has caused epidemics in several South and Central American countries (178,179). Most notable of these were two large outbreaks of groups A and C meningococcal disease in the 1970s in the São Paulo region of Brazil that led to an annual attack rate of 370 cases per 10,000 population (178).

Fever may precede or occur in the absence of lymphadenitis or pneumonia in persons with plague. Imported cases of plague are rare in the United States, perhaps because urban plague has been eliminated in most parts of the world, and U.S. travelers at high risk, such as Peace Corps volunteers and military personnel, often receive immunization (180). The first documented case of imported plague in the United States since 1926 occurred in 1990 (180). A mammalogist who had last been vaccinated 20 years earlier became infected after collecting rodents and crushing their fleas with her fingers in rural Bolivia. There are still active foci of plague in Bolivia, Peru, Ecuador, and Brazil (4). Most human cases have been sporadic and followed contact with wild rodents and their fleas, but small outbreaks due to person-to-person transmission have occurred in the Andean region.

Fever frequently complicates cutaneous anthrax and may be part of a nonspecific illness that precedes the localizing signs of inhalation and gastrointestinal anthrax. Animal anthrax remains a problem in the Caribbean and Latin America where contact with infected carcasses has led to outbreaks of human anthrax (181). Anthrax in the United States is rare and is acquired as a result of contact with imported animal products rather than travel (182). In 1973, a woman living in Florida developed cutaneous anthrax from goatskin drums that she had purchased in Haiti (182).

Tularemia, which is widespread in the northern hemisphere between 30° and 71° latitude, has been reported in Mexico, but not in South America (183). Melioidosis, due to *Pseudomonas pseudomallei*, is rare in the Americas and occurs only between 20° north and south latitude. A fatal case was reported in a Mexican immigrant living in California who presented first with fever and then evidence of pulmonary involvement and bacteremia (184). Melioidosis may develop within several days of exposure to the organism in soil or water or may become manifest after years of silent infection.

Tropical pyomyositis, purulent infection of striated muscle usually due to *Staphylococcus aureus*, is an occasional cause of fever of unknown origin. Although most reports are from tropical Africa and Asia, the disease has been reported in the Caribbean and Latin America and in immigrants from these areas (185).

Rheumatic fever and rheumatic heart disease with the attendant risk of infective endocarditis occur commonly in developing parts of the Americas because of poor and crowded living conditions and perhaps genetic susceptibility (186). In New York City, from 1969 to 1988, over one-half of cases of acute rheumatic fever occurred in Hispanics, many of whom were from families that had immigrated from the Dominican Republic and were living in poor, crowded communities in the city (187).

RICKETTSIAL INFECTIONS

Rickettsial infections are infrequently recognized as a cause of fever in travelers (188). Of the various species that cause human disease, five have been described in Latin America or the Caribbean (Table 2.4) (189). Murine typhus and Q fever are widely distributed throughout the region, while epidemic typhus, trench fever, and tick-borne

Table 2.4   Rickettsial diseases of Latin America and the Caribbean

Disease	*Agent*	*Vector or mode of transmission*	*Distribution*
Murine typhus	*Rickettsia mooseri* (R typhi)	Fleas in rodent-infected houses	Widespread, especially in tropical and urban areas
Epidemic typhus (and Brill-Zinsser disease)	R. *prowazekii*	Body lice in areas where infestation is encouraged by poor living conditions and cool climate	Mountainous areas of Mexico and Guatemala; Andean highlands of South America
Tick-borne spotted fever	R. *rickettsii*	Ixodid ticks	Rural areas of Mexico, Costa Rica, Panama, Colombia, Brazil, and probably elsewhere in Latin America
Trench fever	*Rochalimaea quintana*	Body lice	Mexico; probably in other louse-ridden areas
Q fever	*Coxiella burnetii*	Inhalation of dried infective material from domestic animals; ticks (?)	Widespread; recent outbreaks in meat-processing plants in Uruguay (191)

SOURCE From Reference 189.

spotted fever have a more restricted distribution. The clinical picture of tick-borne spotted fever in Latin America and Rocky Mountain spotted fever in the United States are identical, although the disease has different names, such as São Paulo fever in Brazil or *fiebre manchada* and *fiebre petequial* in Mexico and Colombia (189,190).

PARACOCCIDIOIDOMYCOSIS AND OTHER FUNGAL DISEASES

Undifferentiated fever may be the presenting symptom of initial infection or disseminated disease due to systemic mycoses. Infection with the dimorphic fungus *Paracoccidioides brasiliensis* occurs only in southern Mexico and Central and South America, but has not been reported from the Caribbean (192). In South America, it is most common in Brazil, Colombia, Venezuela, and Argentina, and clinical cases have been seen in all other countries except Chile and the Guayanas (192,193). Disease is most common among male agricultural workers who acquire infection from the soil in warm, humid areas. Imported cases in the United States are often due to reactivation of latent infection acquired years earlier and have been documented in persons with organ transplants and AIDS (192,194,195). Most patients with paracoccidioidomycosis have pulmonary involvement, and the organism can spread to the skin, mucous membranes, lymph nodes, and deep viscera, especially the adrenal glands (193). Diagnosis is made by isolation of the fungus by culture or smear. Serologic tests have been useful in following the response to treatment. Ketoconazole is the treatment of choice, although itraconazole, fluconazole, amphotericin B, and sulfonamides are all active against the fungus (192,196).

Histoplasma capsulatum, but not the African variant *H. capsulatum* var *duboisii*, is found in most, if not all, countries of Latin America and the Caribbean (9). Histoplasmosis is associated with nesting sites of bats, particularly in tropical areas, and outbreaks have occurred among persons who entered caves in Central America and abandoned silver mines in Mexico (9,197). An outbreak of imported histoplasmosis among U.S. soldiers who had been training in Panama was characterized by fever, headache, and malaise but no respiratory symptoms, and the initial diagnosis was arbovirus infection (198). Fever due to reactivated, disseminated histoplasmosis in AIDS patients and other immunocompromised persons has been seen in immigrants from Puerto Rico, the Dominican Republic, and northern South America who did not have a history of travel in endemic areas in the United States (199). Important endemic areas for coccidioidomycosis outside of the southwestern United States include parts of Mexico, Guatemala, Honduras, Venezuela, Paraguay, and Argentina (200). The prevalence of infection is extremely high in frequently visited border towns such as Tijuana (201). Mexicans and blacks have 3.4 and 10 times higher a risk of disseminated disease than whites, and disease complicating HIV infection may also be severe (200). Occasional cases of infection due to *Blastomyces dermatitidis* have been reported from Mexico and Central America (202).

CHAGAS' DISEASE

Fever due to American trypanosomiasis or Chagas' disease occurs only during acute infection or following reactivation of chronic infection in immunosuppressed persons.

Acute Chagas' disease is unlikely to be seen in a traveler, since natural transmission typically requires prolonged rural exposure in a poorly constructed house that is infested with reduviid bugs (203). Moreover, vector control programs in several countries have virtually eliminated insect-mediated transmission (4,204). However, transfusion-induced infection still occurs in many Latin American blood banks that do not screen blood products serologically or treat blood with gentian violet to kill the parasite (203).

Trypanosoma cruzi infection in human beings is reported in all countries in Latin America (4). The majority of the estimated 15 to 20 million infected persons live in Brazil, Venezuela, Chile, Argentina, and Bolivia. Transmission to human beings has not been documented in the Caribbean (4,205). As many as 100,000 chronically infected Latin American immigrants live in the United States, and there have been several transfusion-induced cases (206,207).

Reactivation of chronic Chagas' disease may occur in persons with AIDS, persons who receive heart transplants for chronic Chagas' cardiomyopathy, and other immuno-suppressed individuals (208–210). Parasites become abundant in blood and tissues, and symptoms of localized infection of the central nervous system, skin, or heart may be seen in addition to fever. The diagnosis of acute or reactivated Chagas' disease is made by detecting trypanosomes in the peripheral blood or tissues, and treatment is with nifurtimox or benznidazole.

VISCERAL LEISHMANIASIS

Visceral leishmaniasis or kala-azar is a rare cause of fever in travelers. In the Americas, it is caused by *Leishmania donovani chagasi* and is primarily a disease of undernourished children exposed to the sandfly vector in dry tropical regions of Mexico, Central America, and northern South America (211). It may also occur as an opportunistic infection with atypical manifestations in adults with AIDS and other immunodeficiency states years after leaving an endemic area (211,212). In Honduras, *L. d. chagasi* may cause papular, nonulcerative skin lesions rather than the classic syndrome of prolonged fever, hepatosplenomegaly, and pancytopenia (215). In Brazil, *Leishmania mexicana amazonensis*, which usually causes cutaneous leishmaniasis, has been isolated from patients with classic kala-azar (216). The diagnosis of visceral leishmaniasis is best made by isolating the parasite from bone marrow. The combination of interferon gamma and pentavalent antimony has cured infections that were refractory to antimony alone, but radical cure in patients with AIDS is often not possible (217).

OTHER PROTOZOAL INFECTIONS

Toxoplasmosis is highly prevalent in most countries in the region, especially in low-lying warm and humid areas where the majority of persons become infected by adult-hood, perhaps more often by ingestion of oocysts shed in cat feces than by consumption of poorly cooked meat (218,219). Acute infection of healthy travelers may cause fever and mononucleosis, as occurred in a group of U.S. soldiers several weeks after attending a jungle training course in Panama where they drank water contaminated with oocysts (220). Reactivated infection is not uncommon in immunosuppressed immigrants from tropical areas.

Low-grade fever and flulike symptoms may be associated with the diarrhea of cryptosporidiosis and isosporiasis acquired by healthy travelers (221,222). Cryptosporidiosis is widely distributed throughout the region and may account for 5% to 10% of diarrheal episodes among children in developing countries (223,224). Although less common, *Isospora belli* is also found throughout the region and may cause 15% of cases of chronic diarrhea in AIDS patients in Haiti (225).

Other protozoa that are unusual causes of fever are parasites of lower animals or ones that live free in the environment. The ciliate *Balantidium coli* causes sporadic cases of colitis throughout Latin America, and was responsible for fever and appendicitis in a Hispanic boy seen recently in Los Angeles (226). Babesiosis of cattle and other domestic animals is widespread throughout Latin America and the Caribbean, and human infections have been documented in Mexico (227). Acute amebic meningoencephalitis due to *Naegleria fowleri* has also been reported from several countries in the region (228).

HELMINTHIC INFECTIONS

Helminthic infections are highly prevalent throughout Latin America and the Caribbean, but are unusual causes of fevers in travelers and immigrants. Fever produced by these organisms typically is associated with a peripheral blood eosinophilia and other diagnostic clues.

Acute schistosomiasis with fever, peripheral blood eosinophilia, diarrhea, and cough may develop two to eight weeks after contact with fresh water infested with cercariae of *Schistosoma mansoni* (229). The illness is caused by circulating immune complexes and is recognized most commonly in travelers who are experiencing their first contact with the parasite (230). Foci of transmission are found in Brazil, Suriname, Venezuela, the Dominican Republic, St. Lucia, Montserrat, Guadeloupe, Martinique, Antigua, and Barbuda (4). Control measures and socioeconomic development have decreased the risk of infection in many areas, most notably in Puerto Rico, where active transmission has become rare (4). Rapid improvement of symptoms and cure of infection during acute schistosomiasis is achieved with the combination of corticosteroids and either praziquantel or oxamniquine, but not with antischistosomal agents alone (231). Fever during chronic schistosomiasis *mansoni* is unusual except in the syndrome of prolonged salmonella bacteremia due to bacterial colonization of the gut and tegument of adult worms (72). The clinical picture is one of prolonged fever and weight loss rather than of enteric fever.

Fever, abdominal pain, right lower-quadrant mass, and eosinophilia are the prominent features of abdominal angiostrongylosis due to *Parastrongylus costaricensis*, a roundworm that is unique to this hemisphere (232,233). Infection results from ingestion of infective larvae in the tissues or slime of slugs and has been reported from southern Mexico, several Central and northern South American countries, and Martinique. Eosinophilic meningitis due to *Parastrongylus cantonensis* has been reported in

Cuba, and infected land snails and slugs have been found in Puerto Rico and the Bahamas (234,235).

Lymphatic filariasis due to *Wuchereria bancrofti* is a disease that occurs only after prolonged residence in an endemic area and is unlikely to be seen in short-term travelers (236). "Filarial" fevers, often with retrograde lymphangitis or lymphadenitis, may recur for years after the patient has left an endemic area. Filariasis was formerly widespread throughout the region, but now important foci of transmission are found primarily in Brazil, Guyana, Costa Rica, Haiti, Trinidad, and Tobago (237). A survey of a small town in Haiti showed that 17% of persons had microfilaremia, and, of these, inflammatory lymphadenitis was the most common clinical manifestation (238). In 1981, a survey of Haitian immigrants in Florida showed that 7% had patent infections (239).

Between 1975 and 1989, 26 cases of trichinosis associated with foreign travel were reported in the United States, and 10 followed travel to Mexico (240). Fever occurred in two-thirds of cases, and a history of eating undercooked pork was common. Rates of infection in swine are high in many Latin American and Caribbean countries (241). Geohelminth infections are also common throughout the region, especially in warm rural areas. Over two-thirds of children surveyed in Colombia and St. Lucia had antibodies for *Toxocara*, which causes the visceral larva migrans syndrome with prolonged fever and eosinophilia (242). Fever in association with common intestinal nematodes occurs in special situations, such as disseminated strongyloidiasis in immunosuppressed persons or bacterial liver abscesses, cholangitis, or intestinal perforation complicating chronic ascariasis (243).

Fever may accompany the neurologic symptoms of cysticercosis during massive acute infection when cysts are implanting in the brain or because of meningeal inflammation during chronic infection (244,245). Cysticercosis is a major health problem in swine-rearing areas with poor sanitation, most notably Mexico, but also many parts of Central and South America, Haiti, and the Dominican Republic. Fever, abdominal pain, and eosinophilia may last for weeks during the migratory phase of *Fasciola hepatica* infection, which is found in sheep-raising areas of the region (246).

APPROACH TO THE PATIENT

In view of the lengthy differential diagnosis of fever following travel in Latin America and the Caribbean, evaluation of the patient requires a focused approach. It should be kept in mind that there is a small but real risk of life-threatening infections such as falciparum malaria, typhoid fever, and meningococcemia that can be treated if recognized promptly. Priority also should be given to diseases that cannot be treated but may threaten public health, such as acute hepatitis, dengue, and measles. Exotic life-threatening diseases, including yellow fever, bartonellosis, and the hemorrhagic fevers, are extremely unlikely and need be considered only when there is a suggestive clinical and epidemiologic picture. Fortunately, most febrile episodes in travelers are due to familiar and benign causes and resolve before a diagnosis can be made.

REFERENCES

1   **U.S. Bureau of the Census.** *Statistical abstract of the United States: 1991 (11th edition).* Washington, DC: US Government Printing Office, 1991.

2   **Centers for Disease Control.** Imported dengue—United States, 1990. *MMWR* 1991;40: 519–520.

3   **Centers for Disease Control.** Dengue epidemic—Peru, 1990. *MMWR* 1991;40:145–146.

4   **Pan American Health Organization.** *Health Conditions in the Americas.* 1990 edition, Volume 1, Scientific Publication Number 524. Washington, DC: Pan American Health Organization, 1990.

5   **Communicable Diseases Program, Pan American Health Organization.** Epidemiological stratification of malaria in the region of the Americas. *Epidemiol Bull* 1991;12:1–7.

6   **Centers for Disease Control.** *Malaria Surveillance Annual Summary 1984.* Atlanta, GA: Centers for Disease Control, 1985.

7   **Strickland GT.** Fever in travelers. In: Strickland GT, ed. *Hunter's Tropical Medicine.* 7th ed. Philadelphia: W.B. Saunders, 1991:1023–1031.

8   **Tanowitz HB, Weiss LM, Wittner M.** Diseases of immigrants. In: Strickland GT, ed. *Hunter's Tropical Medicine,* 7th ed. Philadelphia: W.B. Saunders, 1991:1042–1048.

9   **Wilson ME.** *A World Guide to Infections: Diseases, Distribution, Diagnosis.* Oxford: Oxford University Press, 1991.

10   **Liu LX, Weller PF.** Approach to the febrile traveler returning from Southeast Asia and Oceania. In: Remington JS, Swartz MN, eds. *Current Clinical Topics in Infectious Diseases.* Vol. 12. Boston: Blackwell Scientific Publications, 1992;13:138–164.

11   **Salata RA, Olds GR.** Infectious diseases in travelers and immigrants. In: Warren KS, Mahmoud AAF, eds. *Tropical and Geographic Medicine.* 2nd ed. New York: McGraw-Hill, 1990;228–242.

12   **Steffen R, Rickenback M, Urs W, Helminger A, Schär M.** Health problems after travel to developing countries. *J Infect Dis* 1987;156: 84–91.

13   **Hilton E, Edwards B, Singer C.** Reported illness and compliance in US travelers attending an immunization facility. *Arch Intern Med* 1989;178–179.

14   **Kendrick MA.** Study of illness among Americans returning from international travel, July 11–August 24, 1971 (preliminary data). *J Infect Dis* 1972;126:684–685.

15   **Warren KS, Mahmoud AAF.** Appendix 3. Considerations for travelers and immigrants: relative risk and incubation periods. Appendix 4. Exotic communicable diseases: a review by region. In: Warren KS, Mahmoud AAF, eds. *Tropical and Geographic Medicine.* 2nd ed. New York: McGraw-Hill, 1990;1111–1114.

16   **Beal CB, Lyerly WH, Jr.** Global epidemiology of infectious diseases. In: Strickland FT, ed. *Hunter's Tropical Medicine.* 7th ed. Philadelphia: W.B. Saunders, 1991:1048–1074.

17   **Alleyne GAO.** Health and tourism in the Caribbean. *Bull Pan Am Health Organ* 1990; 24:291–300.

18   **Merson MH, Tenney JH, Meyers JD, et al.** Shigellosis at sea: an outbreak aboard a passenger cruise ship. *Am J Epidemiol* 1975;101:165–175.

19   **Spika JS, Dabis F, Hargrett-Bean N, Salcedo J, Veillard S, Blake PA.** Shigellosis at a Caribbean resort. Hamburger and North American origin as risk factors. *Am J Epidemiol* 1987; 126:1173–1180.

20   **Berkelman RL, Cohen ML, Yashuk J, Barrett T, Wells JG, Blake PA.** Traveler's diarrhea at sea: Two multi-pathogen outbreaks caused by food eaten on shore visits. *Am J Public Health* 1983;73:770–772.

21   **Schleck WF 3d, Gorman GW, Payne MC, Broome CV.** Legionnaire's disease in the Caribbean. An outbreak associated with a resort hotel. *Arch Intern Med* 1985;145:2076–2079.

22   **Patterson TF, Bell SR, Bia FJ.** *Vibrio alginolyticus* cellulitis following coral injury. *Yale J Biol Med* 1988;61:507–512.

23   **Steffen R.** Health risks for short-term travelers. In: Steffen R, Lobel HO, Haworth J, Bradley DJ, eds. *Travel Medicine.* Berlin: Springer-Verlog, 1989:27–36.

24   **Escamilla J, Bourgeois AL, Gardiner CH, Kilpatrick ME.** Penicillinase-producing *Neisseria gonorrhoeae* in various seaport cities of Latin America. *Sex Transm Dis* 1988;15:141–143.

25   **Goeman J, Piot P.** The epidemiology of sexually transmitted diseases in Africa and Latin America. *Semin Dermatol* 1990;9:105–108.

26   **Warner DC.** Health issues at the US-Mexican border. *JAMA* 1991;265:242–247.

27   **Centers for Disease Control.** *Health Information for International Travel, 1991.* Atlanta, GA: U.S. Department of Health and Human Services, 1991.

28   **Lobel HO, Campbell CC.** Malaria prophylaxis and distribution of drug resistance. In: Strick-

land GT, ed. *Clinics in Tropical Medicine and Communicable Diseases*. Volume 1. London: W.B. Saunders, 1986:225–242.

29 **Steffen R, Behrens RH.** Traveller's malaria. *Parasitol Today* 1992;8:61–66.

30 **Centers for Disease Control.** Recommendations for the prevention of malaria among travelers. *MMWR* 1990;39(RR-3):1–10.

31 **Phillips-Howard PA, Radalowicz A, Mitchell J, Bradley DJ.** Risk of malaria in British residents returning from malarious areas. *BMJ* 1990;300:499–503.

32 **Lobel HO, Campbell CC, Pappaionou M, Huong AY.** Use of prophylaxis for malaria by American travelers to Africa and Haiti. *JAMA* 1987;257:2626–2627.

33 **Greenberg AE, Lobel HO.** Mortality from *Plasmodium falciparum* malaria in travelers from the United States, 1959–1987. *Ann Intern Med* 1990;113:326–327.

34 **Chia JKS, Nakata MN, Co S.** Smear-negative cerebral malaria due to mefloquine-resistant *Plasmodium falciparum* acquired in the Amazon. *J Infect Dis* 1992;599–600.

35 **Maldonado YA, Nahlen BL, Roberto RR, et al.** Transmission of *Plasmodium vivax* malaria in San Diego County, California, 1986. *Am J Trop Med Hyg* 1990;42:3–9.

36 **Centers for Disease Control.** Mosquito-transmitted malaria—California and Florida, 1990. *MMWR* 1991;40:106–108.

37 **Centers for Disease Control.** Imported malaria associated with malariotherapy of Lyme disease—New Jersey. *MMWR* 1990;39:873–875.

38 **Haworth J.** The global distribution of malaria and the present control effort. In: Wernsdorfer WH, McGregor I, eds. *Malaria: Principles and Practice of Malariology.* Edinburgh: Churchill Livingstone, 1988:1379–1420.

39 **Miller LH, Mason SJ, Clyde DF, McGinniss MH.** The resistance factor to *Plasmodium vivax* in Blacks. *N Engl J Med* 1976;295: 302–304.

40 **Chadee DD.** Imported malaria in Trinidad and Tobago, W.I. (1968–1986). *Ann Trop Med Parasitol* 1989;83:107–114.

41 **Tikasingh E, Edwards C, Hamilton PJJ, Commissiong LM, Draper CC.** A malaria outbreak due to *Plasmodium malariae* on the island of Grenada. *Am J Trop Med Hyg* 1980;29:715–719.

42 **Centers for Disease Control.** *Plasmodium vivax* infection among tourists to Puerto Vallarta and Acapulco, Mexico-New Mexico, Texas. *MMWR* 1985;34:461–462.

43 **Marques AC.** Human migration and the spread of malaria in Brazil. *Parasitology Today* 1987;6:166–170.

44 **Lo SS, Andrade JC, Condino ML, Alves MJ, Semeghini MG, Galvão EC.** Malaria em usarios de drogas de administração endovenosa associado a soropositividade para HIV. *Rev Saude Publica* 1991;25:17–22.

45 **Kremsner PG, Zotter GM, Feldmeier H, et al.** In vitro drug sensitivity to *Plasmodium falciparum* in Acre, Brazil. *Bull World Health Organ* 1989;67:289–293.

46 Drugs for parasitic infections. *Medical Letter* 1992;34:17–24.

47 **Kremsner PG, Zotter GM, Feldmeier H, Graninger W, Westerman RL, Rocha RM.** Clindamycin treatment of falciparum malaria in Brazil. *J Antimicrob Chemother* 1989;23: 275–281.

48 **Collignon P.** Chloroquine resistance in *Plasmodium vivax*. *J Infect Dis* 1991;164:222–223.

49 **Arias AE, Corredor A.** Low response of Colombian strains of *Plasmodium vivax* to classical antimalarial therapy. *Trop Med Parasitol* 1989;40:21–23.

50 **Ryan CA, Hargrett-Bean NT, Blake PA.** *Salmonella typhi* infections in the United States, 1975–1984: increasing role of foreign travel. *Rev Infect Dis* 1989;11:1–8.

51 **Woodruff BA, Pavia AT, Blake PA.** A new look at typhoid vaccination. Information for the practicing physician. *JAMA* 1991;265:756–759.

52 **Goldstein FW, Chumpitaz JC, Guevara JM, Papadopoulou B, Acar JF, Vieu JF.** Plasmid-mediated resistance to multiple antibiotics in *Salmonella typhi*. *J Infect Dis* 1986;153:261–266.

53 **Figueroa JP.** The typhoid fever outbreak in Jamaica. *West Indian Medical J* 1990;39: 201–202.

54 **Morris JG, Ferreccio C, Garcia J, et al.** Typhoid fever in Santiago, Chile: A study of household contacts of pediatric patients. *Am J Trop Med Hyg* 1984;33:1198–1202.

55 **Edelman R, Levine MM.** Summary of an international workshop on typhoid fever. *Rev Infect Dis* 1986;8:329–349.

56 **Hoffman SL.** Typhoid fever. In: Strickland GT, ed. *Hunter's Tropical Medicine*. 7th ed. Philadelphia: W.B. Saunders, 1991:344–359.

57 **Klotz SA, Jorgensen JH, Buckwold FJ, Craven PC.** Typhoid fever. An epidemic with remarkably few clinical signs and symptoms. *Arch Intern Med* 1984;144:533–537.

58 **Gotuzzo E, Frisancho O, Sanchez J, et al.** Association between the acquired immunodeficiency

syndrome and infection with *Salmonella typhi* or *Salmonella paratyphi* in an endemic typhoid area. *Arch Intern Med* 1991;151:581–582.

59 **Baine WB, Farmer JJ III, Gangarosa EJ, Hermann GT, Thornsberry C, Rice PA.** Typhoid fever in the United States associated with the 1972–1973 epidemic in Mexico. *J Infect Dis* 1977;135:649–653.

60 **Cordano AM, Virgilio R.** Tifoidea en Chile. Susceptibilidad de *Salmonella typhi* a cloramfenicol y otras drogas. *Rev Latinoam Microbiol* 1986;28:155–122.

61 **Gotuzzo E, Guerra JC, Benavente L, et al.** Use of norfloxacin to treat chronic typhoid carriers. *J Infect Dis* 1988;157:1221–1225.

62 **Ferreccio C, Morris JG, Valdivieso C, et al.** Efficacy of ciprofloxacin in the treatment of chronic typhoid carriers. *J Infect Dis* 1988; 157:1235–1239.

63 **Swerdlow DL, Ries AA.** Cholera in the Americas. Guidelines for the clinician. *JAMA* 1992;267:1495–1499.

64 **Black RE.** Pathogens that cause travelers' diarrhea in Latin America and Africa. *Rev Infect Dis* 1986;8(suppl 2):s131–s135.

65 **Gorbach SL.** Traveler's diarrhea. In: Gorbach SL, Bartlett JG, Blacklow NR, eds. *Infectious Diseases*. Philadelphia: WB Saunders, 1992: 622–628.

66 **Parsonnet J, Greene KD, Gerber AR, Tauxe RV, Aguilar OJV, Blake PA.** *Shigella dysenteriae* type 1 infections in US travellers to Mexico, 1988. *Lancet* 1989;2:543–545.

67 **Centers for Disease Control.** *Shigella dysenteriae* type 1—Guatemala, 1991. *MMWR* 1991; 40:421, 427–428.

68 **Strockbine NA, Parsonnet J, Greene K, Kiehlbauch JA, Wachsmuth IK.** Molecular epidemiologic techniques in analysis of epidemic and endemic *Shigella dysenteriae* type 1 strains. *J Infect Dis* 1991;163:406–409.

69 **Riley LW, Ceballos BSO, Trabulsi LR, Toledo MRF, Blake PA.** The significance of hospitals as reservoirs for endemic multiresistant *Salmonella typhimurium* causing infection in urban Brazilian children. *J Infect Dis* 1984;150:236–241.

70 **Casner PR, Zuckerman MJ.** *Salmonella arizonae* in patients with AIDS along the U.S.–Mexican border. *N Eng J Med* 1990;323: 198–199.

71 **Centers for Disease Control.** Iguana-associated salmonellosis—Indiana, 1990. *MMWR* 1992; 41:38–39.

72 **Rocha H, Kirk JW, Hearey CD Jr.** Prolonged Salmonella bacteremia in patients with Schisto-

soma mansoni infection. *Arch Intern Med* 1971;128:254–257.

73 **Wignall FS.** Bartonellosis. In: Strickland GT, ed. *Hunter's Tropical Medicine*. 7th ed. Philadelphia: WB Saunders, 1991:426–429.

74 **Mabey DC, Brown A, Greenwood BM.** *Plasmodium falciparum* malaria and *Salmonella* infections in Gambian children. *J Infect Dis* 1987;155:1319–1321.

75 **Wheat LJ, Rubin RH, Harris NL, et al.** Systemic salmonellosis in patients with disseminated histoplasmosis. Case for "macrophage blockade" caused by *Histoplasma capsulatum*. *Arch Intern Med* 1987;147:561–564.

76 **Shaked Y, Maier MK, Samra.** Relapsing fever and salmonella bacteraemia simultaneously affecting a healthy young man. *J Infect* 1986; 13:308–309.

77 **Webb DKH, Serjeant GR.** Systemic *Salmonella* infections in sickle cell anemia. *Ann Trop Paed* 1989;3:169–172.

78 **Katzenstein D, Rickerson V, Braude A.** New concepts of amebic liver abscess derived from hepatic imaging, serodiagnosis, and hepatic enzymes in 67 consecutive cases in San Diego. *Medicine* 1982;61:237–246.

79 **Thompson JE, Forlenza S, Verma R.** Amebic liver abscess: a therapeutic approach. *Rev Infect Dis* 1985;7:171–179.

80 **Greenstein AJ, Barth J, Dicker A, Bottone EJ, Aufses AJ Jr.** Amebic liver abscess: a study of 11 cases compared with a series of 38 patients with pyogenic liver abscess. *Am J Gastroenterol* 1985;6:472–478.

81 **Frachtman RL, Ericsson CD, DuPont HL.** Seroconversion of *Entamoeba histolytica* among short-term travelers to Mexico. *Arch Intern Med* 1982;7:1299.

82 **Gorbach SL, Kean BH, Evans DG, Evans DJ, Bessudo D.** Travelers' diarrhea and toxigenic *Escherichia coli*. *N Engl J Med* 1975; 292:933–936.

83 **Merson MH, Morris GK, Sack DA, et al.** Travelers' diarrhea in Mexico: a prospective study of physicians and family members attending a congress. *N Engl J Med* 1976;294: 1299–1306.

84 **Knoblock J, Mannweiler E.** Development and persistence of antibodies to *Entamoeba histolytica* in patients with amebic liver abscess. *Am J Trop Med Hyg* 1983;32:727–732.

85 **Ravdin JI, Guerrant RL.** Current problems in diagnosis and treatment of amebic infections. *Current Clinical Topics in Infect Dis Vol 7*. New York: McGraw-Hill, 1986; 82–111.

86 Walsh JA. Problems in recognition and diagnosis of amebiasis: estimation of the global magnitude of morbidity and mortality. *Rev Infect Dis* 1986;8:228–238.

87 Martinez-Palomo A, Martinez-Báez M. Selective primary health care: strategies for control of disease in the developing world. X. Amebiasis. *Rev Infect Dis* 1983;5:1093–1102.

88 Williams NP, Hanchard B, Wilks R. Amoebiasis in Jamaica: a forgotten cause of hepatointestinal disease. *WI Med J* 1989;38:159–163.

89 Sargeaunt PG, Jackson TFHG, Simjee A. Biochemical homogeneity of *Entamoeba histolytica* isolates, especially those from liver abscess. *Lancet* 1982;1:1386–1388.

90 Bracha R, Diamond LS, Ackers JP, Burchard GD, Mirelman D. Differentiation of clinical isolates of *Entamoeba histolytica* by using specific DNA probes. *J Clin Microbiol* 1990; 28:680–684.

91 Petri WA, Jackson FHG, Gathhiram V, et al. Pathogenic and nonpathogenic strains of *Entamoeba histolytica* can be differentiated by monoclonal antibodies to the galactose-specific lectin. *Infect Immun* 1990;58:1802–1806.

92 Weinke T, Friedrich-Janicke B, Hopo P, Janitschke K. Prevalence and clinical importance of *Entamoeba histolytica* in two high-risk groups: travelers returning from the tropics and male homosexuals. *J Infect Dis* 1990;161: 1029–1031.

93 Nozaki T, Aca IDS, Okuzawa E, Magalhães M, Tateno S, Takeuchi T. Zymodemes of *Entamoeba histolytica* isolated in the Amazon and the northeast of Brazil. *Trans R Soc Trop Med Hyg* 1990;84:387–388.

94 Okazaki M, Okazaki M, Miranda P, et al. Parasitological and serological studies on amoebiasis and other intestinal parasitic infections in Recife and its suburban area, northeast Brazil. *Rev Inst Med Trop São Paulo* 1988; 30:313–321.

95 DiPerri G, Weinke T, Maurizio S, Sargeaunt P. Distribution of pathogenic zymodemes of *Entamoeba histolytica*. *Trans R Soc Trop Med Hyg* 1988;82:427.

96 Reed SL, Wessel DW, Davis CE. *Entamoeba histolytica* infection and AIDS. *Am J Med* 1991;90:269–271.

97 Centers for Disease Control. *Hepatitis Surveillance Report No. 52*. Atlanta, GA: Centers for Disease Control, 1989.

98 Lemon SL. Type A viral hepatitis. *N Engl J Med* 1985;313:1059–1067.

99 Kilpatrick ME, Escamilla J. Hepatitis A in Peru. The role of children. *Am J Epidemiol* 1986;124:111–113.

100 Ruiz-Gomez J, Bustamante-Calvillo ME. Hepatitis A antibodies: prevalence and persistence in a group of Mexican children. *Am J Epidemiol* 1985;121:116–119.

101 Bensabath G, Hadler SC, Pereira Soares MC, et al. Hepatitis delta infection and Labrea hepatitis. Prevalence and role in fulminant hepatitis in the Amazon basin. *JAMA* 1987;258:479–483.

102 Buitrago B, Hadler SC, Popper H, et al. Epidemiologic aspects of Santa Marta hepatitis over a 40-year period. *Hepatology* 1986; 6:1292–1296.

103 Hadler SC, de Monzon M, Ponzetto A, et al. Delta virus infection and severe hepatitis. An epidemic in the Yupca Indians of Venezuela. *Ann Intern Med* 1984;100:339–344.

104 Torres JR, Mondolfi A. Protracted outbreak of severe delta hepatitis: experience in an isolated Amerindian population of the Upper Orinoco Basin. *Rev Infect Dis* 1991;13:52–55.

105 Koff RS, Pannuti CS, Pereira ML, et al. Hepatitis A and non-A, non-B viral hepatitis in São Paulo, Brazil: epidemiological, clinical, and laboratory comparisons in hospitalized patients. *Hepatology* 1982;2:445–448.

106 Velazquez O, Stetler HC, Avila C, et al. Epidemic transmission of enterically transmitted non-A, non-B hepatitis in Mexico. *JAMA* 1990;263:3281–3285.

107 Bader TF, Krawczynski K, Polish LB, Favorov MO. Hepatitis E in a U.S. traveler to Mexico. *N Engl J Med* 1991;325:1659.

108 Rehle TM. Classification, distribution, and importance of arboviruses. *Trop Med Parasit* 1989;40:391–395.

109 Monath TP. Viral febrile illnesses. In: Strickland GT, ed. *Hunter's Tropical Medicine*. 7th ed. Philadelphia: WB Saunders, 1991: 200–219.

110 Tesh RB. Undifferentiated arboviral fevers. In: Warren KS, Mahmoud AAF, eds. *Tropical and Geographic Medicine*. 2nd ed. New York: McGraw-Hill, 1990;685–691.

111 Monath TP. Venezuelan equine encephalitis (VEE). In: Strickland GT, ed. *Hunter's Tropical Medicine*. 7th ed. Philadelphia: WB Saunders, 1991;226–229.

112 Monath TP. Other arboviral encephalidites. In: Strickland GT, ed. *Hunter's Tropical Medicine*. 7th ed. Philadelphia: WB Saunders, 1991;232–233.

113 Malison MD, Waterman SH. Dengue fever in the United States. A report of a cluster of imported cases and review of the clinical, epidemiological, and public health aspects of the disease. *JAMA* 1983;249:496–500.

114 **Gubler DJ, Casta-Valez A.** A program for prevention and control of epidemic dengue and dengue hemorrhagic fever in Puerto Rico and the U.S. Virgin Islands. *Bull Pan Am Health Organ* 1991;25:237–247.

115 **Gubler DJ.** *Aedes aegypti* and *Aedes aegypti*-borne disease control in the 1990s: top down or bottom up? *Am J Trop Med Hyg* 1989; 40:571–578.

116 *Dengue.* Advisory memorandum no. 94. Atlanta: Department of Health and Human Services, Public Health Service, Centers for Disease Control, 1988.

117 **Dantes HG, Koopman JS, Addy CL, et al.** Dengue epidemics on the Pacific Coast of Mexico. *Int J Epidemiol* 1988;17:178–186.

118 **Figueiredo LT, Cavalcante SM, Simões MC.** Dengue serologic survey of school children in Rio de Janeiro, Brazil, in 1986 and 1987. *Bull Pan Am Health Organ* 1990;24:217–225.

119 **Bustos J, Hamdan A, Lorono MA, Montero MT, Gomez B.** Serologically proven acute rubella infection in patients with clinical diagnosis of dengue. *Epidemiol Infect* 1990; 104:297–302.

120 **Halstead SB.** Pathogenesis of dengue: challenges to molecular biology. *Science* 1988; 239:476–481.

121 **Centers for Disease Control.** Imported and indigenous dengue fever. United States 1986. *MMWR* 1987;33:551–554.

122 **Monath TP.** *Aedes albopictus*, an exotic mosquito vector in the United States. *Ann Intern Med* 1986;105:449–452.

123 **Centers for Disease Control.** Update: *Aedes albopictus* infestation—United States. *MMWR* 1987;36:769–773.

124 **Monath TP.** Yellow fever. In: Strickland GT, ed. *Hunter's Tropical Medicine. 7th ed.* Philadelphia: WB Saunders, 1991;233–238.

125 **Centers for Disease Control.** Summary of notifiable diseases, United States, 1988. *MMWR* 1988;37:55.

126 **Centers for Disease Control.** Yellow fever vaccine: recommendations for the Immunization Practice Advisory Committee (ACIP). *MMWR* 1990;39(No. RR-6):1–6.

127 **Monath TP.** Yellow fever: *Victor, Victoria?* Conqueror, conquest? Epidemics and research in the last forty years and prospects for the future. *Am J Trop Med Hyg* 1991;45:1–43.

128 **Monath TP.** Yellow fever: a medically neglected disease. Report on a seminar. *Rev Infect Dis* 1987;9:165–175.

129 **Vasconcelos PF, Travassos da Rosa JF, Guerreiro SC, Degallier N, Travassos da Rosa ES,** Travassos da Rosa AP. Primeiro registro de epidemias causadas pelo virus Oropouche nos estados do Maranhão e Goias, Brasil. *Rev Inst Med Trop São Paulo* 1989;31:271–278.

130 **Pinheiro FP, Freitas RB, Travassos da Rosa JF, Gabbay YB, Mello WA, LeDuc JW.** An outbreak of Mayaro virus disease in Belterra, Brazil. I. Clinical and virological findings. *Am J Trop Med Hyg* 1981;30:674–681.

131 **Weaver SC, Tesh RB, Guzman H.** Ultrastructural aspects of replication and the New Jersey serotype of vesicular stomatitis virus in a suspected sandfly vector, *Lutzomyia shannoni* (Diptera: Psychodidae). *Am J Trop Med Hyg* 1992;46:201–210.

132 **Iversson LB, Travassos da Rosa AP, Rosa MD.** Ocorrencia recente de infeccão humana por arbovirus Rocio na região do Vale da Ribeira. *Rev Inst Med Trop Med São Paulo* 1989; 31:28–31.

133 **LeDuc JW.** Epidemiology of hemorrhagic fever viruses. *Rev Infect Dis* 1989;11(Supplement):s730–s735.

134 **Salas R, Manzione ND, Tesh RB, et al.** Venezuelan hemorrhagic fever. *Lancet* 1991; 338:1033–1036.

135 **Fisher-Hoch SP.** South American hemorrhagic fevers. In: Strickland GT, ed. *Hunter's Tropical Medicine. 7th edition.* Philadelphia: WB Saunders, 1991:241–244.

136 **Pan American Health Organization.** AIDS surveillance in the Americas. *Epi Bull* 1991; 12:15.

137 **Quinn TC, Narain JP, Zacarias FRK.** AIDS in the Americas: a public health priority for the region. *AIDS* 1990;4:709–724.

138 **Pieniazek D, Peralta JM, Ferreira JA, et al.** Identification of mixed HIV-1/HIV-2 infections in Brazil by polymerase chain reaction. *AIDS* 1991;5:1293–1299.

139 **Kreiss JK, Castro KG.** Special considerations for managing human immunodeficiency virus infection and AIDS in patients from developing countries. *J Infect Dis* 1990;162:955–960.

140 **Morrow RH, Colebunders RL, Chin J.** Interactions of HIV infection with endemic tropical diseases. *AIDS* 1989;3(suppl):s79–s87.

141 **Centers for Disease Control.** Measles—Washington, 1990. *MMWR* 1990;39:473–476.

142 **Markowitz LE, Tomasi A, Hawkins CE, Preblub SR, Orenstein WA, Hinman AR.** International measles importations United States, 1980–1985. *Int J Epidemiol* 1988;17: 187–192.

143 **Borgono JM.** Current impact of measles in Latin America. *Rev Infect Dis* 1983;5:417–421.

144 Centers for Disease Control. International task force for disease eradication. *MMWR* 1990;39:209–211,217.

145 Gibons A. Saying so long to polio. *Science* 1991;251:1020.

146 Centers for Disease Control. Human rabies—Texas, Arkansas, and Georgia, 1991. *MMWR* 1991;40:765–769.

147 Cifuentes EE. Program for elimination of urban rabies in Latin America. *Rev Infect Dis* 1988;10(Suppl):s689–s696.

148 Centers for Disease Control. Rabies surveillance 1986. *MMWR* 1987;36(Suppl 3s): 1S–25S.

149 Lopez A, Miranda P, Tejuda E, Fishbein DB. Outbreak of human rabies in the Peruvian jungle. *Lancet* 1992;15:339:408–411.

150 Smith JS, Fishbein DB, Rupprecht CE, Clark K. Unexplained rabies in three immigrants in the United States. A virologic investigation. *N Engl J Med* 1991;324:205–211.

151 Centers for Disease Control. Tuberculosis among foreign-born persons entering the United States: recommendations of the Advisory Committee for Elimination of Tuberculosis. *MMWR* 1990;39(No RR-18):1–21.

152 Murray CJL, Styblo K, Rouillon A. Tuberculosis in developing countries: burden, intervention and cost. *Bull Int Un Tuberc* 1990; 65:2–20.

153 Centers for Disease Control. Screening for tuberculosis infection in high-risk populations. *MMWR* 1990;39(RR-8):1–7.

154 Scalcini M, Carre G, Jean-Baptiste M, et al. Antituberculous drug resistance in central Haiti. *Am Rev Respir Dis* 1990;142:508–511.

155 Pitchenik AE, Russell BW, Cleary T, Pejovic I, Cole C, Snider DE. The prevalence of tuberculosis and drug resistance among Haitians. *N Engl J Med* 1982;307:162–165.

156 Schiffman PL, Ashkar B, Bishop M, Cleary MG. Drug resistant tuberculosis in a large southern California hospital. *Am Rev Respir Dis* 1977;116:821–825.

157 Shafer RW, Chirgwin KD, Glatt AE, Dahdough MA, Landesman SH, Suster B. HIV prevalence, immunosuppression, and drug resistance in patients with tuberculosis in an area endemic for AIDS. *AIDS* 1991;5:399–405.

158 Cohn DL, Catlin BJ, Peterson KL, Judson FN, Sbarbaro JA. A 62-dose, 6-month therapy for pulmonary and extrapulmonary tuberculosis. *Ann Intern Med* 1990;112:407–415.

159 Chia JKS, Kennedy CA, Ponsillo MA. Fever, hepatosplenomegaly, and pancytopenia in a 39-year-old Hispanic woman. *Rev Infect Dis* 1990;12:636–643.

160 Wise RI. Brucellosis in the United States. Past, present, future. *JAMA* 1980;244:2318–2322.

161 Chusid MJ, Perzigian RW, Dunne WM, Gecht EA. Brucellosis: an unusual cause of a child's fever of unknown origin. *Wis Med J* 1989;88:11–13.

162 Young EJ. Health issues at the US-Mexican border. *JAMA* 1991;265:2066.

163 Taylor JP, Perdue JN. The changing epidemiology of human brucellosis in Texas, 1977–1986. *Am J Epidemiol* 1989;130:160–165.

164 Need JT, Escamilla J. Lyme disease in South America? *J Infect Dis* 1991;163:681–682.

165 Winward KE, Smith J. Ocular disease in Caribbean patients with serologic evidence of Lyme borreliosis. *J Clin Neuro Ophthalmol* 1989;9:65–70.

166 Azulay RD, Azulay-Abulafia L, Sodre CT, Azulay DR, Azulay MM. Lyme disease in Rio de Janeiro, Brazil. *Int J Dermatol* 1991; 30:569–571.

167 St. John RK. Yaws in the Americas. *Rev Infect Dis* 1985;7(suppl):s266–s275.

168 Felsenfeld O. The problem of relapsing fever in the Americas. *Indus Med Surg* 1973;42:7–10.

169 Flanigan TP, Schwan TG, Armstrong C, Van Voris LP, Salata RA. Relapsing fever in the US Virgin Islands: a previously unrecognized focus of infection. *J Infect Dis* 1991;163: 1391–1392.

170 Takafuji ET, Kirkpatrick JW, Miller RN, et al. An efficacy trial of doxycycline chemoprophylaxis against leptospirosis. *N Engl J Med* 1984;310:497–500.

171 Pashkow FJ, Calisher CH, Reller LB, Sulzer CR. Leptospirosis in a traveler from Honduras. *Colo Med* 1981;78:210–212.

172 Gray GC, Johnson AA, Thornton SA, et al. An epidemic of Oroya fever in the Peruvian Andes. *Am J Trop Med Hyg* 1990;42:215–221.

173 Brenner DJ, O'Connor SP, Hollis DG, Weaver RE, Steigerwalt AG. Molecular characterization and proposal of a neotype strain for *Bartonella bacilliformis. J Clin Microbiol* 1991;29:1299–1302.

174 Centers for Disease Control. Brazilian purpuric fever: *Haemophilus aegyptius* bacteremia complicating purulent conjunctivitis. *MMWR* 1986;35:553–554.

175 Centers for Disease Control. Brazilian purpuric fever—Mato Grosso, Brazil. *MMWR* 1990;39:903–905.

176 **Musser JM, Selander RK.** Brazilian purpuric fever: evolutionary genetic relationships of the case clone of *Haemophilus influenzae* biogroup aegyptius to encapsulated strains of *Haemophilus influenzae*. *J Infect Dis* 1990;161:130–133.

177 **Brazilian Purpuric Fever Study Group.** *Haemophilus aegyptius* bacteremia in Brazilian purpuric fever. *Lancet* 1987;2:761–763.

178 **Peltola H.** Meningococcal disease: still with us. *Rev Infect Dis* 1983;5:71–91.

179 **Bryan JP, Silva HR, Tavares A, Rocha H, Scheld WM.** Etiology and mortality of bacterial meningitis in northeastern Brazil. *Rev Infect Dis* 1990;12:128–135.

180 **Centers for Disease Control.** Imported bubonic plague—District of Columbia. *MMWR* 1990;39:895,901.

181 **Harrison LH, Ezzell JW, Abshire TG, Kidd S, Kaufmann AF.** Evaluation of serologic tests for diagnosis of anthrax after an outbreak of cutaneous anthrax in Paraguay. *J Infect Dis* 1989;160:706–710.

182 *Anthrax-Contaminated Goatskin Products from Haiti.* Advisory memorandum No. 61. Atlanta: Department of Health and Human Services, Public Health and Human Services, Public Health Service, Centers for Disease Control, 1981.

183 **Sanford JP.** Tularemia. In: Strickland GT, ed. *Hunter's Tropical Medicine. 7th ed.* Philadelphia: WB Saunders, 1991:416–417.

184 **Barnes PF, Appleman MD, Cosgrove MM.** A case of melioidosis originating in North America. *Am Rev Respir Dis* 1986;134:170–171.

185 **Kennedy CA, Mathisen G, Goetz MB.** Tropical pyomyositis of the abdominal wall musculature mimicking acute abdomen. *West J Med* 1990;152:296–298.

186 **Guilherme M, Weidebach W, Kiss MH, Snitcowsky R, Kalil J.** Association of human leukocyte class II antigens with rheumatic heart disease in a Brazilian population. *Circulation* 1991;83:1995–1998.

187 **Griffiths SP, Gersony WM.** Acute rheumatic fever in New York City (1969 to 1988): a comparative study of two decades. *J Pediatr* 1990;116:882–887.

188 **McDonald JC, MacLean JD, McDade JE.** Imported rickettsial disease: clinical and epidemiologic features. *Am J Med* 1988;85:799–805.

189 **Wisseman CL.** Rickettsial infections. In: Strickland GT, ed. *Hunter's Tropical Medicine. 7th ed.* Philadelphia: WB Saunders, 1991:256–286.

190 **Fuentes L.** Ecological study of Rocky Mountain spotted fever in Costa Rica. *Am J Trop Med Hyg* 1986;35:192–196.

191 **Somma-Moreira RE, Caffarena RM, Somma S, Pérez G, Monteiro M.** Analysis of Q fever in Uruguay. *Rev Infect Dis* 1987;9:386–387.

192 **Sugar AM.** Paracoccidioidomycosis. *Infect Dis Clin North Am* 1988;2:913–925.

193 **Tendrick M, de Luca V, Tourinho EK, et al.** Computed tomography and ultrasonography of the adrenal glands in paracoccidioidomycosis. Comparison with cortisol and aldosterone responses to ACTH stimulation. *Am J Trop Med Hyg* 1991;44:83–92.

194 **Sugar AM, Restrepo A, Stevens DA.** Paracoccidioidomycosis in a renal transplant patient: Report of a case and review of the mycosis in the immunosuppressed host. *Am Rev Respir Dis* 1984;129:340–342.

195 **Goldani LS, Coelho IC, Machado AA, Martinez R.** Paracoccidioidomycosis and AIDS. *Scand J Infect Dis* 1991;23:393.

196 **Diaz M, Negroni R, Montero-Gei F, et al.** A pan-American 5-year study of fluconazole therapy for deep mycoses in the immunocompetent host. *Clin Infect Dis* 1992;14(suppl 1):s68–s76.

197 **Hay RJ.** Histoplasmosis. In: Strickland GT, ed. *Hunter's Tropical Medicine. 7th ed.* Philadelphia: WB Saunders, 1991:523–526.

198 **Burke DS, Churchill FE, Gaydos JC, Kaufman I.** Epidemic histoplasmosis in patients with undifferentiated fever. *Milit Med* 1982, 147:466–467.

199 **Mandel W, Goldberg DM, Neu HC.** Histoplasmosis in patients with the acquired immune deficiency syndrome. *Am J Med* 1986;81:974–976.

200 **Oldfield EC, III.** Coccidioidomycosis. In: Strickland GT, ed. *Hunter's Tropical Medicine. 7th ed.* Philadelphia: WB Saunders, 1991:526–530.

201 **Fredrick BE.** A skin test survey of valley fever in Tijuana, Mexico. *Soc Sci Med* 1989; 29:1217–1227.

202 **Bradsher RW.** Blastomycosis. In: Strickland GT, ed. *Hunter's Tropical Medicine. 7th ed.* Philadelphia: WB Saunders, 1991:530–533.

203 **Schmunis GA.** *Trypanosoma cruzi,* the etiologic agent of Chagas' disease: status in the blood supply in endemic and nonendemic countries. *Transfusion* 1991;31:547–557.

204 **Aquatella H, Catalioti F, Gomez-Mancebo JR, Davalos V, Villalobos L.** Long-term control of Chagas' disease in Venezuela: effects on serologic findings, electrocardio-

graphic abnormalities, and clinical outcome. *Circulation* 1987;76:556–562.

205 Omah-Maharaj IR. Serological investigations for Chagas' disease in Trinidad. *W I Med J* 1991;40:22–25.

206 Kirchhoff LV, Gam AA, Gilliam FC. American trypanosomiasis (Chagas' disease) in Central American immigrants. *Am J Med* 1987; 82:915–920.

207 Grant IH, Gold JWM, Wittner M, et al. Transfusion-associated acute Chagas disease acquired in the United States. *Ann Intern Med* 1989;111:849–851.

208 Gluckstein D, Ciferri F, Ruskin J. Chagas' disease: another cause of cerebral mass in the acquired immunodeficiency syndrome. *Am J Med* 1992;92:429–432.

209 Libow LF, Beltrani VP, Silvers DN, Grossman ME. Post-cardiac transplant reactivation of Chagas' disease diagnosed by skin biopsy. *Cutis* 1991;48:37–40.

210 Stolf NAG, Higushi L, Bocchi E, et al. Heart transplantation in patients with Chagas' disease cardiomyopathy. *J Heart Transplant* 1987;6:307–312.

211 Grimaldi G Jr., Tesh RB, McMahon-Pratt D. A review of the geographic distribution and epidemiology of leishmaniasis in the New World. *Am J Trop Med Hyg* 1989;41: 687–725.

212 Corredor A, Gallego JF, Tesh RB, et al. Epidemiology of visceral leishmaniasis in Colombia. *Am J Trop Med Hyg* 1989;40: 480–486.

213 Badaró R, Carvalho EM, Rocha H, Queiroz AC, Jones TC. *Leishmania donovani:* an opportunistic microbe associated with progressive disease in three immunocompromised patients. *Lancet* 1986;1:647–648.

214 Peters BS, Fish D, Golden R, Evans DA, Bryceson ADM, Pinching AJ. Visceral leishmaniasis in HIV infection and AIDS: clinical features and response to therapy. *Quart J Med* 1990;283:1101–1111.

215 Ponce C, Ponce E, Morrison A, et al. *Leishmania donovani chagasi:* new clinical variant of cutaneous leishmaniasis in Honduras. *Lancet* 1991;337:67–70.

216 Barral A, Badaró R, Barral-Netto M, Grimaldi G Jr., Momen H, Carvalho EM. Isolation of *Leishmania mexicana amazonensis* from the bone marrow in a case of American visceral leishmaniasis. *Am J Trop Med Hyg* 1986;35:732–734.

217 Badaró R, Falcoff E, Badaró FS, et al. Treatment of visceral leishmaniasis with penta-

valent antimony and interferon gamma. *N Engl J Med* 1990;322:16–21.

218 Sousa OE, Saenz RE, Frenkel JK. Toxoplasmosis in Panama: a 10-year study. *Am J Trop Med Hyg* 1988;38:315–322.

219 Ruiz OJ, Arjona AC, Moreno GSM. *Toxoplasmosis en Colombia.* 2nd ed. Bogotá: Ministerio de Salud, 1988:1–67.

220 Benenson MW, Takafuji ET, Lemon SM, Greenup RL, Sulzer AJ. Oocyst-transmitted toxoplasmosis associated with ingestion of contaminated water. *N Engl J Med* 1982; 307:666–669.

221 Ma P, Helmick CG, D'Souza AJ, Navin TR. Cryptosporidiosis in tourists returning from the Caribbean. *N Engl J Med* 1985; 312:647–648.

222 Godiwala T, Yaeger R. Isospora and traveler's diarrhea. *Ann Intern Med* 1987;106:908–909.

223 Ungar BLP, Gilman RH, Lanata CF, Perez-Schael I. Seroepidemiology of cryptosporidium infection in two Latin American populations. *J Infect Dis* 1988,157:551–556.

224 Cruz JR, Floridalma C, Cáceres P, Chew F, Pareja G. Infection and diarrhea caused by *Cryptosporidium* sp. among Guatemalan children. *J Clin Microbiol* 1988;26:88–91.

225 DeHowitz JA, Pape JW, Boncy M, Johnson WD. Clinical manifestations and therapy of *Isospora belli* infection in patients with the acquired immunodeficiency syndrome. *N Engl J Med* 1986;315:87–90.

226 Dodd LG. *Balantidium coli* infestation as a cause of acute appendicitis. *J Infect Dis* 1991;163:1392.

227 Ruebush TK III. Human babesiosis. *Trans Roy Soc Trop Med Hyg* 1980;74:149–152.

228 Duma RJ. Primary amebic meningoencephalitis. In: Warren KS, Mahmoud AAD, eds. *Tropical and Geographic Medicine.* 2nd ed. New York: McGraw-Hill, 1990:321–327.

229 Clark WD, Cox PM Jr., Ratner LH, Correa-Coronas R. Acute schistosomiasis *mansoni* in 10 boys. An outbreak in Caguas, Puerto Rico. *Ann Intern Med* 1970;73:379–385.

230 Hiatt RA, Sotomayor ZR, Sanchez G, Zambrana M, Knight WB. Factors in the pathogenesis of acute schistosomiasis mansoni. *J Infect Dis* 1979;139:659–666.

231 Lambertucci JR. A new approach to the treatment of acute schistosomiasis. *Mem Inst Oswaldo Cruz* 1989;84(suppl 1):23–30.

232 Loría-Cortés R, Lobo-Sanahuja JF. Clinical abdominal angiostrongylosis. A study of 116 children with intestinal eosinophilia granu-

loma caused by *Angiostrongylus costaricensis*. *Am J Trop Med Hyg* 1980;29:538–544.

233 Morera P. Abdominal angiostrongyliasis: a problem of public health. *Parasitol Today* 1985;1:173–175.

234 Cross JH. Public health importance of *Angiostrongylus cantonensis* and its relatives. *Parasitol Today* 1987;3:367–369.

235 Kliks MM, Palumbo NE. Eosinophilic meningitis beyond the Pacific Basin: the global dispersal of a peridomestic zoonosis caused by *Angiostrongylus cantonensis*, the nematode lungworm of rats. *Soc Sci Med* 1992;34:199–212.

236 Ottesen EA. The filariases and tropical eosinophilia. In: Warren KS, Mahmoud AAD, eds. *Tropical and Geographic Medicine. 2nd ed.* New York: McGraw-Hill, 1990:407–429.

237 Nathan MB, Stroom V. Prevalence of *Wuchereria bancrofti* in Georgetown, Guyana. *Bull Pan Am Health Organ* 1990; 24:301–306.

238 Raccurt CP, Mojon M, Hodges WH. Parasitological, serological, and clinical studies of *Wuchereria bancrofti* in Limbe, Haiti. *Am J Trop Med Hyg* 1984;33:1124–1129.

239 Yangco BG, Vincent AL, Vickery AC, Nayar JK, Saverman DM. A survey of filariasis among refugees in South Florida. *Am J Trop Med Hyg* 1984;33:246–251.

240 McAuley JB, Michelson MK, Schantz PM. Trichinella infection in travelers. *J Infect Dis* 1991;164:1013–1016.

241 Schenone H. El problema de la triquinosis humana y animal en America Latina. *Bol Chil Parasitol* 1984;39:47–53.

242 Schantz PM. *Toxocara* larva migrans now. *Am J Trop Med Hyg* 1989;41:21–34.

243 Pawlowski ZS. Soil-transmitted helminthiases. *Clin Trop Med Comm Dis* 1986;1:617–642.

244 Nash TE. Diagnosis and treatment of cysticercosis. In: Remington JS, Swartz MN, eds. *Current Clinical Topics in Infectious Diseases. Vol 7.* New York: McGraw-Hill, 1986;297–310.

245 McCormick GP, Zee C, Heiden J. Cysticercosis cerebri. Review of 127 cases. *Arch Neurol* 1982;39:534–539.

246 Bunnag D, Bunnag T, Goldsmith R. Liver fluke infections. In: Strickland GT. *Hunter's Tropical Medicine. 7th ed.* Philadelphia: WB Saunders, 1991:818–822.

Fever in a recent visitor to the Middle East

CHARLES N. OSTER
EDMUND C. TRAMONT

So long as the Middle East remains a strategic economic force and the spiritual home to three major religions, many foreigners will visit this region. In general, infectious disease threats to visitors are similar to those of the so-called Third World countries. Additional unique risks include leishmaniasis, schistosomiasis, sand fly fever, and Congo-Crimean hemorrhagic fever (CCHF) (Tables 3.1, 3.2).

The Middle East is a large area which in total constitutes a land mass about the size of the continental United States (Figure 3.1). Much of the land mass is desert, forcing the people to live crowded along the seacoasts and in river and mountain valleys that have enough water to support agriculture. With the exception of language and religion, almost all of the people have the same culture. A visitor finds little difference, for example, between life in Iran and life in Egypt. Israel is the chief exception. The total population is approximately 200 million.

Disease risks vary depending upon the area visited. For example, the risk of acquiring an infectious disease in Israel is no different than in Italy or Greece. Similarly, the new and modern cities of Saudi Arabia are quite safe. The situation in the less-developed countryside or in the older cities is quite different. The breakdown of sanitation, overcrowding, and malnutrition attendant to any armed conflict, a common intrusion into the lives of those living in the Middle East for many years, predisposes inhabitants and visitors alike to infectious diseases. In these settings, diseases such as food and waterborne illnesses, typhoid fever, cholera, epidemics of meningococcal disease, malaria, and parasitic infections are common.

Experiences related to Desert Shield/Desert Storm

During Desert Shield/Desert Storm, the influx of over 600,000 foreign troops gave the Western world another glimpse at potential infectious diseases threats. However, this buildup lasted only eight months and took place during the fall and winter; the

Table 3.1   Endemic diseases of the Middle East

Viral
Viral hepatitis
Sand fly fever
Congo-Crimean hemorrhagic fever
Rift Valley fever
West Nile fever
Rabies

Bacterial
Shigellosis
Escherichia coli gastroenteritis
   Enterotoxigenic
   Enteroinvasive
   Enteroadhesive
Salmonellosis (enteric fever)
Tuberculosis
Meningococcal disease
Brucellosis
Anthrax
Cholera
Bejel

Parasitic
Leishmaniasis
Giardiasis
Malaria
   Plasmodium falciparum
   Plasmodium vivax
Intestinal helminthic infection
Schistosomiasis
Amebiasis
Filariasis
Echinococcus disease

Rickettsial
Typhus
   Endemic
   Epidemic
Q fever

increased incidence of those infectious diseases attendant to the summer months did not materialize in the foreign troops. Nevertheless, important lessons were relearned; diarrhea illnesses and dysentery were the most common problems, and leishmaniasis was troublesome, while hepatitis, malaria, and sand fly fever caused fewer problems than were anticipated (1,2,3, James Brien, DO (Doctor of Osteopathy) personal communication).

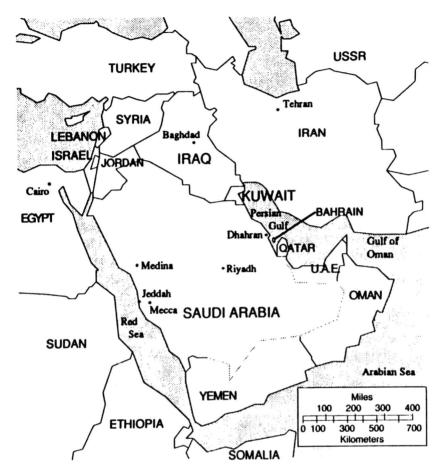

Figure 3.1   The Middle East.

INFECTIOUS DISEASES OF HIGH PREVALENCE

Diarrhea/acute gastroenteritis

Diarrhea and/or acute gastroenteritis are predictable and common occurrences whenever individuals travel and reside outside of their own geographical environment and partake of local foodstuffs and water. The Middle East is no exception. Virtually all etiologic agents, viral, bacterial, and parasitic, have been isolated at one time or another (1,4,5). During Desert Shield/Desert Storm, enterotoxigenic *Escherichia coli* and *Shigella* were the most prevalent (4), but the most unique aspect of gastrointestinal illnesses was the high prevalence of antibiotic resistance among the bacterial causes (Table 3.3). Two out of three bacterial pathogens were resistant to trimethoprim-sulfamethoxozole or tetracycline, and one out of three was resistant to ampicillin.

Table 3.2 Endemic diseases of the Middle East that may present after returning home

---

0–10 days after return
Diarrhea
Enteric fever
Malaria (*Plasmodium falciparum*)
Congo-Crimean hemorrhagic fever
Epidemic typhus
Meningococcal disease
Acute hepatitis
Sand fly fever
Anthrax

Greater than 10 days after return
Leishmaniasis (cutaneous, visceral, viscerotropic)
Hepatitis
Enteric fever
Malaria (*P. vivax, P. falciparum*)
Tuberculosis
Giardiasis
Amebiasis
Congo-Crimean hemorrhagic fever (convalesence)
Sand fly fever (convalescence)
Brucellosis
Anthrax
Q fever
Typhus (endemic, epidemic)

Table 3.3 Enteric pathogens isolated from United States military personnel in Desert Shield/Desert Storm, September 1990–March 1991*

Enteric pathogen	*Percent*
Enterotoxigenic *E. coli* Heat labile, heat stable	21.1
Enteroinvasive *E. coli*	0.7
Shigella	19.0
Mixed *E. coli* and *Shigella*	6.9
Salmonella	1.6
Campylobacter	0.5
Norwalk agent[†]	3.4
Giardia lamblia[‡]	2.1

*432 personnel tested.
[†]Only 87 specimens tested.
[‡]422 personnel tested.
SOURCE Adapted from References 3, 4.

Fortunately, all strains isolated (before 1991) were sensitive to the quinolone antibiotics norfloxacin and ciprofloxacin (4, 5).

As with all causes of diarrhea, fluid and salt replacement constitutes the cornerstone of treatment. Although antibacterial treatment carries with it the risk of prolonging the carrier state, the treatment is advisable whenever there is fever and/or evidence of tissue invasion (blood and/or polymorphonuclear cells on staining of a stool specimen). Loperamide will reduce the duration of diarrhea but should always be given with an antibiotic when dysentery is present.

Cutaneous leishmaniasis

Endemic cutaneous leishmaniasis due to *Leishmania tropica* and *Leishmania major* is present throughout the Middle East, including Saudi Arabia, Oman, Kuwait, and Iraq. These diseases are transmitted by the bite of infected phlebotomine sand flies. After an incubation period of two to eight weeks, a papule appears which then gradually enlarges and ulcerates. The lesions will heal spontaneously within weeks to months in nearly all cases; relapses or persistence of Old World cutaneous leishmaniasis lesions are very uncommon.

Diagnosis depends upon demonstration of the parasite. This can be accomplished by visualization of amastigotes in lesion aspirates or biopsies after staining with Giemsa or fluorescein-tagged genus-specific monoclonal antibodies (6) or by culturing the promastigote stage of the parasite from aspirates or biopsies in Schneider's medium (7). Diagnosis based on the clinical presentation alone will often be erroneous; therefore, all suspected cases should be referred to hospitals with the capability of making a parasitological diagnosis. There are no serological methods available that can reliably confirm the diagnosis.

Treatment of Old World cutaneous leishmaniasis is not required in the majority of the cases, since the lesions will heal spontaneously in several weeks to months. However, treatment should be considered in patients with large lesions, those that are cosmetically disfiguring, and those that compromise function.

Standard treatment is sodium stibogluconate (Pentostam, Burroughs Wellcome, England), 20 mg/kg/day intravenously for 20 days (8). The ulcers will start to heal during treatment, with reduction of the induration of the ulcer margin and re-epithelialization of the ulcer. Most patients will not be completely healed by the end of treatment; however, nearly all will go on to complete healing. The occasional patient who has not fully healed a month after treatment may be offered a second course of sodium stibogluconate.

Sodium stibogluconate causes many side effects. Myalgias and arthralgias occur in nearly all patients and may be disabling. Elevations of aspartate aminotransferase (AST) and alanine aminotransferase (ALT) up to five times normal occur in 50% of patients (8); these abnormalities generally peak in the second or third week of therapy and thereafter have a trend toward normal, even with continued administration of the drug. Minor electrocardiogram (ECG) abnormalities, including nonspecific ST and T wave changes, occur in a dose-dependent manner and are not a reason to interrupt therapy as long as the daily dose of 20 mg/kg is not exceeded (9). Finally, elevations of serum amylase and lipase are seen in nearly all patients and may be associated with clinical pancreatitis in some (10). The development of clinical pancreatitis requires discontinuation of therapy, but the proper management of patients who develop biochemical pancreatitis has not been defined.

Because of the toxicities of sodium stibogluconate, careful consideration of the risk/benefit ratio for each patient is mandatory; only the most serious cases should be treated with this drug. Patients with lesions that are not functionally disabling or cosmetically disfiguring are best followed without specific therapy and allowed to heal spontaneously. Despite the fact that adjunctive interferon-Y therapy is beneficial in visceral leishmaniasis (10a), there are no proven alternative therapies for Old World cutaneous leishmaniasis. Although ketoconazole, 600 mg/day for 28 days, cured 76% of patients with New World cutaneous leishmaniasis (11), and Pentamidine, 2 mg/kg every other day for 7 injections cured 96 patients in Central America (11a), this regimen has not been tried with Old World cutaneous disease.

Experience related to Desert Storm   Since movement of nonimmune populations into areas endemic for cutaneous leishmaniasis may lead to large outbreaks (12), deployment of about 600,000 American and allied military personnel to the Middle East had been expected to lead to a large number of cases of cutaneous leishmaniasis. Contrary to these expectations, only 17 proven cases were diagnosed in American personnel. These 17 were probably only a small fraction of the people infected, but were those with the most severe and/or persistent disease, which forced them to seek medical attention. Seven leishmanial isolates were obtained from these 17 patients for speciation; six isolates speciated to date (Spring 1992), and three have been L. *tropica* and three L. *major* (M. Grogl, personal communication).

Visceral leishmaniasis

Visceral leishmaniasis, caused by *Leishmania donovani*, occurs only in isolated areas of the Middle East, including sporadic cases in Oman, the southwestern provinces of Saudi Arabia, and the central and northern provinces of Iraq. Transmission occurs through the bite of an infected phlebotomine sand fly, although there are rare reports of transmission from a patient to his sexual partner (13), from mother to baby (14) and from blood donor to recipient (15).

Visceral leishmaniasis presents as a chronic wasting disease with fever, weight loss, hepatosplenomegaly, pancytopenia, and hypergammaglobulinemia. The disease is progressive and ends fatally without treatment. The diagnosis must be confirmed by demonstrating parasites in tissue histopathologically or by culturing parasites from these tissues. Parasites can be demonstrated in the spleen in over 95% of cases, the bone marrow in 85% to 90%, and the liver in 75% to 90% (16).

After the diagnosis is confirmed by demonstration of parasites, patients should be treated with sodium stibogluconate, 20 mg/kg/day, for 30 days. Prompt clinical improvement is seen after starting therapy, with lysis of fever and increased appetite and sense of well-being occurring after only two to three days of treatment. Complications of treatment are similar to those seen with the use of sodium stibogluconate for the treatment of cutaneous leishmaniasis (vide supra). Pentamidine and amphotericin B have also been used to treat visceral leishmaniasis, although experience with these drugs is limited (17,18). The addition of gamma interferon to pentavalent antimony may improve the response in those patients who do not respond to the antimony alone (18).

Experience related to Desert Storm   During Desert Shield/Desert Storm, the U.S. and allied military personnel were stationed in northeast Saudi Arabia and then moved north into Kuwait and southern Iraq. Since these areas were not known to be endemic for visceral leishmaniasis, no cases of this parasitic disease were expected. However, at least seven men were diagnosed with a systemic form of leishmaniasis after returning to the United States. They were diagnosed by culturing the organism from bone marrow aspirates (3). Five of these leishmanial isolates were identified by isoenzyme analysis (19,20), and were found to be *L. tropica*, the causative agent of Old World cutaneous leishmaniasis. It was because of this finding that blood donations by Desert Shield/ Storm veterans were withheld for 15 months after returning to the USA.

Six of these seven men were symptomatic; the seventh, asymptomatic person was identified when his unit was screened because of another symptomatic case. Five of the six were febrile. Four had an acute syndrome with high fever (103.0°F to 105.6°F), rigors, and malaise. The other two symptomatic patients had low-grade fever, nausea, watery diarrhea, and abdominal pain. One patient had mild hepatosplenomegaly, two had generalized lymphadenopathy (one of these patients was found to be coinfected with human immunodeficiency virus (HIV), and two developed mild splenomegaly. None of these patients had skin lesions. Six of the seven patients had mild elevations of AST and/or ALT, and three were mildly anemic. No patient had leukopenia, thrombocytopenia, or hypergammaglobulinemia.

Five of these patients who were still symptomatic when diagnosed were treated with sodium stibogluconate. In two patients (including the HIV-positive patient), the treatment was stopped after eight and 18 days because of thrombocytopenia; the other three completed the recommended 30-day course of treatment. All five were well three to 12 months after therapy.

This form of disseminated leishmaniasis is distinct from classical visceral leishmaniasis and has therefore been called viscerotropic leishmaniasis to avoid confusion. It is caused by *L. tropica*, not *L. donovani*. The illness associated with viscerotropic leishmaniasis is milder than that associated with classic visceral leishmaniasis; none of these patients had markedly enlarged livers or spleens, and none had pancytopenia, hypergammaglobulinemia, or wasting, which are commonly seen with visceral leishmaniasis.

This diagnosis should be considered in any person who has been in the Middle East and develops an unexplained systemic illness that is persistent for several weeks, especially if the person has been febrile or develops mild enlargement of the liver, spleen, or lymph nodes. Diagnosis requires demonstration of the parasite in the bone marrow, liver, spleen, or lymph nodes. Amastigotes can be seen in touch preparations of these tissues after staining with fluorescein-conjugated, genus-specific monoclonal antibodies (6). Promastigotes can be cultured from these biopsies using Schneider's or biphasic blood agar media (21,22).

Viral hepatitis

Hepatitis A, B, C, D, and E are all endemic to the Middle East (23–28). Ninety-six percent of adult Saudis have been reported to have antibodies to hepatitis A (24). The prevalence of hepatitis B surface antigen was 17% (27), and the prevalence of hepatitis D antibody (delta hepatitis) was 32% (29). The influx of a large number of guest workers has resulted in a change in the epidemiology of acute hepatitis; both hepatitis C and E have increased to high levels (R. Edelman, M.D., personal communications, 27).

Immune serum globulin (ISG) obtained from Western donors will be effective in preventing symptomatic acute hepatitis A but will be less effective as prophylaxis against the other forms of viral hepatitis. Completing the three-dose immunization regimen for hepatitis B will prevent greater than 90% of cases of hepatitis B (and delta hepatitis), while receiving fewer doses will afford proportionately less protection (30). A hepatitis A vaccine should be available by 1994.

Sand fly fever

Sand fly fever (31–34), also known as *Phlebotomus* fever, *pappataci* fever, and three-day fever, was first recognized as an illness caused by a filterable agent transmitted by the sand fly *Phlebotomus pappataci* in 1909 (35). There are two major virus types, the Naples virus and the Sicilian virus, and they are phleboviruses of the family Bunyaviridae (Table 3.4).

Table 3.4   Vector-borne viral diseases endemic in the Middle East

Disease	Agents	Ecology and transmission	Disease pattern/ annual incidence	Major clinical features
Sand fly fever	Phlebovirus	Sand fly (*Phlebotomus*)	Spring–summer	Febrile illness; frontal headache, back pain
Congo-Crimean hemorrhagic fever (CCHF)	Nairoviruses	*Hyalomma* ticks; hares, domestic animals; tick bite, contact with blood of man or domestic animals	Spring–summer	Hepatitis with major blood loss
Rift Valley fever (RVF)	Phlebovirus	*Aedes* mosquitos; mosquito bite, contact with infected domestic animals	Infrequent epidemics; heavy rains promote	Retinitis, encephalitis, fulminant hemorrhagic hepatitis
West Nile fever	Flavivirus	*Culex* mosquitos; mosquito bite	Spring–summer	Febrile illness (rash); encephalitis

Sand flies, which also transmit *Leishmania*, are tiny (2–3 mm by 0.5–1 mm), nocturnal, biting midges that are particularly abundant from June to August and are closely associated with human and animal habitation. Because sand flies require a humid microenvironment, sand fly fever is most prevalent along the coasts and in the fertile land areas.

The site of the bite usually becomes a tiny hemorrhagic spot with surrounding erythema. After an incubation period of three to six days, there is commonly an abrupt onset of fever as high as 40°C (104°F), which is sometimes biphasic and is often associated with severe frontal headaches, retroorbital pain, severe myalgias, especially of the lower back, and sometimes nausea, vomiting, and abdominal pain (34). Conjunctival suffusion with prominent facial flushing, photophobia, and ocular pain accompanying eye movement can be striking physical findings.

The illness lasts two to four days, but convalescence can be complicated by depression, fatigue, and generalized weakness that can last for months (36). Mortality is nil.

The diagnosis can be made by viral isolation in acute cases but is most commonly made by serologic testing (Division of Vector-Borne Diseases, Centers for Disease Control (CDC), Ft. Collins, CO 80522; United States Army Medical Research Institute for Infectious Diseases (USAMRIID), Ft. Dietrick, MD 21702).

OTHER VIRAL INFECTIONS UNIQUE TO OR PREVALENT IN THE MIDDLE EAST

Congo-Crimean hemorrhagic fever

Congo-Crimean hemorrhagic Fever is caused by a nairovirus and is transmitted by the bite of ticks of the genus *Hyalomma*. Serologic surveys have suggested that CCHF is quite prevalent in local animals throughout the Middle East, especially, in the northern areas of Iraq and southern Turkey (37–41). Human infections are common among those in close contact with domestic animals and occur primarily from June to September.

Of particular concern is secondary household and nosocomial transmission. Exposure to infected blood appears to be the risk factor (42).

The initial clinical presentation is quite similar to sand fly fever (see above) but quickly progresses to a hemorrhagic fever illness with hepatitis. The incubation period tends to be longer than that for sand fly fever (six to 14 days), the patient appears toxic, nausea and vomiting is more common, abdominal pain and repeated vomiting can be striking features, and, in severe cases, disseminated intravascular coagulation will develop (Table 3.5). Death will occur in 13% to 50% of cases (43).

The illness runs a 10 to 14-day course with a convalescence that can last several weeks. If the diagnosis of CCHF is considered, strict precautions must be used in handling laboratory specimens, and the patient should be isolated, with blood and body fluid precautions. Serologic tests are available through the CDC and USAMRIID (see above).

There are no proven treatment regimens. However, as with other hemorrhagic fever

Table 3.5 Congo-Crimean hemorrhagic fever

	Percent
Symptoms	
Fever	100
Anorexia	100
Bleeding tendency	100
Headache	90
Abdominal pain	90
Backache	90
Arthralgia/myalgia	70
Diarrhea	40–50
Photophobia	50
Cough (nonproductive)	16–40
Chest pain	20
Sore throat	16
Signs	
Fever to 40°C (104°F)	100
Skin hemorrhages (petechiae, purpura)	100
Jaundice	25–100
Hematuria	90
Tachycardia	70–90
Hypotension	70–90
Oliguria	80
Hepatomegaly	80–100
Disturbed consciousness	80
Gastrointestinal bleeding (hematemesis or melena)	70
Epistaxis	50
Vaginal bleeding (women)	50
Edema	50
Meningeal irritation	40
Bleeding gums	40
Relative bradycardia	20
Conjunctival injection	20
Palmar erythema	20
Gingival ulcers	
Laboratory findings	
Hematologic	
Anemia (as condition deteriorates)	75–100
Leukopenia	60
Thrombocytopenia	100
Atypical lymphocytes	60
Coagulation studies	
Prolonged bleeding time	100
Prolonged prothrombin time	75
Prolonged partial thromboplastin time	67
Diminished fibrinogen	100
Increased fibrin split products	60
Chemistries	
Hyperbilirubinemia	75–100
Elevated transaminases	90
Urinalysis	
Hematuria	90
Proteinuria	90
Serology	
(IgM, IgG)	100

viruses, ribavirin is effective in vitro. A loading dose of 2 g IV followed by 1 g every eight hours for four days, then 500 mg every eight hours for six days, is the suggested regimen (44,45). Immune convalescent serum has also been recommended but is not readily available (46).

Rift Valley fever

Like sand fly fever, Rift Valley fever (Table 3.4) is caused by phlebovirus. It is transmitted by *Aedes* mosquitos and is most prominent in the Middle East along the Nile River. The mosquito eggs can remain dormant in soil for years, hatching during heavy rains and irrigational flooding. Thus, the illness occurs in epidemics. Rift Valley fever infections usually cause an undifferentiated febrile illness but can cause a fulminant hepatitis, DIC, and, in up to 20% of patients, retinitis and vasculitis which can cause permanent blindness (47). The diagnosis can be made during the acute phase by isolation of the virus on tissue culture or in mice and serologically in the convalescent phase (CDC, USAMRIID).

West Nile fever

West Nile fever (48) is a mosquito-borne (*Culex* genus) flaviviral disease that clinically resembles sand fly fever (Table 3.4). Clinically, a high fever develops, accompanied by a macular rash on the trunk and limbs, nausea, abdominal pain, diarrhea, headache, conjunctival injection, periocular pain, myalgias, and arthralgias. The typical disease is self-limited, although convalescence can be prolonged. The diagnosis can be made by virus isolation and serologic testing (CDC, USAMRIID).

Hantaanlike hemorrhagic fever

Sporadic cases of Hantaan hemorrhagic fever with renal syndrome (HFRS) occur, but, unless the patient has had close contact with rodents, it is a very minor threat to visitors (49). The disease occurs in the fall and winter when rodents seek warm shelter.

Rabies

Rabies is present in the Middle East. Vaccination of domestic animals is rare, and only visitors bitten by stray animals are at risk.

BACTERIAL DISEASES PREVALENT IN THE MIDDLE EAST

There are a number of other bacterial infections that are prevalent in the Middle East. These illnesses are likely to remain a problem for as long as certain Middle East customs remain, whereby domesticated animals, especially goats, sheep and dogs, virtually share the same living quarters with humans, open privies are commonplace, and no running water is available.

Brucellosis

Brucellosis, a zoonotic disease contracted by the inhalation of infectious aerosols, ingestion of contaminated meat or dairy products, or direct contact with contaminated tissues, is endemic in the Middle East (50–52).

Clinical manifestations are protean and resemble those of extrapulmonary tuberculosis. A history of ingestion of unpasteurized milk or milk products, especially cheese, or contact with livestock or uncooked meat suggest exposure. Many local inhabitants feel that pasteurizing milk removes its "goodness" and, indeed, prefer drinking it when it is so fresh as to be still warm. Clinical disease may first become manifest acutely or recur months to years after exposure, especially as an FUO (Table 3.2). The diagnosis is made by isolation of the pathogen, a very high IgM *Brucella* titer ($\geq$1:160) during the acute illness, and an elevated IgG titer in late disease. Because pigs are forbidden in the Middle East for religious reasons, *Brucella suis* is not isolated. *Brucella melitensis* predominates, but brucellosis due to *Brucella abortus* does occur.

Although many antibiotic regimens have been used to treat patients successfully, doxycycline, 100 mg b.i.d., plus rifampin 600 mg/day for six weeks is the current recommended regimen. This will result in a cure rate of up to 95% of patients; a second course is indicated in those who fail the initial course. Drug resistance has not yet been reported.

Mycobacterium

As in other parts of the world where overcrowding, poor sanitation, and poor nutrition exist, tuberculosis is widespread in certain areas of the Middle East. Of particular concern is the prevalence of resistance to the more commonly used chemotherapeutic agents: isoniazid (20%), rifampin (10%), streptomycin (5%), and ethambutol (4%) (53,54). Therefore, other antituberculous drugs should be instituted in infected patients until the sensitivity patterns are known.

Other

Plague is also an endemic zoonotic disease, especially in the southern portion of the Arabian peninsula. However, the last case was reported from this area during the 1970s.

Sporadic cases of enteric fever, typhoid fever and cholera continue to be reported from the Middle East, especially among guest workers (55). *Salmonella typhi* was the most frequent bacterial isolate from the blood in a study from Bahrain (56), but whether this is a common or unique situation reflecting the Western-style medicine practiced in this small, but wealthy, country is unknown. The clinical manifestations, the diagnosis and treatment are similar to those in other parts of the world. A high index of suspicion should be maintained whenever a patient presents with the appropriate constellation of signs and symptoms, especially the "neuropsychiatric" type of illness. The reader is referred to standard texts for a more complete discussion of typhoid fever.

Because of the likelihood of antimicrobial-resistant *Salmonella* species, initial treatment with ciprofloxacin (750 mg q 12 h) or ceftriaxone (2 g IV) is suggested. Severe cases should receive dexamethasone (3 mg/kg initially, followed by 1 mg/kg every six hours for eight doses) (57). Any person presenting with *Salmonella* bacteremia should be evaluated for concomitant schistosomiasis.

Outbreaks of Group A meningococcal disease have been reported in pilgrims to Mecca after they have returned home (58,59). The clinical manifestations, diagnosis, and treatment are the same as for *Neisseria meningitidis* infections acquired elsewhere.

Although rare, anthrax is another endemic zoonotic illness of Middle Eastern countries. Anthrax spores are capable of surviving in the soil for years. Direct contact with or inhalation of spores carried on contaminated hides or undercooked meats are the principle modes of transmission. Tourist items made of hides or hair are particularly dangerous.

Characteristic cutaneous lesions, the most common clinical manifestation (95% of cases), begin as small, commonly pruritic, papules that in 24 to 72 hours enlarge into painless ulcers surrounded by vesicles. A characteristic black necrotic eschar follows. Local edema can be striking. The lesions occur most often in exposed areas. Mortality is about 20% in untreated cases.

Inhalation anthrax is difficult to diagnose and carries with it a high mortality rate. The disease begins after an incubation period varying from one to six days, presumably dependent upon the dose of inhaled organisms. Onset is gradual and nonspecific, with fever, malaise, and fatigue, sometimes in association with a nonproductive cough and mild chest discomfort. In some cases, there may be a short period of improvement. The initial symptoms are followed in two to three days by the abrupt development of severe respiratory distress with dyspnea, diaphoresis, stridor, and cyanosis. Physical findings may include evidence of pleural effusions, edema of the chest wall, and mediastinitis. Chest radiographs usually reveal a dramatically widened mediastinum, often with pleural effusions, but typically without infiltrates. The pleural fluid may be hemorrhagic. A hemorrhagic anthrax meningitis may develop rapidly. Shock and death usually follow within 24 to 36 hours of the onset of respiratory distress.

Bacillus anthracis is easily isolated on routine culture media. Gram stains of clinical specimens are often positive, and specific IFA staining can establish the diagnosis. The laboratory should be made aware whenever the diagnosis of anthrax is being considered so that the appropriate precautions can be taken to avoid secondary, laboratory-acquired cases.

Historically, penicillin has been regarded as the drug of choice, but penicillin-resistant strains have been isolated and implicated in human cases. Ciprofloxacin has been shown to be an effective alternative in in vitro studies, and, because of the biological warfare threat, this drug was stocked for this purpose by the U.S. military during Desert Storm. Doxycycline, erythromycin, and the aminoglycosides are alternative antibiotics. A licensed vaccine is available.

Bejel, nonvenereal syphilis, occurs primarily among the local nomads or Bedouins (14% to 21% seropositive) (60) but should pose little risk to visitors.

RICKETTSIAL DISEASES PREVALENT IN THE MIDDLE EAST

Typhus

Both epidemic (louse-borne) and endemic (flea-borne) typhus are found in the Middle East. These illnesses present with similar manifestations, although epidemic typhus is more severe and may be fatal. Patients will have fever, headache, malaise, and myalgia. Most will develop a rash by the fifth to seventh day of illness, but some will not. Treatment must be initiated on clinical grounds alone, since the diagnosis can only be confirmed serologically. Tetracycline or chloramphenicol is effective for these illnesses, but relapses have been reported after chloramphenicol treatment (61). A single oral dose of doxycycline, 200 mg, is sufficient to cure louse-borne typhus, but 100 mg b.i.d. for 7 to 15 days, or until the patient has been afebrile for three days, is preferred for flea-borne typhus (62). Ciprofloxacin may also be effective, but experience is limited (63,64). Q fever has also been reported in the Middle East.

PARASITIC DISEASES (PREVALENT IN THE MIDDLE EAST)

Malaria

Endemic malaria persists in Yemen, Oman, the United Arab Emirates, northern Iraq, and western Saudi Arabia. Malaria has been eradicated from eastern Saudi Arabia, Qatar, Bahrain, and Kuwait, although imported cases in guest workers and the presence of Anopheles vectors make transmission in these areas possible. *Plasmodium falciparum* infections are most common, but *Plasmodium vivax* also occurs and accounts for up to 25% of malaria infections in the region. Through 1991, *P. falciparum* has remained susceptible to chloroquine throughout most of the Middle East, although cases resistant to chloroquine have been reported from Oman, Yemen, and Saudi Arabia (65,66). Patients with *P. vivax* infections should be treated with chloroquine plus primaquine to prevent relapses. The reader is referred to standard texts for a more complete description of malaria.

Schistosomiasis

Both *Schistosoma mansoni* and *Schistosoma haematobium* are found in Oman, Egypt, and Saudi Arabia, and *S. haematobium* is found near the Tigris and Euphrates Rivers in Iraq. Infection occurs after contact with contaminated fresh water. When infection occurs in an individual who has not previously been infected with schistosomiasis, an acute febrile illness can develop four to six weeks after exposure. Patients with acute schistosomiasis, also known as Katayama fever, have an abrupt onset of hectic fever, malaise, headache, abdominal pain, diarrhea, anorexia, nausea, and vomiting. Patients often have tender hepatomegaly and occasionally have splenomegaly. All patients will have eosinophilia and elevated IgE levels. Diagnosis is confirmed by finding *S. mansoni* eggs in the stool or rectal biopsy. Treatment with praziquantel, 40 mg/kg in a single dose, is effective in eradicating the adult worms, but does little to modify the course of acute schistosomiasis, which is felt to be due to immune complexes (67). This syndrome usually resolves within two to four weeks without sequelae, although paraplegia has been reported with acute schistosomiasis (68,69).

REFERENCES

1 Hyams KC, Bourgeois AL, Merrell BR, et al. Diarrheal disease during operation Desert Shield. N Eng J Med 1991;325:1423–1428.

2 Malone JD, Paparello DO, Thornton S, Mapes T, Haberberger R, Hyams KC. Parasitic infections in troops returning from operation Desert Storm. N Eng J Med 1991;325:1448.

3 CDC. Viscerotropic leishmaniasis in persons returning from Operation Desert Storm—1990–1991. MMWR 1992;41:131–134.

4 Oldfield EC III, Wallace MR, Hyams KC, Yousif AA, Lewis DE, Bourgeois AL. Endemic infectious diseases of the Middle East. Rev Infect Dis 1991;13:Suppl 3:S199–S217.

5 Gasser RA, Magill AJ, Oster CN, Tramont EC. The threat of infectious diseases in Americans returning from operation Desert Storm. N Eng J Med 1991;324:859–863.

6 Anthony RL, Grogl M, Sacci JB, Ballou WR. Rapid detection of Leishmania amastigotes in fluid aspirates and biopsies of human tissues. Am J Trop Med Hyg 1987;37:271–276.

7 Hendricks L, Wright N. Diagnosis of cutaneous leishmaniasis by in vitro cultivation of saline aspirates in Schneider's Drosophila medium. Am J Trop Med Hyg 1979;28:962–964.

8 Ballou WR, McClain JB, Gordon DM, et al. Safety and efficacy of high-dose sodium stibogluconate therapy of American cutaneous leishmaniasis. Lancet 1987;ii:13–16.

9 Chulay JD, Spencer HC, Mugambi M. Electrocardiographic changes during treatment of leishmaniasis with pentavalent antimony (sodium stibogluconate). Am J Trop Med Hyg 1985;34:702–709.

10 Gasser RA, Magill AJ, Oster CN. Pentavalent antimonials induce pancreatitis in patients with leishmaniasis [abstract no. 228]. Proceedings of the American Society of Tropical Medicine and Hygiene. Seattle, 1992.

11 Saenz RE, Paz H, Berman JD. Efficacy of ketoconazole against Leishmania braziliensis panamensis cutaneous leishmaniasis. Am J Med 1990;89:147–155.

12 Naggan L, Gunders AE, Dizian R, et al. Ecology and attempted control of cutaneous leishmaniasis around Jericho, in the Jordon Valley. J Infect Dis 1970;121:427–432.

13 Symmers WSC, Bell MD. Leishmaniasis acquired by contagion: a case of marital infection in Britain. Lancet 1960;i:127–132.

14 Nyakundi PM, Muigai R, Were JBO, Oster CN, Gachihi GS, Kirigi G. Congenital visceral leishmaniasis: case report. Trans R Soc Trop Med Hyg 1988;82:564.

15 Chung HL, Chow HK, Lu JP. The first two cases of transfusion kala-azar. Chin Med J 1948;66:325–326.

16 Kager PA, Rees PH. Splenic aspiration: review of the literature. Trop Geogr Med 1983;35:111–124.

17 Bryceson ADM, Chulay JD, Mugambi M, et al. Visceral leishmaniasis unresponsive to antimonial drugs. II. Response to high dosage sodium stibogluconate or prolonged treatment with pentamidine. Trans R Soc Trop Med Hyg 1985;79:705–714.

18 Badaro R, Falcoff E, Badaro FS, et al. Treatment of visceral leishmaniasis with pentavalent antimony and interferon gamma. N Engl J Med 1990;322:16–21.

19 Kreutzer RD, Christensen HA. Characterization of Leishmania spp. by isozyme electrophoresis. Am J Trop Med Hyg 1980;29:199–208.

20 Kreutzer RD, Souralyn N, Semko ME. Biochemical identities and differences among Leishmania species and subspecies. Am J Trop Med Hyg 1987;36:22–32.

21 Hendricks LD, Wood DE, Hajduk ME. Hemoflagellates: commercially available liquid media for rapid cultivation. Parasitol 1978;76:309–316.

22 Grogl M, et al. Leishmania spp.: development of Pentostam-resistant clones in vitro by discontinuous drug exposure. Exp Parasitol 1989;69:78–90.

23 Szmuness W, Dienstag JL, Purcell RH, et al. The prevalence of antibody to hepatitis A antigen in various parts of the world: a pilot study. Am J Epidemiol 1977;106:392–398.

24 El-Hazmi MA. Hepatitis A antibodies: prevalence in Saudi Arabia. *J Trop Med Hyg* 1989;92:427–430.

25 El-Hazmi MA. Hepatitis B virus in Saudi Arabia. *J Trop Med Hyg* 1989;92:56–61.

26 Al-Kandari S, Nordenfelt E, Al-Nakib B, et al. Acute non-A, non-B hepatitis in Kuwait. *Scand J Infect Dis* 1987;19:611–616.

27 Shobokshi OA, Serebour FE. The aetiology of acute viral hepatitis in the western region of Saudi Arabia. *Trans R Soc Trop Med Hyg* 1987;81:219–221.

28 Khuroo MS. Study of an epidemic of non-A, non-B hepatitis: possibility of another human hepatitis virus distinct from post-transfusion non-A, non-B type. *Am J Med* 1980;68:8181–8124.

29 Famia S, el-Hazmi MA, Vivian PA, et al. Delta agent infection in Riyadh, Saudi Arabia. *Trans R Soc Trop Med Hyg* 1987;81:317–318.

30 Hilleman MR. Vaccine perspectives from the vantage of hepatitis B. *Vac Res* 1992;1:1–15.

31 Sadi S, Tesh R, Javadian E, et al. Studies on the epidemiology of sand fly fever in Iran. II. The prevalence of human and animal infection with five phlebotomus fever virus serotypes in Isfahan province. *Am J Trop Med Hyg* 1977;26:288–293.

32 Javadian E, Tesh R, Saidi S, et al. Studies on the epidemiology of sand fly fever in Iran. Host-feeding patterns of *Phlebotomus papatasi* in an endemic area of the disease. *Am J Trop Med Hyg* 1977;26:294–298.

33 Tesh RB, Saidi S, Gajdamovic SJ, et al. Serological studies on the epidemiology of sandfly fever in the Old World. *Bull World Health Organ* 1976;54:663–674.

34 Bartelloni PJ, Tesh RB. Clinical and serologic responses of volunteers infected with phlebotomus fever virus (Sicilian type). *Am J Trop Med Hyg* 1976;25:456–462.

35 Sabin AB, Philip CB, Paul JR. Phlebotomus (pappataci or sand fly) fever. A disease of military importance. Summary of existing knowledge and preliminary report of original investigations. *JAMA* 1944;125:603–606.

36 Eitrem R, Vene S, Niklasson B. Incidence of sand fly fever among Swedish United Nations soldiers on Cyprus during 1985. *Am J Trop Med Hyg* 1990;43:207–211.

37 Hoogstraal H. The epidemiology of tick-borne Crimean-Congo hemorrhagic fever in Asia, Europe, and Africa. *J Med Entomol* 1979;15:307–417.

38 Al-Tikriti SK, Al-Ani F, Jurji FJ, Tantawi H, et al. Congo/Crimean haemorrhagic fever in Iraq. *Bull World Health Organ* 1981;59:85–90.

39 Suleiman MNEH, Muscat-Baron JM, Harries JR, et al. Congo/Crimean haemorrhagic fever in Dubai. An outbreak at the Rashid hospital. *Lancet* 1980;2:939–941.

40 Al-Nakib W, Lloyd G, El-Mekki A, et al. Prelimary report on arbovirus-antibody prevalence among patients in Kuwait: evidence of Congo/Crimean virus infection. *Trans Soc Trop Med Hyg* 1984;78:474–476.

41 Al-Tikriti SK, Hassan FK, Moslih JM, et al. Congo/Crimean haemorrhagic fever in Iraq: A seroepidemiological survey. *J Trop Med Hyg* 1981:84:117–120.

42 Burney MI, Ghafoor A, Saleen M, et al. Nosocomial outbreak of viral haemorrhagic fever caused by Crimean hemorrhagic fever-Congo virus in Pakistan, January 1976. *Am J Trop Med Hyg* 1980:29:941–947.

43 Swanepoel R, Gill DE, Shepherd AJ, et al. The clinical pathology of Crimean-Congo hemorrhagic fever. *Rev Infect Dis* 1989;11 (suppl 4):S794–800.

44 Watts DM, Ussery MA, Nash D, et al. Inhibition of Crimean Congo hemorrhagic fever viral infectivity yields in vitro by ribavirin. *Am J Trop Med Hyg* 1989;41:581–585.

45 Huggins JW, Hsiang CM, Cosgriff TM, et al. Prospective, double blind concurrent, placebo-controlled clinical trial of intravenous ribavirin therapy of hemorrhagic fever with renal syndrome. *J Inf Dis* 1991;164:1119–1127.

46 Vassilenko SM, Vassilev TL, et al. Specific intravenous immunoglobulin for Crimean-Congo haemorrhagic fever. *Lancet* 1990;335:791–792.

47 Abdel-Wahab KSE-D, El Baz LM, El Tayeb EM, et al. Rift Valley fever virus infections in Egypt: pathological and virological findings in man. *Trans Roy Soc Trop Med Hyg* 1978;72:392.

48 Marburg K, Goldblum H, Sterk VV, et al. The natural history of West Nile fever. Clinical observations during an epidemic in Israel. *Am J Hyg* 1956;64:259.

49 LeDuc JW, Smith GA, Johnson KM. Hantaan-like viruses from domestic rats captured in the United States. *Am J Trop Med Hyg* 1984;33:992.

50 Arrighi M. Brucellosis surveillance in Saudi Arabia's eastern province. *Annals of Saudi Medicine* 1986;6(suppl):5–10.

51 Kiel FW, Khan MY. Analysis of 506 consecutive positive serologic tests for brucellosis in Saudi Arabia. *J Clin Microbiol* 1987;25:1384–1387.

52 Kiel FW, Khan MY. Brucellosis in Saudi Arabia. *Soc Sci Med* 1989;29:999–1001.

53 al-Orainey IO, Saeed ES, el-Kassimi FA, al-Shareet N. Resistance to antituberculosis drugs in Riyadh, Saudi Arabia. *Tubercle* 1989;70: 207–210.

54 Schiott CR, Engbaek HC, Vergmann B, et al. Incidence of drug resistance amongst isolates of *Mycobacterium tuberculosis* recovered in the Gizan area, Saudi Arabia. *Saudi Med J* 1985;6:375–378.

55 Elhag KM, Mustafa AK, Sethi SK. Septicaemia in a teaching hospital in Kuwait-I: incidence and aetiology. *J Infect* 1985;10: 17–24.

56 Kumar S, Al-Hilli F. Bacteremia in Bahrain. A study of aetiological conditions, clinical presentation and antibiotic therapy. *Bahrain Medical Bulletin* 1988;10:130–140.

57 Hoffman SL, Punjabi NH, Kumala S, et al. Reduction of mortality in chloramphenicol-treated severe typhoid fever by high-dose dexamethasone. *N Engl J Med* 1984;310:82–88.

58 Moore PS, Harrison LH, Telzak EE, et al. Group A meningococcal carriage in travelers returning from Saudi Arabia. *JAMA* 1988;260: 2686–2689.

59 Moore PS, Reeves MW, Schwartz B, et al. Intercontinental spread of an epidemic group A *Neisseria meningitidis* strain. *Lancet* 1980;2: 260–263.

60 Csonka G, Pace J. Endemic nonvenereal treponematosis (Bejel) in Saudi Arabia. *Rev Infec Dis* 1985;7(suppl 2):S260–265.

61 Shaked Y, Samra Y, Maier MK, et al. Relapse of rickettsial Mediterranean spotted fever and murine typhus after treatment with chloramphenicol. *J Infect* 1989;18:35–37.

62 Raoult D, Drancourt M. Antimicrobial therapy of rickettsial diseases. *Antimicrob Agents Chemother* 1991;35:2457–2462.

63 Eaton M, Cohen MT, Shlim DR, et al. Ciprofloxacin treatment of typhus. *J Am Med Assoc* 1989;262:772–773.

64 Strand O, Stromberg A. Ciprofloxacin treatment of murine typhus. *Scand J Infect Dis* 1990;22:503–504.

65 Division of Control of Tropical Diseases. World malaria situation, 1988. *World Health Stat Q* 1990;43:68–78.

66 el-Sibae MM. A case of chloroquine resistant falciparum malaria in Saudi Arabia. *J Egypt Soc Parasitol* 1991;21:591–592.

67 Hiatt RA, Ottesen EA, Sotomayor ZR, et al. Serial observations of circulating immune complexes in patients with acute schistosomiasis. *J Infect Dis* 1980;142:665–670.

68 CDC. Acute schistosomiasis with transverse myelitis in American students returning from Kenya. *MMWR* 1984;33:445–447.

69 Haribhai HC, Bhigjee AI, Bill PL, et al. Spinal cord schistosomiasis. A clinical, laboratory and radiological study, with a note on therapeutic aspects. *Brain* 1991;114:709–726.

Fluconazole and itraconazole: Current status and prospects for antifungal therapy

ALAN M. SUGAR

INTRODUCTION

The field of antifungal chemotherapy for invasive mycoses began in the 1950s with the introduction of amphotericin B. This drug has been the major single agent used for the treatment of serious invasive fungal infections. It has been considered the "gold standard" against which all new antifungals have been compared. Amphotericin B also has the reputation of being a toxic compound, and the problems with its use have been well documented (1).

During the following decades, fungal infections became more than mere curiosities and rare medical problems. In fact, within the last five years, infection due to various species of *Candida* has become an increasingly common cause of hospital-acquired bloodstream infection (2,3). Moreover, infection caused by heretofore unrecognized fungi is becoming increasingly common, often requiring intensive therapy to eradicate or suppress fungal growth (4). The increasing numbers of patients infected with the human immunodeficiency virus (HIV) have resulted in a marked increase of both pulmonary and extrapulmonary disease caused by the endemic mycoses, especially histoplasmosis and coccidioidomycosis. This enormous increase in the number of patients with mycotic diseases and in the different pathogens encountered in the course of modern medical practice has resulted in an acute need for new, broad-spectrum, less toxic antifungal drugs. Ability to administer oral medications and to avoid the problems inherent with chronic intravenous administration of amphotericin B has also become an important facet in the approach to the treatment of many mycotic infections.

The first major advance, providing an alternative to amphotericin B, was the introduction into clinical practice of ketoconazole, an imidazole derivative (Figure 4.1). Ketoconazole could be given orally and was clinically useful in the treatment of the endemic mycoses, various forms of candidiasis, and other infections. However, many nonalbicans species of *Candida*, aspergillosis, and mucormycosis remained resistant to this drug and treatable only with regimens based on amphotericin B. Certain problems have become apparent as physicians have gained experience with the use of ketocona-

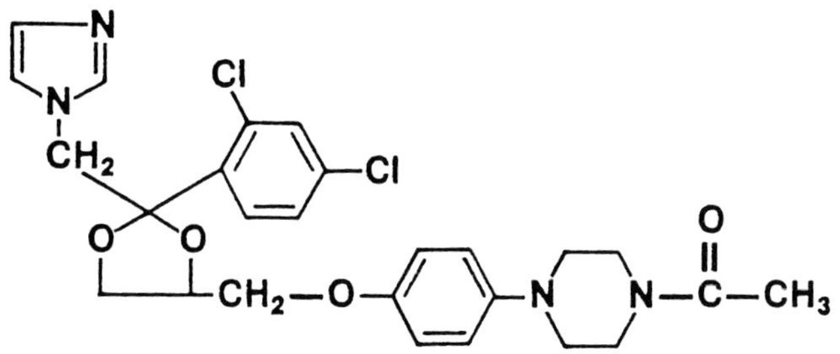

KETOCONAZOLE

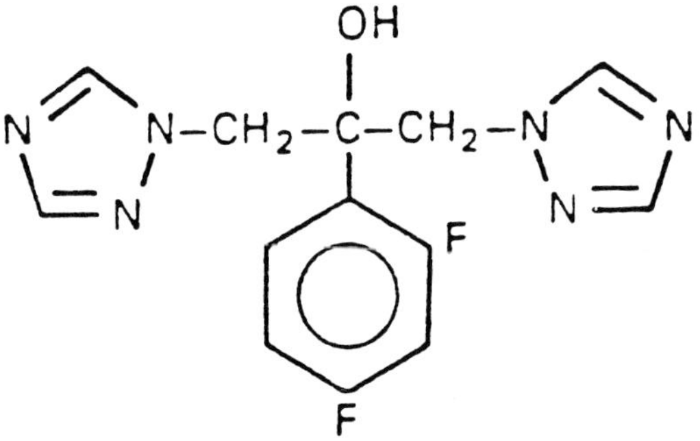

FLUCONAZOLE

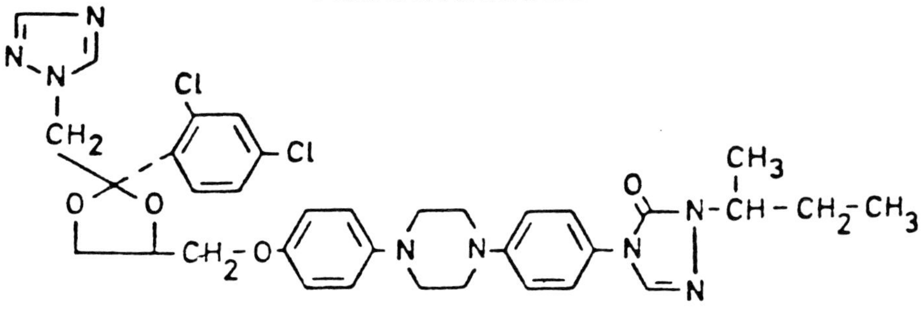

ITRACONAZOLE

Figure 4.1 Structures of ketoconazole (an imidazole derivitive) and of triazole derivatives, fluconazole and itraconazole.

zole. While the drug is very safe to use, idiosyncratic hepatitis has occurred (5), which necessitates the monitoring of liver function tests throughout the course of therapy. Absorption of ketoconazole has also been problematic, and the importance of an acidic environment in the stomach for adequate drug absorption is now well understood (6). Finally, the use of ketoconazole to treat infection in immunosuppressed patients (e.g., patients with leukemia, malignancies, or acquired immunodeficiency syndrome (AIDS)) has met with little success. Thus, while ketoconazole was a welcome addition to the antifungal armamentarium, areas were still amenable to improvement.

Against this background, the triazoles, fluconazole and itraconazole, were synthesized and studied. Both drugs have been approved in various countries throughout the world; fluconazole has been approved for use in the United States, and the approval for itraconazole is under review at the time of this writing. Several symposia reviewing both drugs have already been published and provide a preliminary indication of the utility of these agents (7–9). The purpose of this chapter is to focus on new information about fluconazole and itraconazole and to provide preliminary indications of their potential places in the antifungal armamentarium.

CHEMISTRY

Both fluconazole and itraconazole are classified as triazole derivatives; the important determinant of activity is a triazole moiety (Figure 4.1). However, the physicochemical properties of these two drugs are remarkably different (Table 4.1). Fluconazole is water soluble and miminally protein bound in the circulation, whereas itraconazole is essentially insoluble in aqueous media and is highly protein bound in the bloodstream. Fluconazole is available as a tablet and as an aqueous solution for intravenous administration. Itraconazole is currently dispensed as a lactose bead-encapsulated capsule. A new liquid formulation using hydroxypropyl-β-cyclodextrin appears to offer more reliable absorption and near-total bioavailability of the drug (10). As a result of these properties, fluconazole distributes throughout body water, and itraconazole is found concentrated in lipid-rich tissues. Because of the excellent bioavailability of oral fluconazole, intravenous fluconazole can be reserved for patients unable to tolerate an orally administered medication. There is currently no intravenous preparation of itraconazole, and the drug must be given orally.

MECHANISM OF ACTION

The primary mechanism of action of all the azoles is thought to be inhibition of ergosterol biosynthesis, the major molecular target of the azoles being inhibition of 14-methylation of lanosterol (Figure 4.2). As a result, 14-methylated ergosterol precursors accumulate in the cell membrane, which presumably destabilizes the cell membrane and leads to inhibition of cell growth and, eventually, cell death (11).

Structure activity relationship studies have been done, and the important part of the molecule has been identified as the unsubstituted nitrogen of the azole moiety (11). It

Table 4.1   Comparison of fluconazole and itraconazole

	Fluconazole	Itraconazole
Water solubility	Excellent	Poor
Requires low gastric pH for absorption	No	Yes*
IV preparation available	Yes	No
Renal excretion	Yes	No
Hepatic excretion	No	Yes
Penetrates into CSF and other body water compartments	Yes	No
Half-life	24 h	24 h
Spectrum of activity		
Candida albicans	Good	Good
Nonalbicans *Candida*	Fair–poor	Fair–poor
Aspergillus species	Poor†	Good
Cryptococcus neoformans	Good	Good
Blastomyces dermatitidis	Fair	Good
Coccidioides immitis	Good	Good
Histoplasma capsulatum	Good	Good
Paracoccidioides brasiliensis	Good	Good
Sporotthrix schenkii	Fair	Good
Agents of mucormycosis	Unknown	Unknown
Dematiaceous fungi	Fair	Good
Toxicity		
GI side effects	Rare	Rare
Hepatotoxicity	Rare	Rare
Endocrine effects		
Cortisol	No	Some
Testosterone	No	No
Mineralocorticoidlike	No	Yes

*Best absorption of itraconazole occurs when the pill is taken just after a meal.
†In currently approved doses, fluconazole is not active against species of *Aspergillus*.

is this nitrogen (N-4) that binds to the heme iron of cytochrome P450 enzymes. Individual azole derivatives exhibit differing affinities for binding to their target enzymes and thus differ in their ability to inhibit enzyme activity. Presumably, this differential affinity for human cytochrome P450 enzymes explains the propensity for the azoles to cause certain toxicities. This is especially true for endocrine-mediated side effects: Binding of the antifungal to mammalian enzymes will cause inhibition of the corresponding hormone (e.g., testosterone). Thus, ketoconazole, which has a much greater affinity for enzymes responsible for human steroid hormone synthesis than do fluconazole or itraconazole, produces more clinically evident endocrinologic toxicity than either of the newer agents. Indeed, in experimental studies, 25 and 50 mg/day of fluconazole had no effect on circulating testosterone levels, and in vitro exposure of rat

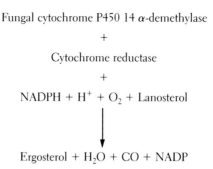

(Reaction blocked by the azole antifungals)

Figure 4.2   Major mechanism of action of fluconazole and itraconazole.

Leydig cells to 10 μg/mL fluconazole had no effect on testosterone production (12). Clinical experience with doses of fluconazole up to 400 mg/day confirms this lack of effect on testosterone in larger numbers of patients.

Itraconazole interacts in vitro in a highly specific manner with fungal cytochrome P450 enzymes compared to the human enzymes. For example, 7×10^{-6} M itraconazole resulted in 50% inhibition of rat liver 14 alpha demethylase. To completely block ergosterol production in *Candida albicans*, only 5×10^{-9} M itraconazole was required (reviewed in 11). In vivo adrenal response to corticotropin was not adversely affected in patients receiving 100 to 400 mg/day. However, detailed studies of testosterone biosynthesis and effects on mineralocorticoid synthesis have not been published. Clinical studies have documented the presence of certain side effects that may be endocrine mediated and are worthy of further study. For example, hypertriglyceridemia and hypokalemia have been found in 9% and 6% of patients, and 1% of the 189 patients reviewed were found to have edema, decreased libido, or gynecomastia. Most of these patients were treated with 400 mg/day (167), five received 200 mg/day, six, received 100 mg/day, and two received 50 mg/day. For the most part, the toxicities noted in this study were not specifically correlated to the doses of itraconazole taken by each patient. Since endocrine-mediated toxicity is likely to be dose dependent, this information is critical to proper interpretation of toxicity data. At 600 mg/day, hypertension and hypokalemia each developed in five of eight patients (13). One patient taking this dose developed reversible adrenal insufficiency. Thus, the maximum tolerated dose of itraconazole appears to be 400 mg/day in most patients.

While the major mechanism of action of azoles undoubtedly is the inhibition of fungal ergosterol synthesis, recent data on the interactions of amphotericin B, which binds to ergosterol, and azoles suggest that there may be additional cellular and biochemical events leading to antifungal effects. For example, in a recent study in murine-disseminated candidiasis, additive or synergistic effects were seen when mice were treated with amphotericin B in combination with SCH 39304, an experimental triazole derivative (14). Similar results have been obtained in a murine model of cryptococcal meningitis (15). If there was a decrease in ergosterol in the fungal cell membrane, one might expect to see less of an effect of the amphotericin B component of the regimen. That this was not the case suggests that other events may contribute to the antifungal effects of both polyenes and azoles, especially when the two classes of agents are used together.

PHARMACOLOGY

The pharmacology of fluconazole differs from that of ketoconazole and itraconazole by virtue of the water solubility of fluconazole. Bioavailability of fluconazole exceeds 80%, and the drug is minimally protein bound. In contrast to ketoconazole, gastric acid is not required for its absorption (16). The drug is distributed throughout body water (1 l/kg). Thus, free, and presumably active, drug is present throughout tissues in virtually the entire body (17). High concentrations of fluconazole in the urine and cerebrospinal fluid (CSF) make this drug highly promising for treating fungal infections in these locations (18–20). While the achievement of high concentrations of fluconazole in the CSF may be intuitively satisfying, it is important to realize that the critical parameter for the treatment of certain mycoses, such as cryptococcal meningitis, is probably the concentration of drug that penetrates into the brain itself. Experience with the satisfactory results obtained using amphotericin B or itraconazole support this concept. Neither of these drugs achieves significant concentrations within the CSF, yet most patients treated with either of these agents will respond to such treatment.

Fluconazole achieves high concentrations in peritoneal fluid in patients treated with continuous ambulatory peritoneal dialysis (CAPD) (21, 22), with levels in peritoneal fluid reaching over 60% of serum levels. Daily administration of 200 to 400 mg/day, depending on the clinical situation, should be adequate to treat most patients with *Candida* peritonitis. A study of low doses of fluconazole (50 mg/day) in patients undergoing hemodialysis indicated that about 38% of the daily dose of fluconazole was removed during a three-hour dialysis session. This is not surprising, and, for the treatment of fungal infections in the hemodialysis patient, a usual dose of the drug should be given after each dialysis.

Fluconazole has also been detected in what should be effective concentrations in the eye, and experimental and human endophthalmitis have been successfully treated with fluconazole (23–26). However, experience with treating *Candida* and other fungal endophthalmitis with fluconazole is limited, and patients treated with this drug should be closely followed for evidence of response. As one might imagine, considerable controversy exists concerning the relative merits and risks of using amphotericin B, with or without flucytosine, or fluconazole for these devastating infections.

The terminal half-life of fluconazole is approximately 24 hours and, without a loading dose, steady state concentrations are reached in about five days. Optimal dosing depends on the indication with doses ranging from 50 to 400 mg given once daily. Intravenous drug can be reserved for patients unable to take medications by mouth or who have problems with absorption of material through their gastrointestinal tract. Fluconazole can be taken without regard to food intake, and gastric pH is not a variable in determining optimal absorption of the drug.

In doses of 200 to 400 mg/day, fluconazole has been noted to interact with several drugs. Phenytoin serum concentrations can increase to toxic levels (reviewed in 17). Cyclosporine concentrations have also been elevated, but not always with concomitant nephrotoxicity (27–29). Potentiation of warfarin effects on the prothrombin time have been noted (30). Rifampin has been reported to induce the metabolism of fluconazole; however, the clinical implications of this finding are not clear (31). Antipyrine metabolism in mice was also found to be reduced, indicating that fluconazole is an inhibitor of cytochrome P450 enzymes in these animals; this may explain the increases in serum concentrations of some drugs (32).

Itraconazole, like ketoconazole, is highly lipophilic and essentially insoluble in aqueous solutions at neutral pH. Absorption following oral administration requires the presence of food, and a low pH also aids in maximizing concentration of itraconazole in the blood (33–35). Bradford et al. have indicated that, in cases of apparent failure of itraconazole therapy, measurement of serum concentrations of the drug may be helpful in determining the cause of lack of response (36). Itraconazole is highly protein bound (>99%) to plasma proteins, and concentrations of itraconazole in body fluids are low. However, when itraconazole is assayed in tissues, concentrations two to five times those found in blood are regularly obtained (37). Thus, itraconazole appears to reach potential sites of infection in concentrations that should be conducive to an antifungal effect.

Itraconazole is extensively metabolized in the liver, and at least one of the metabolites may have antifungal effects. This may explain the discrepancies observed when comparing measurement of itraconazole levels in serum by bioassay or high-pressure liquid chromatography (HPLC). Levels determined by bioassay have been in the μg/mL range, whereas HPLC routinely delivers concentrations in the ng/mL range. The difference may be the detection of bioactive metabolites of itraconazole by bioassay. Drugs that induce liver enzymes may decrease serum itraconazole concentrations. Antituberculous medications may be particularly problematic (38). Rifampin may be the most important in this regard: Up to four weeks may be required after discontinuation of rifampin in order to achieve detectable serum levels of itraconazole (DA Stevens and AM Sugar, personal observations). Itraconazole has also been noted to increase digoxin concentrations (39), and, as is the case with fluconazole, a possible interaction with cyclosporine has been noted, but not all researchers agree (40–43). It would be prudent to closely follow cyclosporine blood concentrations and renal function in patients who are also receiving itraconazole. No interactions between itraconazole and warfarin, insulin, or antipyrine have been described.

There have been no published data on the pharmacokinetics of itraconazole in patients with renal or hepatic insufficiency. However, the itraconazole investigational brochure cites work performed at Janssen Pharmaceutica indicating that itraconazole is not dialyzable and plasma protein binding is unchanged in patients with renal insufficiency. The major drawbacks to this study are the small number of patients evaluated, seven in each group, and the fact that only a single dose of itraconazole was administered before serum levels were determined. Thus, dosage of itraconazole does not need to be modified in patients with renal insufficiency or in patients treated with hemodialysis or CAPD. The measurement of serum itraconazole concentrations would be useful in such patients to insure adequate (not too low) absorption. In the presence of liver failure, serum concentrations may be higher due to a decrease in first pass metabolism. This study, too, involved only six healthy patients and 12 with cirrhosis of the liver. A single dose of 100 mg was administered to the patients, and 50 mg was given to the healthy volunteers. Further information on the pharmacokinetics in patients with renal insufficiency would be useful in the development of guidelines for its use in this patient population.

SPECTRUM OF ACTIVITY

One of the major problems confronting the clinician in the choice of antifungal agents for the treatment of a particular mycosis is the lack of a suitably standardized and clinically relevant in vitro antifungal susceptibility testing system. Decisions to develop new antifungals have often been based on the results of treatment of experimental mycoses in various animal models of infection. Correlation of in vitro results with clinical response to therapy, particularly with the azoles, has been poor. A subcommittee of the National Committee for Clinical Laboratory Standards has been tackling the myriad problems in order to develop a standardized method for the determination of in vitro susceptibility of yeasts to various antifungals (44). A standard method has now been agreed upon, following years of intense work in this area (manuscript in preparation). However, clinical correlations are still lacking. Therefore, antifungal susceptibility testing remains a research tool and can not be relied upon to provide clinically useful information. The physician must rely upon accumulated experience with these drugs for guidance in most clinical situations.

The use of animal models of mycotic diseases in the development and evaluation of new antifungal drugs has been discussed at length and will not be discussed in this chapter (45). However, the correlations between efficacy in these animal models and subsequent experience in humans has been quite good, and these models remain a useful preclinical tool for evaluation of potentially useful compounds as antifungal drugs and for the study of new indications for established antifungals.

The antifungal susceptibility data presented in Table 4.1 are derived from studies in animal models and experience treating human infections. From existing information, it appears that the maximal tolerated dose of itraconazole is 400 mg/day. However, higher doses of fluconazole have been studied (up to 2,000 mg/day; E Anaissie, personal communication) and toxicity has been minimal. Thus, with fluconazole, additional indications may evolve as dosages are increased. Indeed, dose-finding studies are currently underway in the treatment of several mycoses, including cryptococcal meningitis, to investigate whether doses in excess of 400 mg/day confer any therapeutic advantage.

CLINICAL USES

Cryptococcosis

Cryptococcosis has become an important cause of morbidity and mortality as a result of the burgeoning of the AIDS epidemic. Much effort in the evaluation of fluconazole has been directed towards establishing its role in this serious infection. Preliminary work suggested that fluconazole would be useful in AIDS patients as primary or maintenance therapy of this mycosis (46, 47). Several major studies have appeared that provide some data from which conclusions may be drawn (48, 49).

In a large, multicenter, comparative study of amphotericin B versus fluconazole as primary therapy of cryptococcal meningitis in patients with AIDS, the two drugs yielded comparable results. Patients in both groups were similar in all demographic and clinical parameters evaluated. Amphotericin B was given at a mean dose of 0.4 to 0.5 mg/kg/day. Of the 63 patients receiving amphotericin B, only nine also received flucytosine. Fluconazole was initiated at a dose of 200 mg/day. Eighty-three of the 141 fluconazole recipients took this dose. The other 48 patients had the dosage increased to 400 mg/day. Interestingly, the outcome of the patients receiving either 200 or 400 mg/ day was the same.

Of the amphotericin-B-treated patients, 25 of 63 (40%) were successfully treated, that is, they had improvement or complete resolution of their clinical symptoms and two negative cultures of their CSF, at least one week apart, by the end of therapy (Table 4.2). Any other extrameningeal culture-positive sites also had to have been sterilized. Forty-four of the 131 fluconazole-treated patients (34%) also were successfully treated. This difference was not statistically significant. Patients failing therapy were similar in the two groups: 38 (60%) of the amphotericin-B-treated patients and 87 (66%) of the fluconazole-treated patients. Failure was defined in four ways: quiescent disease, disease progression, toxic reaction, and death. Quiescent disease represents an important category of response in AIDS patients, since most studies of the different treatment regimens yield similar percentages of patients in this classification. These patients are clinically cured or improved but have persistently positive cultures of the CSF. About one-quarter of patients receiving either drug fell into this group. Finally, the percentage of patients dying during the 10-week trial was the same: 14% versus 18% in the amphotericin B and fluconazole groups, respectively.

The time to negative CSF cultures was different in the two groups. Patients treated with amphotericin B had a median time to negative CSF culture of 42 days (95%

Table 4.2 Fluconazole versus amphotericin B in the treatment of acute cryptococcal meningitis: outcome at 10 weeks of therapy

Outcome	Amphotericin B No. of patients (%)	Fluconazole No. of patients (%)
Successful treatment	25 (40)	44 (34)
Treatment failure	38 (60)	87 (66)
Quiescent disease	17 (27)	34 (26)
Disease progression	7 (11)	26 (20)
Toxicity	5 (8)	3 (2)
Death	9 (14)	24 (19)

SOURCE Adapted from Reference 110.

confidence interval (CI): 28 to 71 days). The median time to negative CSF culture in the fluconazole-treated patients was 64 days (95% CI: 53 to 67 days). The clinical implications of the slower CSF sterilization with fluconazole are not clear and require further study.

One conclusion that can be made from this study is that treatment of cryptococcal meningitis in patients with AIDS is frustratingly difficult. Only a minority of patients have their CSF sterilized, and about two-thirds will have less than an optimal response. This may very well be secondary to the low doses of both drugs used in this study. In fact, Larsen et al. suggest that fluconazole, 400 mg/day, is inferior to amphotericin B, 0.7 mg/kg/day, plus flucytosine, 150 mg/kg/day. In that small study, eight of 14 patients treated with fluconazole failed therapy, whereas all six amphotericin B/flucytosine patients responded successfully (50). In addition, anecdotal evidence suggests that doses of amphotericin B of 0.7–1.0 mg/kg/day, perhaps with the addition of lower doses of flucytosine (e.g., 50–75 mg/kg/day), or higher doses of fluconazole, 600–800 mg/day, may be more efficacious. Particularly interesting is a brief report of the combined use of fluconazole and flucytosine resulting in response rates similar to those obtained with higher doses of combined amphotericin B/flucytosine therapy. Further work along these lines is clearly indicated.

The general consensus that patients successfully treated for cryptococcal meningitis require lifelong maintenance therapy was confirmed in a placebo-controlled trial (51). In that study, fluconazole was found to be more effective than placebo in preventing relapse of cryptococcal disease at any site: one of 34 patients versus 10 of 27 relapsed, respectively. Survival and toxicity of the regimens were similar in both groups.

A larger study of the relative efficacy and toxicity of amphotericin B 1 mg/kg/wk, versus fluconazole, 200 mg/day, in patients successfully treated for acute cryptococcal meningitis with amphotericin B further demonstrated the utility of maintenance therapy. Of the evaluable patients, 14 of 78 (18%) receiving amphotericin B and two of 111 (2%) receiving fluconazole suffered relapses of cryptococcal disease. Patients receiving amphotericin B had significantly more bacterial infections and bacteremias, presumably secondary to the long-term intravenous catheterization required for amphotericin B infusions, and toxicity due to the medication occurred more frequently in patients taking amphotericin B. Thus, fluconazole has emerged as an effective and safe drug for the suppression of cryptococcal meningitis in patients previously treated for acute cryptococcal meningitis. One point that deserves some attention, however, is whether successful primary therapy of acute cryptococcal meningitis with fluconazole results in the same clinical situation as that following amphotericin B therapy. Studies to date have evaluated maintenance therapy only after amphotericin B treatment. Extrapolation of the data to CSF culture-negative patients following fluconazole therapy may not be appropriate, and future studies will have to address the nature and timing of "maintenance" therapy in AIDS patients with cryptococcal meningitis who have received fluconazole as their only antifungal therapy.

Some patients with cryptococcal meningitis will have residual foci in the prostate gland following successful therapy of the meningitis (52). Fluconazole has been used to eradicate the fungus from the prostate in an attempt to further reduce the risk of reactivation of the central nervous system infection. In a small study, seven of 14 such patients receiving fluconazole had eradication of *Candida neoformans* from the prostate after a median of four weeks. The two patients who had a relapse of cryptococcal meningitis both had *C. neoformans* persistently recovered from the urine. The authors suggested that higher doses of fluconazole might be indicated in patients with continued isolation of the fungus from the urine, since one patient with multiple, large prostatic abscesses had sterilization of these while taking 600 mg/day of fluconazole, and none of four patients taking 100 mg/day had sterilization of the urine.

Uncontrolled experience using fluconazole in doses in excess of 400 mg/day has accumulated slowly over the past several years. One such published study of eight patients who failed all previous therapy for cryptococcal meningitis and who received fluconazole, 800 mg/day, showed that four responded satisfactorily to therapy (53). Seven patients died, but only three of the seven had active cryptococcosis at the time of death. The sole survivor had sterilization of the CSF only after the fluconazole dose was increased to 800 mg/day.

Other manifestations of cryptococcosis, such as focal osteomyelitis, have been successfully treated with fluconazole (54). Problems with this approach to therapy have been discussed and include questions about the most appropriate dose and duration of therapy, need for maintenance therapy in different patient populations, and the role of combination therapy with flucytosine or other drugs (55). However, fluconazole appears to be one possible option for treating patients with these rarer forms of cryptococcosis.

Itraconazole has also been evaluated in AIDS patients with cryptococcal meningitis; however, comparative data with amphotericin B or fluconazole are not available. Nonrandomized, open studies have shown that itraconazole induces a clinical response in 50% to 60% of patients treated (56–59). Approximately 25% of patients continue to grow the fungus from the CSF, yet are clinically well. This percentage is identical to that seen in patients treated with amphotericin B or fluconazole (48). While the anecdotal information is promising, the relative benefits versus risks of itraconazole compared to amphotericin B or fluconazole remain unexplored. Further comparative studies are clearly justified in order to answer the many questions concerning the most appropriate agent for use in any given clinical situation.

Itraconazole has also been used successfully in a case of presumed cryptococcal endophthalmitis (60) and in other miscellaneous presentations of the disease (61). There are no guidelines to help physicians decide whether itraconazole, fluconazole, or amphotericin B is the drug of choice in any given patient. Degree of illness, concomitant medications, renal and hepatic function, need for intravenous administration, and severity of the infection may be important considerations as such decisions are formulated.

Attention of investigators treating patients with cryptococcal meningitis with azoles has focused on patients with AIDS, and very little information exists about the role of these drugs in treating non-AIDS patients with cryptococcal disease. Many feel that fluconazole and itraconazole should work in this setting; however, serious questions have been raised concerning duration of therapy, need for long-term suppressive therapy (especially in organ transplant recipients), and appropriate daily dose of the azole compounds in the therapy of the non-AIDS patient with cryptococcosis.

Aspergillosis

Fluconazole has not been systematically studied in patients with aspergillosis. Data obtained from a rabbit model of invasive aspergillosis suggest that doses in excess of 800 mg per day will be needed if any anti-*Aspergillus* effect is to be expected (62).

Much more work has been done with itraconazole treatment of various manifestations of invasive aspergillosis. Unfortunately, the data are in the form of uncontrolled open studies; trials comparing the relative efficacies and toxicities of amphotericin B and itraconazole in patients with aspergillosis have not yet begun.

Viviani and colleagues reported on 20 patients with aspergillosis who were treated with itraconazole (56). Ten of these had tissue-invasive aspergillosis; three had cystic fibrosis complicated by bronchopulmonary aspergillosis; one had chronic necrotizing pulmonary aspergillosis associated with pulmonary alveolar proteinosis; two patients had aspergillomas; and one each had *Aspergillus* empyema, peritoneal aspergillosis, and surgical wound infection with *Aspergillus*. Overall, 14 of the 20 were deemed to have responded to therapy and were classified as being in remission or markedly improved. Three of four patients who showed moderate clinical improvement continued to have positive cultures, and two patients failed to respond to therapy. Details of the individual cases are presented in that report, but this preliminary evidence indicates that itraconazole can be used to satisfactorily treat patients with aspergillosis.

This same group published an updated report of their experience with itraconazole, with eight of the 34 patients with aspergillosis reported in the earlier study. Itraconazole, 100 to 400 mg was administered once daily to patients. Of 18 with invasive aspergillosis, 15 were considered cured, one was thought to have manifested moderate improvement, and two failed therapy. Only one of five patients with cystic fibrosis complicated by aspergillosis failed to respond.

Similar results have been obtained by other investigators in open label studies (63, 64). Dupont reported the results of treatment of 49 patients with various forms of aspergillosis, the majority of whom responded favorably to itraconazole (64). Of particular note in that study were the 14 patients with aspergillomas, of whom two were cured and eight symptomatically improved. Should itraconazole be shown to be effective in the treatment of patients with aspergillomas, this would constitute a major advance in the management of patients, especially those with symptomatic aspergillomas (e.g., hemoptysis, cough).

One other intriguing possible use of itraconazole is in patients with allergic bronchopulmonary aspergillosis (65). Six such patients were treated with 200 mg twice daily, and all experienced improvement in pulmonary function during the trial. Sputum cultures of two of three patients became negative during therapy. Previously, antifungal therapy had not been successful in treating this manifestation of aspergillosis. Successful application of itraconazole in this setting would be a major benefit to patients with this disease.

Miscellaneous cases of extrapulmonary aspergillosis successfully treated with itraconazole have been reported, adding to the anecdotal evidence that itraconazole has an important role in the treatment of patients with invasive aspergillosis (66–69).

The general impression gleaned from the literature on the use of itraconazole in treating various forms of invasive aspergillosis is that this drug represents an alternative to amphotericin B in many patients. Acute primary therapy and longer-term "maintenance" or suppressive therapy both appear to be possible with itraconazole. The National Institutes of Health Mycoses Study Group is about to embark on a multicenter comparative study of itraconazole versus amphotericin B in the treatment of invasive aspergillosis. Results of this ambitious project are eagerly awaited.

Candidiasis

The bulk of information concerning the utility of azoles in the treatment of candidiasis can be found in papers focusing on mucocutaneous candidiasis. Comparative studies of the therapeutic role of fluconazole or itraconazole in treating candidemia or invasive candidiasis have not yet been published.

It is clear that both fluconazole and itraconazole are effective agents for the treatment of oral or vaginal candidiasis. Fluconazole in a dose of 50 or 100 mg/day has been shown to be effective in the treatment of oral candidiasis in patients with AIDS (70, 71). Other options have been explored, including a single 150- or 400-mg dose of fluconazole (72, 73) and maintenance therapy with daily or intermittent doses of fluconazole (74). A single dose of 100 mg of fluconazole resulted in clinical resolution in all of 16 patients and 75% mycological cure at two weeks posttreatment, as compared with 65% and 20% of 17 patients treated with clotrimazole troches (5/day for 14 days) (75). With any of the treatment regimens, response to therapy is usually rapid, with clinical and mycological improvement seen within three to five days. Not surprisingly, a large minority of patients continues to have positive cultures at the end of therapy, and relapse is virtually certain at some point once primary therapy is discontinued. Most relapses will occur within 30 days of discontinuing therapy. Some form of maintenance therapy may be required to minimize the morbidity of multiple frequent relapses. In patients with underlying predisposing factors other than infection with HIV, once the predisposition is ameliorated, recurrence of thrush is uncommon and maintenance therapy is usually not required.

Occasional patients with thrush do not respond to usual doses of fluconazole. One such patient who did not improve after 200 or 400 mg/day of fluconazole has been reported (76). This patient eventually responded to 800 mg/day of the drug. Anecdotal experience supports this approach in selected patients. Other theoretically appealing strategies include combination therapy with fluconazole and flucytosine or amphotericin B. However, many of these patients with recalcitrant oral candidiasis who do not have responsive disease have severe immunosuppression, which presumably is the primary reason for the failure of therapy to eradicate or diminish the numbers of organisms in the mouth. Overall prognosis is not good for these patients, and the least toxic option with the best clinical results should be chosen on an individual basis.

Oropharyngeal and esophageal candidiasis in the neutropenic patient have also been treated successfully with fluconazole (77). Of note, a shift has occurred from C. albicans to other less common and probably more azole-resistant strains of Candida isolated from patients who were treated with fluconazole. As will be discussed below, Candida krusei is becoming increasingly recognized as a common Candida isolate in such patients.

Candida vaginitis is also amenable to treatment with fluconazole. In fact, studies have shown that a single 150-mg dose of fluconazole is clinically effective in close to 100% of patients so treated, and mycological response one to two months following the single dose occurred in about three-fourths of the patients (78, 79). Fluconazole has emerged as an effective, safe, and convenient option for the treatment of this common condition. Itraconazole has also been used to treat vaginal candidiasis in regimens of one to five days, with results slightly less encouraging than those obtained with single-dose fluconazole (80, 81).

Two studies have reported on the successful use of fluconazole in patients with hepatosplenic candidiasis, also known as chronic disseminated candidiasis (82, 83). This infection, typically seen in the leukemic patient in remission, following an episode of chemotherapy-induced neutropenia, has been difficult to treat with amphotericin B, often requiring many months and many grams of drug. Symptomatic improvement occurred in six of six fluconazole-treated patients in the first study (82) and in 14 of 16 patients in the second (83). Although randomized trials have not been done and are probably not feasible because of the relative rarity of this disease, it appears that results using fluconazole for this indication are excellent, and fluconazole can be considered as first-line therapy for this form of candidal infection.

Two small studies of the use of fluconazole in the treatment of patients with candidemia have been published (84, 85). In the first, 34 episodes of candidemia in 24 children with various immunosuppressive illnesses were studied. Oral or intravenous fluconazole at a dose of 6 mg/kg/day was given. Clinical and mycological success was achieved in 30 of the 34 episodes (88%). Of potential concern, only one of the four failures was due to *C. albicans*. *C. krusei* and two unspeciated *Candida* isolates were responsible for the infections. Two patients developed a rise in liver transaminases, but the drug was otherwise well tolerated. This study illustrates one major problem in the interpretation of the results. Of the 34 episodes of candidiasis, 17 were oral thrush, a very responsive form of candidiasis. Four patients were said to be multiply colonized, nine had *Candida* in the urine, two had "septicemia," and one each had "otitis" and subhepatic abscess. Thus, most of the patients had easily treated infections, some had infections of uncertain significance, and only a minority had true invasive disease. The overall response rate of 88% must not be extrapolated to seriously ill patients with documented invasive candidiasis.

The other study was of six nonneutropenic, critically ill, postsurgical patients who were in the intensive care unit and who received fluconazole, 200 mg/day (84). These six patients had 12 episodes of candidemia. Two patients had peritoneal infection with *Candida*, and two were thought to have intravenous catheter related candidemia. All were classified as cured after 13 to 38 days of fluconazole therapy. Three isolates of *C albicans* were recovered from blood cultures: two were *Candida tropicalis*, and one was *Candida parapsilosis*. Unfortunately, this is a sketchy report, and critical data, such as the renal function of patients (which allows one to estimate what the dose should be to be equivalent to that in a person with normal renal function), the APACHE II score (which permits an estimate of the degree of organ system dysfunction present in the patients), and the number of blood cultures positive for the organism at the start of therapy, and the number of blood cultures and the results during and after therapy, are missing.

Because of fluconazole's attractive pharmacokinetics, safety, and relatively broad spectrum of activity, prophylaxis of mycoses with this drug in immunosuppressed patients has generated some interest. Two such studies have been published (86, 87). Wingard et al. performed a retrospective review of patients on the bone marrow transplantation service and adult leukemia services using 1989 and 1990. Various regimens of antifungal prophylaxis were used during this time period: miconazole (35% of patients), fluconazole (18%), amphotericin B (2%), or ketoconazole (0.4%). Thirty-five percent of patients did not receive antifungal prophylaxis, and, in 10% of cases, the type of prophylaxis was unknown. In the 419 patients whose antifungal prophylaxis was known, there were 36 cases of fungemia. No cases of C. albicans or C. tropicalis infections occurred in the 84 patients receiving fluconazole, whereas, of the patients receiving some other regimen (or no antifungal prophylaxis), there were 10 cases of C. albicans and 10 cases of C. tropicalis infections. Of particular note was the occurrence of seven cases of C. krusei infection in fluconazole recipients (8% of patients), compared with four (1%) in the other group. This difference was highly significant. When odds ratios for C. krusei colonization were determined in patients receiving fluconazole, there was a 3.5 times increased risk of colonization (95% CI: 2.1 to 6.0) and a 7.2 times increased risk of infection (95% CI: 2.1 to 25.3). The authors also demonstrated a slightly increased risk for C. krusei colonization, but not infection, in patients receiving norfloxacin. In addition to C. krusei, colonization with Torulopsis glabrata and Candida lambica was also found. Approximately half of patients in the fluconazole and the no-fluconazole groups were colonized with C. albicans during the study. Fortunately, the C. krusei infections were responsive to therapy with amphotericin B and flucytosine.

A second large study in bone marrow transplant patients has also been published (87). Fluconazole, 400 mg/day, was compared with placebo in patients with neutrophil counts less than $1,000/mm^3$. Two-thirds of the 177 patients in the placebo group had positive surveillance fungal cultures, compared with one-third of the patients receiving fluconazole. Superficial infections occurred in one-third of the placebo group and in only 8% of the fluconazole group. There was also a difference in the occurrence of systemic fungal infection in the two groups: 16% versus 3% in the placebo and fluconazole groups, respectively. The five patients on fluconazole prophylaxis with systemic fungal infections had infections with C. krusei ($n = 3$), and one patient each developed aspergillosis or mucormycosis. No infections occurred with any other species of Candida.

In both of those prophylaxis studies, fluconazole was well tolerated and decreased the risk of colonization and infection with most species of Candida. However, the emergence of C. krusei in two different institutions using fluconazole, 400 mg/day, is reminiscent of the shift in fungi that occurred when ketoconazole was the prophylactic agent under study. The lesson seems to be that, if a suitable niche for proliferation of fungi exists, previously uncommon strains, less susceptible to the antifungal employed, will become more prominent. It may be unreasonable to expect a single antifungal drug to adequately protect against every possible fungal pathogen. Differences in susceptibility of different fungi to various antifungal agents are to be expected, and previously unrecognized organisms will become more prominent in areas where antifungal prophylaxis is routinely employed.

Fluconazole, 100 mg/day, has also been shown to prevent thrush in AIDS patients, when compared with placebo in a double-blind study (88). In this small study, eight of 13 placebo recipients and none of 12 fluconazole recipients developed thrush over the 12-week duration of therapy. This study raises the possibility that mucocutaneous candidiasis can be prevented in AIDS patients. A natural extension of this concept is whether other, more invasive mycoses can be prevented. Surely, the prevention of cryptococcosis, histoplasmosis, coccidioidomycosis, and other less common fungal infections would decrease morbidity if a safe and cheap agent could be found. Long-term administration of fluconazole appears to be safe. Proper doses of the drug for adequate prophylaxis are not yet known. The potential for development of resistant organisms once large numbers of patients begin to take this drug also is of some concern. Studies addressing this issue have been proposed, and an AIDS Clinical Trial Group (ACTG) study comparing fluconazole with clotrimazole troches in prevention of thrush and other fungal infections is still underway at the time of this writing.

Fluconazole has been used in other forms of candidiasis (89, 90), but simple case reports are difficult to interpret and utilize in the formulation of guidelines for the appropriate use of the drug. Ongoing multicenter studies of fluconazole in various serious manifestations of candidiasis, such as candidemia in immunocompetent and neutropenic patients, should provide some guidance in the most appropriate use of the drug.

There is less in the published literature on the use of itraconazole for treating invasive candidal infections (91). As noted above, mucocutaneous candidiasis is usually responsive to itraconazole therapy, but single-dose therapy, as employed with fluconazole, for treating vaginal candidiasis does not seem to be as efficacious. Interpretation of anecdotal reports of the use of any drug in invasive candidiasis is always hampered by the problem of definition of disease and whether isolation of *Candida* represented invasion of tissue, contamination, or just colonization.

In a small randomized trial, van't Wout et al. compared itraconazole, 200 mg twice daily, with amphotericin B, 0.6 mg/kd/day or 0.3 mg/kg/day in combination with flucytosine, in neutropenic patients with proven or suspected systemic fungal infections (92). Sixteen patients in each group were evaluable. Patients on itraconazole therapy received the drug for a median of 20 days, whereas amphotericin B was administered for a median of 13 days. Response to therapy was similar in both groups: 10 of 16 and 9 of 16 demonstrated a clinical response, as defined by total or >50% resolution of the initial signs of infection, respectively. As in other studies, recovery of circulating neutrophils was critical to responding to antimicrobial therapy: 13 of 15 with neutrophil recovery during treatment responded clinically, while only six of 17 patients with neutrophil counts persistently below 500/mm^3 demonstrated a response to therapy. Interestingly, only two of six patients with definite, probable, or possible candidiasis (all but one due to *C. albicans*) responded to itraconazole, but six of eight patients with definite or probable aspergillosis responded. These are encouraging results of the use of itraconazole in seriously ill patients and support the use of larger comparative trials in immunosuppressed patients with invasive mycoses, especially aspergillosis.

Endemic mycoses

Histoplasmosis   Interestingly, current research in the United States into the role of azoles in the treatment of histoplasmosis has focused on disseminated histoplasmosis in patients with AIDS. Studies of fluconazole in this population are just being started at the time of this writing. One disturbing report, in German, describes a patient with sarcoidosis who was treated with steroids and who died with disseminated histoplasmosis despite treatment with fluconazole, 400 mg/day, and then over 1 g of amphotericin B (93). Perhaps higher doses of fluconazole will be needed in the treatment of the endemic mycoses, but this can only be determined by direct clinical trials.

Preliminary results with itraconazole suggest that it is very effective and well tolerated as long-term maintenance therapy (94). Studies are in progress to assess the efficacy and safety of itraconazole as primary therapy of acute histoplasmosis in AIDS patients. Results of these studies will lead to further trials comparing the various agents with each other. Meanwhile, patients should be encouraged to participate in ongoing clinical trials of antifungals for these diseases.

Negroni et al. have reported on 32 patients with histoplasmosis who completed six months of therapy with itraconazole (95). Twenty-nine of these patients had chronic disseminated histoplasmosis. Relatively low doses were used: 100 mg/day for two months, then 50 mg/day for four months. Of the 32 patients, 29 were said to have been cured clinically. In 23 patients followed for longer than one year, no relapses were identified. These authors concluded that itraconazole appears to be the drug of choice in the treatment of histoplasmosis. Given the fact that it has a better safety profile and less erratic absorption than ketoconazole, itraconazole may become the oral drug of choice for treating histoplasmosis in both the immunocompetent and immunosuppressed patient. The roles of fluconazole and other azoles will still need further evaluation.

Coccidioidomycosis   Most forms of clinically evident acute pulmonary coccidioidomycosis do not require therapy. However, anecdotal reports indicate that ketoconazole and the newer azoles are being used to treat patients who, in the past, had spontaneously resolving pneumonitis. The wisdom of this approach is uncertain, but prospective identification of the very small percentage of patients who will develop some form of disseminated coccidioidomycosis is not yet possible. The relative merits of using ketoconazole, fluconazole, or itraconazole have not been determined for this indication. The scant published literature focuses on more severe manifestations of the disease.

The early experience using fluconazole, 50 to 100 mg/day, in the treatment of different forms of coccidioidomycosis was disappointing: Responses were infrequent and relapses common (96). However, as doses of the drug were increased to higher levels, responses were seen, and even patients with coccidioidal meningitis responded to therapy (97, 98). Unfortunately, there is little published literature at present upon which to base informed decisions about azole therapy of coccidioidomycosis in any of its forms. In areas of the country where clinical trials are underway, every effort should be made to enter suitable patients into these studies in order to answer questions about the most appropriate agent and the most efficacious and least toxic dose.

Several publications attest to the potential of itraconazole in the treatment of coccidioidomycosis (99–101). The majority of patients with nonmeningeal coccidioidomycosis responds to therapy. However, due to differences in assessing responses from study to study and from earlier studies of ketoconazole, it is impossible to compare the results obtained with itraconazole to those obtained with any other therapy. In a relatively large open trial with this drug, 25 of 44 patients (57%) with various forms of coccidioidomycosis achieved remission, and of these 25, relapse later occurred in four. These results are similar to those obtained with ketoconazole and demonstrate once again the difficulty in achieving satisfactory response in this extremely recalcitrant mycotic disease. It is the preliminary impression of physicians with experience with azole therapy of coccidioidomycosis that itraconazole may be better than any other agent for the chronic therapy of chronic forms of coccidioidomycosis (102).

Ten patients with coccidioidal meningitis who have been treated with itraconazole have been reported (99). They received itraconazole, 300 to 400 mg/day, for a median of 10 months. Eight of the patients were evaluable, and five received itraconazole as the sole medication to treat the meningitis; four of these patients responded to therapy and had no clinical evidence of active disease at the time of the publication. Duration of therapy is certainly an important, but as yet unanswered, question (98). Obviously, more work needs to be done to expand on these preliminary, very promising findings.

Blastomycosis   Even less is known about the utility of these new azoles in the treatment of blastomycosis. Preliminary review of data obtained during the course of pilot studies conducted under the auspices of the Mycoses Study Group suggests that fluconazole in doses of less than 400 mg/day is not satisfactory in the treatment of pulmonary or extrapulmonary blastomycosis. Further studies of higher doses are warranted to evaluate the role of fluconazole in this potentially serious disease.

In contrast, itraconazole induced a 90% response rate in over 90% of patients treated with 200 to 400 mg/day of this drug (WE Dismukes et al., manuscript submitted for publication). Itraconazole was well tolerated and, when approved by the US Food and Drug Administration (FDA), will probably become the drug of choice for treating patients with forms of blastomycosis that require medical therapy.

Paracoccidioidomycosis   This disorder, rarely seen in the United States, is a common invasive mycosis diagnosed in South and Central America. Preliminary results are available for both fluconazole and itraconazole. Among 29 patients with pulmonary or extrapulmonary paracoccidioidomycosis treated with fluconazole, 27 responded to 200 to 400 mg/day, usually within one month after beginning therapy (103). Only seven patients were followed for more than a year, and one relapsed. The authors noted that most of the patients who appeared clinically cured had durable remissions, but longer followup is necessary to document permanent cure of previously chronic infection.

Negroni et al. treated 25 patients with chronic disseminated paracoccidioidomycosis with itraconazole, 50 mg daily for six months (104). Nineteen of these patients were clinically cured, and the response of an additional six was described as "striking improvement." Two patients sustained a relapse of their disease and were retreated with itraconazole, again for six months. This second treatment course was successful.

Restrepo et al. also reported preliminary results in 16 patients with paracoccidioido-mycosis who were treated with itraconazole, 100 mg daily for six months (105). Twelve of these patients had disseminated and four had only pulmonary disease. Thirteen patients completed therapy and were evaluated. All patients improved: 11 with major and two with minor improvement, as defined by a scoring system. In seven patients followed for more than six months posttherapy, no relapses were seen. The impression from this early experience with itraconazole therapy of paracoccidioidomycosis is that this drug is highly efficacious and well tolerated and may represent an improvement over ketoconazole.

Sporotrichosis There is very little experience with using fluconazole as therapy for patients with sporotrichosis. More uncontrolled experience with itraconazole has been reported in the literature (102), and results with this drug are highly encouraging. Saturated solution of potassium iodide (KI) still remains a first-line agent in treating patients with typical lymphocutaneous sporotrichosis. If this is not tolerated, itracona-zole appears to be a useful alternative, since the experience with ketoconazole has been mixed and there just is not enough known about fluconazole for its routine use in this infection.

Given the serious nature of disseminated sporotrichosis, including pulmonary sporo-trichosis, and the lack of experience with azoles in this form of the disease, amphoteri-cin B remains the drug of choice. However, as additional patients are treated with the azoles, it would not be surprising to see itraconazole emerge as an alternative to amphotericin B in patients with this severe form of sporotrichosis. While KI is the traditional first-line treatment of lymphocutaneous disease, itraconazole would appear to be a useful alternative, if cost of therapy is not a problem.

Miscellaneous infections Early experience with itraconazole in the treatment of patients with chromomycosis due to *Cladosporium* spp or *Fonsecaea pedrosoi* has indicated that many patients, especially those infected with *F. pedrosoi*, may be cured with long-term therapy. This would represent a major advance in the treatment of these patients with disfiguring and progressive disease.

The anecdotal evidence suggests that fluconazole may be less effective in these infections, although very few patients have received this agent in appropriate doses, i.e., 400 to 800 mg/day.

TOXICITY

Azole antifungal drugs have proven to be relatively safe antimicrobial compounds. Certainly compared to the well-appreciated, and often formidable, toxicities of ampho-tericin B, azoles are easily administered and well tolerated. While remarkably safe, even for long durations of administration, adverse side effects due to these drugs have been reported, and unique toxicities for both fluconazole and itraconazole have been recognized.

The most common complaints voiced by patients taking these drugs are related to gastrointestinal upset. Nausea, vomiting, and diarrhea are reported to occur in about 5% of patients taking either drug. Since fluconazole can be taken without regard to relationship to food consumption, taking the pills with food may decrease the upper gastrointestinal effects. On the other hand, itraconazole must be taken with food in order to optimize its absorption. Thus, there is no effective strategy to decrease nausea or vomiting due to this drug. Fortunately, patients with gastrointestinal complaints may improve even as therapy is continued.

The concern that fluconazole or itraconazole would be as hepatotoxic and prone to endocrinologic effects as ketoconazole has not been realized. However, both drugs have been noted to produce hepatotoxicity in a very small number of patients. There is little information concerning the likelihood of patients who experience hepatotoxicity with one azole developing hepatotoxicity to another. Since the reaction is thought to be idiosyncratic and not dose related, there may be reason to suspect that cross-sensitivity to these drugs would not occur. We have treated one patient who had a history of liver function abnormalities with ketoconazole therapy (so severe that ketoconazole was discontinued) with fluconazole, SCH 39304 (an investigational triazole no longer available), and currently with itraconazole for recalcitrant chromoblastomycosis. This patient has never developed any further signs of hepatic dysfunction while on any of these newer azole drugs. Since many patients may need to be treated for long durations for chronic, slowly responsive mycoses, and since development of clinical resistance to therapy may occur, it is imperative that the safety of the different azoles be verified.

Rare side effects reported with fluconazole include anaphylaxis (106), Stevens-Johnson syndrome (107), and thrombocytopenia (108). These reactions have been rare, with only one or slightly more cases individually reported in the literature. However, since these side effects may be serious, patients should be followed closely when taking fluconazole.

CONCLUSIONS AND FUTURE PROSPECTS

The introduction of fluconazole and itraconazole into clinical practice has provided the physician with viable alternatives to amphotericin B for the treatment of many mycoses. However, due to the enormous difficulties in rigorously studying many fungal infections, the indications for use of these agents in any particular situation are often not known. Certainly, one would want to know the relative efficacy of either of these azoles compared to amphotericin B and their relative efficacy and toxicity compared to each other, but this information is simply not known. As is to be expected with any new drug, reports of the failure of fluconazole have appeared in the literature (89, 109). It is noteworthy that, in both of these papers, the doses of fluconazole have been on the low side, even though, for the most part, the doses employed fell within accepted guidelines. As higher doses of fluconazole are used, one can expect differences in response rates to appear. Once itraconazole is approved for use in the United States, and as the drug becomes more widely prescribed, publications will also begin to define its limitations.

For certain mycoses, e.g., the endemic mycoses, invasive aspergillosis, and various manifestations of candidiasis, studies are in progress or will begin in the near future.

Results of these clinical trials will begin to address these critical issues that presently defy rational solution. In the meantime, case-by-case review of each clinical situation, often in consultation with experts in the management of patients with invasive mycoses, will have to serve as the best alternative for treating these increasingly common infections.

REFERENCES

1 Gallis HA, Drew RH, Pickard WW. Amphotericin B: 30 years of clinical experience. *Rev Infect Dis* 1990;12:308–329.

2 Wey SB, Mori M, Pfaller MA, Woolson RF, Wenzel RP. Risk factors for hospital-acquired candidemia: A matched case-control study. *Arch Intern Med* 1989;149:2349–2353.

3 Komshian SV, Uwaydah AK, Sobel JD, Crane LR. Fungemia caused by *Candida* species and *Torulopsis glabrata* in the hospitalized patient: Frequency, characteristics, and evaluation of factors influencing outcome. *Rev Infect Dis* 1989;11:379–390.

4 Anaissie E. Opportunistic mycoses in the immunocompromised host: Experience at a cancer center and review. *Clin Infect Dis* 1992;14 (Suppl. 1):S43–53.

5 Lewis JH, Zimmerman HJ, Benson GD, Ishak KG. Hepatic injury associated with ketoconazole therapy: analysis of 33 cases. *Gastroenterology* 1984;86:503.

6 Lake-Bakaar G, Tom W. Gastropathy and ketoconazole malabsorption in the acquired immunodeficiency syndrome. *Ann Intern Med* 1988;15:471–473.

7 Bennett JE. Fluconazole: A novel advance in therapy for systemic fungal infections. *Rev Infect Dis* 1990;12:S263–389.

8 Cauwenbergh G, Degreef H. Clinical use of itraconazole in fungal infections. *J Am Acad Dermatol* 1990;23:549–614.

9 Hay RJ, Dupont B, Graybill JR. First International Symposium on Itraconazole. *Rev Infect Dis* 1987;9:S1–S152.

10 Hostetler JS, Hanson LH, Stevens DA. Effect of cyclodextrin on the pharmacology of antifungal oral azoles. *Antimicrob Agents Chemother* 1992;36:477–480.

11 Vanden Bossche H. Itraconazole: A selective inhibitor of the cytochrome p-450 dependent ergosterol biosynthesis. In: Fromtling RA, ed. *Recent Trends in the Discovery, Development, and Evaluation of Antifungal Agents.* J.R. Prous Science Publishers, 1987:207–221.

12 Hanger DP, Jevons S, Shaw JTB. Fluconazole and testosterone: in vivo and in vitro studies. *Antimicrob Agents Chemother* 1988;32:646–648.

13 Sharkey PK, Rinaldi MG, Dunn JF, Hardin TC, Fetchick RJ, Graybill JR. High-dose itraconazole in the treatment of severe mycoses. *Antimicrob Agents Chemother* 1991;35:707–713.

14 Sugar AM. Interactions of amphotericin B and SCH 39304 in the treatment of experimental murine candidiasis: lack of antagonism of a polyene-azole combination. *Antimicrob Agents Chemother* 1991;35:1669–1671.

15 Albert MM, Graybill JR, Rinaldi MG. Treatment of murine cryptococcal meningitis with an SCH 39304-amphotericin B combination. *Antimicrob Agents Chemother* 1991;35:1721–1725.

16 Blum RA, D'Andrea DT, Florentino BM, et al. Increased gastric pH and the bioavailability of fluconazole and ketoconazole. *Ann Intern Med* 1991;114:755–757.

17 Grant SM, Clissold SP. Fluconazole: A review of its pharmacodynamic and pharmacokinetic properties, and therapeutic potential in superficial and systemic mycoses. *Drugs* 1990;39: 877–916.

18 Brammer KW, Coakley AJ, Jezequel SG, Tarbit MH. The disposition and metabolism of [^{14}C] fluconazole in humans. *Drug Metab and Disp* 1991;19:764–767.

19 Tucker RM, Williams PL, Arathoon EG, et al. Pharmacokinetics of fluconazole in cerebrospinal fluid and serum in human coccidioidal meningitis. *Antimicrob Agents Chemother* 1988;32:369–373.

20 Arndt CAS, Walsh TJ, McCully CL, Balis FM, Pizzo PA, Poplack DG. Fluconazole penetration into cerebrospinal fluid: Implications for treating fungal infections of the central nervous system. *J Infect Dis* 1988;157:178–180.

21 Levine J, Bernard DB, Idelson BA, Saunders C, Sugar AM. Fungal peritonitis complicating continuous ambulatory peritoneal dialysis: Successful treatment with fluconazole, a new orally active antifungal agent. *Am J Med* 1989;86:825–827.

22 Debruyne D, Ryckelynck J-P, Moulin M, Ligny BHD, Levaltier B, Bigot M-C. Pharmacokinetics of fluconazole in patients undergoing continuous ambulatory peritoneal dialysis. *Clin Pharmacokinet* 1990;18:491–498.

23 Walsh TJ, Foulds G, Pizzo PA. Pharmacokinetics and tissue penetration of fluconazole in rabbits. *Antimicrob Agents Chemother* 1989;33: 467–469.

24 Filler SG, Crislip MA, Mayer CL, Edwards JE Jr. Comparison of fluconazole and amphotericin B for treatment of disseminated candidiasis and endophthalmitis in rabbits. *Antimicrob Agents Chemother* 1991;35:288–292.

25 Cruciani M, Di Perri G, Concia E, et al. Fluconazole and fungal ocular infection. *J Antimicrob Chemother* 1990;25:718–720.

26 Savani DV, Perfect JR, Cobo LM, Durack DT. Penetration of new azole compounds into the eye and efficacy in experimental *Candida* endophthalmitis. *Antimicrob Agents Chemother* 1987;31:6–10.

27 Sugar AM, Saunders C, Idelson BA, Bernard DB. Interaction of fluconazole and cyclosporine. *Ann Intern Med* 1989;110:844.

28 Canafax DM, Graves NM, Hilligoss DM, Carleton BC, Gardner MJ, Matas AJ. Interaction between cyclosporine and fluconazole in renal allograft recipients. *Transplantation* 1991; 51:1014–1018.

29 Torregrosa V, De la Torre M, Campistol JM, et al. Interaction of fluconazole with cyclosporin A. *Nephron* 1992;60:125–126.

30 Lazar JD, Wilner KD. Drug interactions with fluconazole. *Rev Infect Dis* 1990;12:s327–333.

31 Apseloff G, Hilligoss DM, Gardner MJ, et al. Induction of fluconazole metabolism by rifampin: In vivo study in humans. *J Clin Pharmacol* 1991;31:358–361.

32 La Delfa I, Zhu QM, Mo Z, Blaschke TF. Fluconazole is a potent inhibitor of antipyrine metabolism in vivo in mice. *Drug Metab and Disp* 1989;17:49–53.

33 Van Peer A, Woestenborghs R, Heykants J, Gasparini R, Gauwenbergh G. The effects of food and dose on the oral systemic availability of itraconazole in healthy subjects. *Eur J Clin Pharmacol* 1989;36:423–426.

34 Heykants J, Van Peer A, Van de Velde V, et al. The clinical pharmacokinetics of itraconazole: An overview. *Mycoses* 1989;32 (Suppl. 1):67–87.

35 Hardin TC, Graybill JR, Fetchick R, Woestenborghs FR, Rinaldi MG, Kuhn JG. Pharmacokinetics of itraconazole following oral administration to normal volunteers. *Antimicrob Agents Chemother* 1988;32:1310–1313.

36 Bradford CR, Prentice AG, Warnock DW, Copplestone JA. Comparison of the multiple dose pharmacokinetics of two formulations of itraconazole during remission induction for acute myeloblastic leukemia. *J Antimicrob Chemother* 1991;28:555–560.

37 Van Cutsem J, Van Gerven F, Janssen PAJ. Activity of orally, topically, and parenterally administered itraconazole in the treatment of superficial and deep mycoses: Animal models. *Rev Infect Dis* 1987;9:s15–32.

38 Blomlcy M, Teare EL, De Belder A, Thway Y, Weston M. Itraconazole and antituberculosis drugs. *Lancet* 1990;336:1255.

39 Rex J. Itraconazole-digoxin interaction. *Ann Intern Med* 1992;116:525.

40 Novakova I, Donnelly P, De Witte T, De Pauw B, Boezeman V. Itraconazole and cyclosporin nephrotoxicity. *Lancet* 1987;2:920–921.

41 Shaw MA, Gumbleton M, Nicholls PJ. Interaction of cyclosporin and itraconazole. *Lancet* 1987;2:637.

42 Kwan JTC, Foxall PJD, Davidson DGC, Bending MR, Eisinger AJ. Interaction of cyclosporin and itraconazole. *Lancet* 1987;2:282.

43 Lewiston NJ, Stevens DA, Theodore J. Cyclosporine and itraconazole interaction in heart and lung transplant recipients. *Ann Intern Med* 1990;113:327–329.

44 Pfaller MA, Rinaldi MG, Galgiani JN, et al. Collaborative investigation of variables in susceptibility testing of yeasts. *Antimicrob Agents Chemother* 1990;34:1648–1654.

45 Ryley JF. Screening and evaluation in vivo. In: Ryley JF, ed. *Chemotherapy of Fungal Diseases*. 1st ed. Berlin: Springer-Verlag, 1990:129–147. (*Handbook of Experimental Pharmacology*; 96).

46 Stern JJ, Hartman BJ, Sharkey P, et al. Oral fluconazole therapy for patients with acquired immunodeficiency syndrome and cryptococcosis: experience with 22 patients. *Am J Med* 1988;85:477–480.

47 Sugar AM, Saunders C. Oral fluconazole as suppressive therapy of disseminated cryptococcosis in patients with acquired immunodeficiency syndrome. *Am J Med* 1988;85:481–489.

48 Saag MS, Powderly WG, Cloud GA, et al. Comparison of amphotericin B with fluconazole in the treatment of acute AIDS-associated cryptococcal meningitis. *N Engl J Med* 1992; 326:83–89.

49 Powderly WG, Saag MS, Cloud GA, et al. A Controlled trial of fluconazole or amphotericin B to prevent relapse of cryptococcal meningitis in patients with the acquired immunodeficiency syndrome. *N Engl J Med* 1992;326:793–798.

50 Larsen RA, Leal MAE, Chan LS. Fluconazole compared with amphotericin B plus flucytosine for cryptococcal meningitis in AIDS. A randomized trial. *Ann Intern Med* 1990;113:183–187.

51 Bozzette SA, Larsen RA, Chiu J, et al. A placebo-controlled trial of maintenance therapy with fluconazole after treatment of cryptococcal meningitis in the acquired immunodeficiency syndrome. *N Engl J Med* 1991;324:580–584.

52 Larsen RA, Bozzette S, McCutchan JA, et al. Persistent *Cryptococcus neoformans* infection of the prostate after successful treatment of meningitis. *Ann Intern Med* 1989;111:125–128.

53 Berry AJ, Rinaldi MG, Graybill JR. Use of high-dose fluconazole as salvage therapy for cryptococcal meningitis in patients with AIDS. *Antimicrob Agents Chemother* 1992;36:690–692.

54 Jamil S, Brennessel D, Pessah M, Hilton E. Fluconazole treatment of cryptococcal osteomyelitis. *Program and Abstracts of the 31st ICAAC* 1992;1:115–117.

55 Sugar AM. Commentary: Fluconazole for cryptococcosis. *Infect Dis Clin Pract* 1992;1:118.

56 Viviani MA, Tortorano AM, Langer M, et al. Experience with itraconazole in cryptococcosis and aspergillosis. *J Infect* 1989;18:151–165.

57 Denning DW, Tucker RM, Hanson LH, Stevens DA. Itraconazole in opportunistic mycoses: cryptococcosis and aspergillosis. *J Am Acad Dermatol* 1990;23:602–607.

58 Denning DW, Tucker RM, Hanson LH, Hamilton JR, Stevens DA. Itraconazole therapy for cryptococcal meningitis and cryptococcosis. *Arch Intern Med* 1989;149:2301–2308.

59 Viviani MA, Tortorano AM, Pagano A, et al. European experience with itraconazole in systemic mycoses. *J Am Acad Dermatol* 1990;23:587–593.

60 Denning DW, Armstrong RW, Fishman M, Stevens DA. Endophthalmitis in a patient with disseminated cryptococcosis and AIDS who was treated with itraconazole. *Rev Infect Dis* 1991;13:1126–1130.

61 Denning DM, Tucker RM, Hanson LH, Stevens DA. Itraconazole in opportunistic mycoses: Cryptococcosis and aspergillosis. *J Am Acad Dermatol* 1990;23:602–607.

62 Patterson TF, Miniter P, Andriole VT. Efficacy of fluconazole in experimental invasive *Aspergillosis. Rev Infect Dis* 1990;12:S281–285.

63 Denning DW, Tucker RM, Hanson LH, Stevens DA. Treatment of invasive aspergillosis with itraconazole. *Am J Med* 1989;86:791–800.

64 Dupont B. Itraconazole therapy in aspergillosis: Study in 49 patients. *J Am Acad Dermatol* 1990;23:607–614.

65 Denning DW, Van Wye JE, Lewiston NJ, Stevens DA. Adjunctive therapy of allergic bronchopulmonary aspergillosis with itraconazole. *Chest* 1991;100:813–819.

66 Phillips P, Bryce G, Shepherd J, Mintz D. Invasive external otitis caused by aspergillus. *Rev Infect Dis* 1990;12:277.

67 Sachs MK, Paluzzi RG, Moore JH Jr, Fraimow HS, Ost D. Amphotericin-resistant *Aspergillus* osteomyelitis controlled by itraconazole. *Lancet* 1990;335:1475.

68 Kloss S, Schuster A, Schroten H, Lamprecht J, Wahn V. Control of proven pulmonary and suspected CNS *Aspergillus* infection with itraconazole in a patient with chronic granulomatous disease. *Eur J Pediatr* 1991;150:483–485.

69 Van't Wout JW, Raven EJM, Van der Meer JWM. Treatment of invasive aspergillosis with itraconazole in a patient with chronic granulomatous disease. *J Infect* 1990;20:147–150.

70 Dupont B, Drouhet E. Fluconazole in the management of oropharyngeal candidosis in a predominantly HIV antibody-positive group of patients. *J Med Veterin Mycol* 1988;26:67–71.

71 Cirelli A, Rossi F, Ciardi M. Treatment of oropharyngeal and esophageal candidiasis with a new antifungal agent, fluconazole, in HIV-infected patients. *Curr Ther Res* 1990;47:81–87.

72 Chave JP, Cajot A, Bille J, Glauser MP. Single-dose therapy for oral candidiasis with fluconazole in HIV-infected adults: a pilot study. *J Infect Dis* 1989;159:806–807.

73 Chave J-P, Francioli P, Hirschel B, Glauser MP. Single-dose therapy for esophageal candidiasis with fluconazole. *AIDS* 1990;4:1034–1035.

74 Esposito R, Castagna A, Foppa CU. Maintenance therapy of oropharyngeal candidiasis in HIV-infected patients with fluconazole. *AIDS* 1990;4:1033–1034.

75 Koletar SL, Russell JA, Fass RJ, Plouffe JF. Comparison of oral fluconazole and clotrimazole troches as treatment for oral candidiasis in patients infected with human immunodeficiency virus. *Antimicrob Agents Chemother* 1990;34:2267–2268.

76 Ansari AM, Gould IM, Douglas JG. High dose oral fluconazole for oropharyngeal candidosis in AIDS. *J Antimicrob Chemother* 1990;25:720–721.

77 Kremery V Jr, Koza I, Hornikova M, et al. Fluconazole in the treatment of mycotic oropharyngeal stomatitis and esophagitis in neutropenic cancer patients. *Chemotherapy* 1991;37:343–345.

78 Adetoro OO. Comparative trial of a single oral dose of fluconazole (150 mg) and a single

intravaginal tablet of clotrimazole (500 mg) in the treatment of vaginal candidiasis. *Curr Ther Res* 1990;48:275–281.

79 Andersen GM, Barrat J, Bergan T, Brammer KW, Cohen J, Dellenbach P. A comparison of single-dose oral fluconazole with 3-day intravaginal clotrimazole in the treatment of vaginal candidiasis. *Br J Obstetrics Gynaecol* 1989;96: 226–232.

80 Sanz Sanz F, Del Palacio Hernanz A. Randomized comparative trial of three regimens of itraconazole for treatment of vaginal mycoses. *Rev Infect Dis* 1987;9 (Suppl. 1):S139–42.

81 Calderon-Marquez JJ. Itraconazole in the treatment of vaginal candidosis and the effect of treatment on the sexual partner. *Rev Infect Dis* 1987;9 (Suppl. 1):S143–145.

82 Kauffman CA, Bradley SF, Ross SC, Weber DR. Hepatosplenic candidiasis: Successful treatment with fluconazole. *Am J Med* 1991;91: 137–141.

83 Anaissie E, Bodey GP, Kantarjian H, et al. Fluconazole therapy for chronic disseminated candidiasis in patients with leukemia and prior amphotericin B therapy. *Am J Med* 1991;91: 142–150.

84 Nolla-Salas J, Leon C, Torres-Rodriguez JM, Martin E, Sitges-Serra A. Treatment of candidemia in critically ill surgical patients with intravenous fluconazole. *Clin Infect Dis* 1992; 14:952–954.

85 Viscoli C, Castagnola E, Fioredda F, Ciravegna B, Barigione G, Terragna A. Fluconazole in the treatment of candidiasis in immunocompromised children. *Antimicrob Agents Chemother* 1991;35:365–367.

86 Wingard RJ, Merz WG, Rinaldi MG, Johnson TR, Karp JE, Saral J. Increase in *Candida krusei* infection among patients with bone marrow transplantation and neutropenia treated prophylactically with fluconazole. *N Engl J Med* 1991;325:1274–1277.

87 Goodman JL, Winston DJ, Greenfield RA, et al. A controlled trial of fluconazole to prevent fungal infections in patients undergoing bone marrow transplantation. *N Engl J Med* 1992; 326:845–851.

88 Stevens DA, Greene SI, Lang OS. Thrush can be prevented in patients with acquired immunodeficiency syndrome and the acquired immunodeficiency syndrome-related complex: Randomized, double-blind, placebo-controlled, study of 100-mg oral fluconazole daily. *Arch Intern Med* 1991;151:2458–2464.

89 McIlroy MA. Failure of fluconazole to suppress fungemia in a patient with fever, neutropenia, and typhlitis. *J Infect Dis* 1991;163:420–421.

90 Isalska BJ, Stanbridge TN. Fluconazole in the treatment of candidal prosthetic valve endocarditis. *Br Med J* 1988;297:178–179.

91 Cauwenbergh G, De Doncker P, Stoops K, De Dier A-M, Goyvaerts H, Schuermans V. Itraconazole in the treatment of human mycoses: Review of three years of clinical experience. *Rev Infect Dis* 1987;9 (Suppl. 1):S146–152.

92 van't Wout JW, Novakova I, Verhagen CAH, Fibbe WE, De Pauw BE, Van der Meer JWM. The efficacy of itraconazole against systemic fungal infections in neutropenic patients: a randomized comparative study with amphotericin B. *J Infect* 1991;22:45–52.

93 Tornieporth N, Disko R, Seeliger HPR, Emslander HP. Disseminated histoplasmosis after a visit to a tropic country in a man with known sarcoidosis. *Dtsch Med Wochenschr* 1989;114:1744.

94 Wheat LJ. Histoplasmosis in Indianapolis. *Clin Infect Dis* 1992;14 (Suppl. 1):S91–99.

95 Negroni R, Robles AM, Arechavala A, Taborda A. Itraconazole in human histoplasmosis. *Mycoses* 1989;32:123–130.

96 Catanzaro A, Fierer J, Friedman PJ. Fluconazole in the treatment of persistent coccidioidomycosis. *Chest* 1990;97:666–669.

97 Classen DC, Burke JP, Smith CB. Treatment of coccidioidal meningitis with fluconazole. *J Infect Dis* 1988;158:903–904.

98 Dewsnup DH, Graybill JR, Stevens DA. Is it ever safe to stop oral azole therapy of *Coccidiodes immitis* meningitis? *Program and Abstracts of the 31st ICAAC 1991*. Chicago, IL: McCormick Place, abstract 1156.

99 Tucker RM, Denning DW, Dupont B, Stevens DA. Itraconazole therapy for chronic coccidioidal meningitis. *Ann Intern Med* 1990;112:108–112.

100 Graybill JR, Stevens DA, Galgiani N, Dismukes WE, Cloud GA, NAIAD Mycoses Study Group. Itraconazole treatment of coccidioidomycosis. *Am J Med* 1990;89:282–290.

101 Diaz M, Puente R, De Hoyos LA, Cruz S. Itraconazole in the treatment of coccidioidomycosis. *Chest* 1991;100:682–684.

102 Graybill JR. Future directions of antifungal therapy. *Clin Infect Dis* 1992;14:s170–181.

103 Diaz M, Negroni R, Montero-Gei F, et al. A Pan-American 5-year study of fluconazole therapy for deep mycoses in the immunocompetent host. *Clin Infect Dis* 1992;14 (Suppl. 1):S68–76.

104 Negroni R, Palmieri O, Koren F, Tiraboschi IN, Galimberti RL. Oral treatment of paracoccidioidomycosis and histoplasmosis with

itraconazole in humans. *Rev Infect Dis* 1987;9 (Suppl. 1):S47–50.

105 Restrepo A, Gomez I, Robledo J, Patino MM, Cano LE. Itraconazole in the treatment of paracoccidioidomycosis: A preliminary report. *Rev Infect Dis* 1987;9 (Suppl. 1):S51–6.

106 Neuhaus G, Pavic N, Pletscher M. Anaphylactic reaction after oral fluconazole. *Br Med J* 1991;302:1341.

107 Gussenhoven MJE, Haak A, Peereboom-Wynia JDR, Van't Wout JW. Stevens-Johnson syndrome after fluconazole. *Lancet* 1991; 338:120.

108 Agarwal A, Sakhuja V, Chugh KS. Fluconazole-induced thrombocytopenia. *Ann Intern Med* 1990;113:899.

109 Evans TG, Mayer J, Cohen S, Classen D, Carroll K. Fluconazole failure in the treatment of invasive mycoses. *J Infect Dis* 1991; 164:1232–1235.

Genital warts: diagnosis, treatment, and counseling for the patient

JUDITH L. STEINBERG
LAURENCE J. CIBLEY
PETER A. RICE

Infection with human papillomavirus (HPV), the etiologic agent of genital warts, has increased ten-fold in prevalence in the United States over the last 15 years, making condyloma acuminata the most commonly diagnosed sexually transmitted disease in the United States (1). The last decade has seen a marked increase in our understanding of HPV infection. With the application of techniques of molecular biology to the study of HPV, over 60 genotypes of the virus have been identified. Detection of HPV DNA in tissue has shown that infection with this agent is frequently subclinical or latent, thereby emphasizing the inadequacies of current diagnostic modalities. Moreover, a link between HPV infection and the development of anogenital carcinoma has been demonstrated. Once simply a cosmetic problem, the scope and implications of HPV infection have been broadened, and the need for treatment and prevention have become more acute. The current management of HPV infection must be founded upon an understanding of the extent and limitations of diagnostic and treatment methods, the natural history and transmission of infection, and modes of prevention. The following chapter will focus on these issues and will present recommendations for management, given our current understanding of HPV infection.

VIROLOGY AND PATHOGENESIS

The human papillomavirus is a nonenveloped, double-stranded DNA virus that has an icosahedral capsid. The genome, composed of 7,900 base pairs, is divided into three domains, an early (E) region that encodes transformation, replication, and regulatory functions, a late (L) region, encoding the major and minor viral capsid proteins, and a long control region (LCR), which contains transcription regulatory sequences and the origin of replication (2). HPV is typed based on DNA homology; variants with less than 50% homology are classified as different genotypes. Presently, over 60 HPV genotypes have been identified, and at least 20 have been associated with genital warts, including

HPV 6, 11, 16, 18, 31, 33, 35, 39, 41 to 45, 51 to 56, and 59 (3). HPV 6 and 11 are the most common genotypes associated with anogenital infection.

Papillomaviruses (PV) are species specific and have tropisms both for certain cell types and for specific anatomic sites (2). HPV infects the basal layer of squamous or transitional cell epithelium. The virus gains entry, presumably as a result of trauma. Productive viral replication occurs only in fully differentiated superficial epithelial cells. However, HPV DNA may persist indefinitely in basal cells in a nonreplicating or latent state (4). This may account for the finding of HPV DNA in histologically normal-appearing tissue and recurrence of disease following presumably successful treatment (4, 5). Perhaps because terminally differentiated keratinocytes, the cell line used for tissue culture, are difficult to maintain, HPV has not been successfully cultivated in vitro.

The infected basal layers of epithelium are stimulated to grow as a result of HPV infection. Hyperplastic proliferation of the epidermis (termed acanthosis) occurs often in association with an increased superficial keratin layer (hyperkeratosis). Parakeratosis, the persistence of nuclei in the superficial layer, may also be present.

The host response to HPV infection is poorly understood, but an intact immune system is important in the control of this infection. Patients with immunological disorders, such as Wiskott-Aldrich syndrome, common variable immunodeficiency, human immunodeficiency virus (HIV) infection, lymphoproliferative diseases, and those receiving immunosuppressive therapy, such as renal allograft recipients, are subject to more frequent and severe HPV infection (6). Nevertheless, most patients with HPV infection do not exhibit any consistent identifiable immune defect (6).

HUMAN PAPILLOMAVIRUS INFECTION: DIAGNOSIS

The diagnosis of HPV infection includes inspection, visualization under magnification, and cytologic or histopathologic examination of the target tissues. DNA and immuno-histochemical detection methods may serve as adjunctive diagnostic modalities.

Clinical manifestations

The typical appearance of condyloma acuminata, one of the most commonly detected forms of HPV infection, is that of an exophytic lesion, a sessile, or a pedunculated tumor (Figure 5.1). Condylomata are often multiple and are located at areas of increased friction which in men most often include the glans penis, prepuce, coronal sulcus, urethral meatus of the penile shaft; and in women, the labia, vaginal introitus, and perianal area (4). Condylomata may occur internally in the vagina or on the cervix, but HPV infection is more commonly subclinical in these areas. Cervical condylomata appear as papillary epithelial elevations; underlying irregular vascular loops are often apparent (7). In the vagina, condylomata may appear as raised, small white elevations that are composed of small asperities or contain central capillary loops, or they may appear as raised, nonvascular, keratotic plaques (7). Condylomata may also be located at less frequently inspected sites such as the anal canal, the urethra, and, less commonly, the bladder.

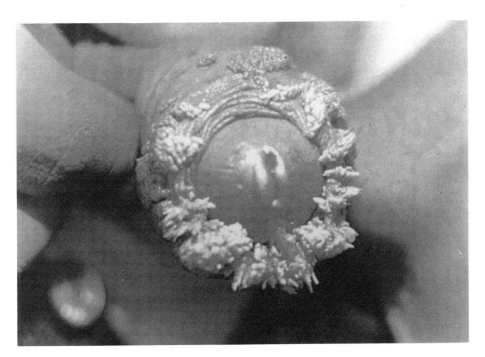

Figure 5.1 Extensive exophytic penile condylomata. (Reprinted by permission of David Oriel from: Oriel D. Genital human papillomavirus infection. In: Holmes KK, Mardh P, Sparling PF, Wiesner PJ, et al., eds. *Sexually Transmitted Diseases. Second ed.* New York: McGraw-Hill, 1990.)

Other clinically evident manifestations of HPV infection include papular warts, which are usually small, multiple, keratotic, and less papillary. These are often similar in appearance to verruca vulgaris and occur on nonmucosal areas such as the penile shaft in men or the labia majora and perineum in women. Bowenoid papulosis appears as multiple small papules or plaques which are sometimes pigmented. These are usually located on the glans penis, vaginal introitus, or labia (4). On histologic examination, these lesions may reveal intraepithelial neoplasia, termed "vulvar intraepithelial neoplasia" (VIN) in women, and may progress to advanced neoplasia. Lastly, the Buschke-Löwenstein tumor is a rare, giant condyloma that is locally invasive and destructive. Histologically, it appears benign; however, transformation into a metastasizing squamous cell carcinoma has been reported (8).

More commonly, HPV infection is subclinical. Detection of subclinical lesions may be accomplished by soaking the suspected area with 3% to 5% acetic acid for two to five minutes or longer (9), followed by examination either directly or under magnification, using a hand-held lens or colposcope. Subclinical lesions appear as flat or slightly raised, shiny, "aceto"-whitened areas (Figure 5.2a,b); intraepithelial neoplasia will often appear as dull gray or white. Under magnification, subclinical lesions may show varying degrees of vascular changes, such as punctation or mosaicism (Figure 5.3) (10).

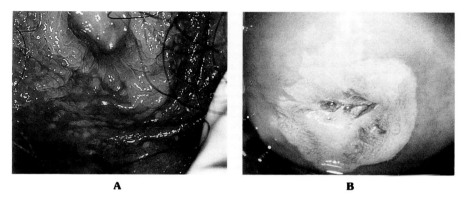

A   **B**

Figure 5.2   (a).   Whitening of vulva following acetic acid application. (b) Aceto-whitened area of the cervix, visualized with a colposcope, under a green filter. (Reprinted by permission of David Oriel from: Oriel D. Genital human papillomavirus infection. In: Holmes KK, Mardh P, Sparling PF, Wiesner PJ, et al., eds. *Sexually Transmitted Diseases. Second ed.* New York: McGraw-Hill, 1990.)

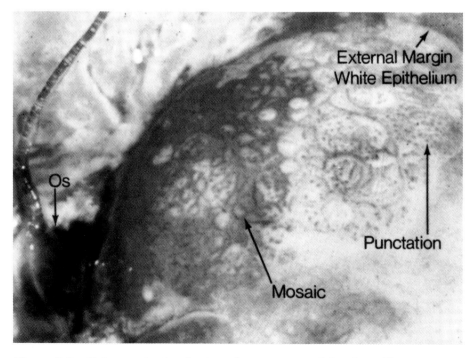

Figure 5.3   Colposcopic visualization of severe cervical dysplasia. Punctation, mosaicism, and white epithelium are apparent. (Reprinted by permission of David Oriel from: Oriel D. Genital human papillomavirus infection. In: Holmes KK, Mardh P, Sparling PF, Wiesner PJ, et al., eds. *Sexually Transmitted Diseases. Second ed.* New York: McGraw-Hill, 1990.)

Areas of "reversed punctation"—a mass of aceto-white flecks against a background of normal pink mucosa—may be seen in the vagina (7).

Colposcopy has traditionally been used in the evaluation of female patients; more recently, its use in male patients with condylomata or male contacts of women with condylomata has been advocated (11–13), but the hand-held lens remains more practical. In male contacts of women with condylomata, the use of colposcopy to guide biopsies has resulted in a three- to twelvefold increased level of detection of HPV infection, compared with diagnosis by the presence of grossly visible or exophytic lesions (11–13). Nevertheless, the use of colposcopy to closely examine aceto-whitened areas may sometimes overestimate the presence of HPV infection. Reports of histologic confirmation of colposcopically directed biopsy specimens have ranged from 53% to 88% in studies of patients with external genital warts or their sexual contacts (12–15). Operator skill is essential in the accurate use of the colposcope to prevent needless multiple biopsies, which may be unacceptable to patients.

A recent diagnostic technique for the detection of HPV-associated lesions of the cervix, including neoplasia, is cervicography. In this technique, acetic acid is applied to the cervix, and a photograph is taken which can be reviewed as a slide that, with projection on a screen, provides approximately ×16 magnification. If abnormalities are found, then colposcopy is performed. Sequential cervicography can be used to follow progression of abnormalities. Studies have shown that cervicography is more sensitive, but less specific, than cytologic screening (16,17). Another limitation is that cervicography can only detect lesions on the ectocervix.

Presently, the most widely available and preferred method for diagnosing HPV infection is detection of specific histopathologic or cytologic changes in tissue specimens (4). In addition, this is the only method that will determine the degree of epithelial abnormality. The classic cytologic finding is the koilocyte, a squamous cell with a hyperchromatic nucleus that is surrounded by a perinuclear clear zone. Koilocytes are present in the more superficial epithelial layers. Multinucleated cells may also be present; prominent acanthosis, papillomatosis, and elongated rete pegs present in histological specimens indicate HPV infection. (Chronic inflammatory changes in the submucosa may also be seen (Figure 5.4) (4).)

Determining the accuracy of cytologic screening and histopathology in detecting HPV infection has been difficult because an adequate gold standard is lacking. As newer DNA detection methods are utilized to diagnose HPV infection (see below), the sensitivities of cytology and histopathology have been called into question. Ten percent or more of tissue specimens from women with normal cervical Papanicolau (Pap) smears may contain HPV DNA (18). Variability in Pap smear detection rates may be due, at least in part, to the sampling method and pathologic criteria used. In one study of Pap-smear-negative women with external genital warts (19), HPV DNA was detected by in situ hybridization in 31% of cervical biopsy samples taken from these women, compared with 43% of biopsy specimens that were histologically typical of HPV infection. Using the combination of histology and DNA detection, 55% of this entire group of women had evidence of cervical HPV infection. In other studies (20–24), HPV DNA has been detected in up to 45% of cervical biopsy specimens that lacked the histological features of HPV infection. Because these studies often lack a gold standard

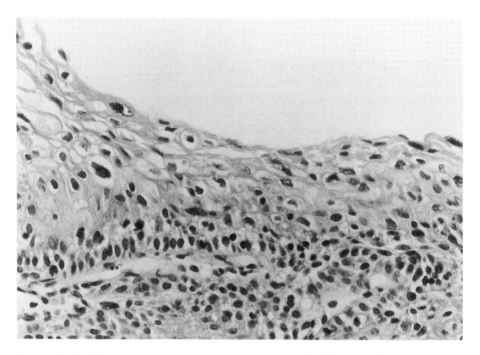

Figure 5.4 Condyloma of uterine cervix (flat lesion). There is mild thickening of the squamous epithelium (acanthosis). Most of the squamous cells in upper and middle thirds show koilocytosis. The koilocyte nuclei are enlarged compared with the normal basal cells, show considerable variation in size from one to another, and have variably irregular nuclear shapes, with prominent irregularity of the nuclear membrane. There is associated clearing of the cytoplasm around the nuclei (perinuclear halo). The submucosa shows associated chronic inflammation (lymphocytes and plasma cells). Hematoxylin and eosin, original magnification × 200. (Courtesy of J.C. O'Keane, M.D.)

with which to compare DNA detection methods, the immediate clinical significance of detecting viral DNA sequences in normal tissue is not clear.

Nucleic acid hybridization techniques are highly sensitive diagnostic methods that can be used in a type-specific manner. Approaches to DNA (or RNA) detection in tissue specimens or cell scrapings include Southern (or Northern) blot hybridization, dot blot techniques, in situ filter techniques, and in situ tissue hybridization. Estimates of sensitivity range from detection of 0.01 to 0.1 of a HPV genome copy per cell for Southern blot hybridization to one to 10 copies per cell for dot blot techniques (4). Although Southern blotting is the most sensitive and has served as the gold standard of hybridization techniques, it is least amenable to clinical use because it is slow and difficult to perform. Both the Southern and dot blot methods require extraction and separation of viral DNA from the specimen. Southern blotting requires an additional electrophoresis step. The in situ filter technique is the simplest method but can be applied only to the analysis of cell scrapings; its sensitivity is 0.1 genome copy per cell (4). In situ tissue hybridization, performed on fixed, paraffin-embedded specimens, offers correlation of viral detection with pathologic findings (Figure 5.5). Both the dot blot and tissue in situ hybridization techniques are commercially available.

The Southern blot method can detect HPV DNA in up to 90% of biopsy specimens that are histopathologically consistent with HPV infection and 70% to 95% of specimens that reveal cervical intraepithelial neoplasia (CIN) or invasive cervical carcinoma (4,25). In situ tissue hybridization techniques offer sensitivity that ranges from 40% to 90% (13, 25–27). Diminished sensitivity of DNA hybridization techniques in specimens that are histologically typical for HPV infection may result from: (a) sampling errors in biopsying and microscopic visualization of tissues; (b) infection by HPV genotypes not recognized by the DNA probes; (c) limitations in the sensitivities of the DNA probe assays; and/or (d) non-HPV related pathologic processes (4). The specificity of these procedures, compared to a gold standard of histopathology, is approximately

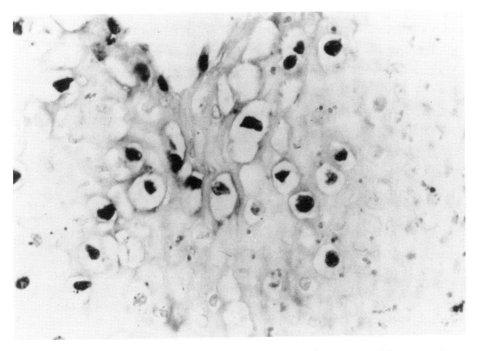

Figure 5.5   HPV 6 infection of a vulvar condyloma demonstrated by tissue in situ hybridization, using a biotinylated HPV 6 probe. The darkly staining nuclei of many koilocytic cells are positive for HPV 6. (Reprinted by permission of Attila T, Lorincz AT from: Lorincz AT. Human papillomavirus detection tests. In: Holmes KK, Mardh P, Sparling PF, Wiesner PJ, et al. *Sexually Transmitted Diseases. Second ed.* New York: McGraw-Hill, 1990.)

90%, according to one study (4,28). "False-positive" hybridization probe tests may result from insufficient stringency in carrying out the reactions; however, specific binding with HPV DNA in correctly performed tests represents latent infection in histologically normal tissues (4).

The polymerase chain reaction (PCR) technique has recently been applied to the diagnosis of HPV infection. It is at least 10^3 times more sensitive than other DNA hybridization techniques and is theoretically capable of detecting a single copy of HPV DNA in the entire sample of the specimen being tested (4). Using histopathology as a gold standard, PCR has a sensitivity of 90% to 100% (4,27,29). Although PCR is intrinsically highly specific, false positives may occur secondary to laboratory contamination or surface contamination of uninfected tissue following sexual contact (4). PCR is not yet commercially available.

Immunohistochemical techniques may also be applied to cytologic and tissue specimens. Detection of genus-specific antigen is accomplished using antisera raised to bovine papillomavirus structural proteins. The antiserum is coupled with horseradish peroxidase or biotin to allow for staining of specimens. Using this technique, detection rates range from 40% to 80% (29). Although specificity is excellent (4), higher-grade neoplastic lesions are less likely to yield positive results. Last, this technique is unable to distinguish between genotypes. Thus, although commercially available, immunohistochemistry does little to facilitate diagnosis.

More recently, investigation has centered around the development of genotype-specific monoclonal and polyclonal antisera that can be used to detect specific HPV types in tissue. Antisera are raised to bacterial/HPV fusion proteins that have been recovered using recombinant DNA techniques. Recent studies (30,31), however, have documented low detection rates with these methods.

Diagnostic recommendations

Patients with clinically evident condylomata, their sexual contacts, and patients at high risk for sexually transmitted diseases should be screened for the presence of HPV infection using acetic acid application. Ideally, examination should be performed under magnification. Exophytic warts and aceto-whitened areas can be treated, but atypical lesions that are pigmented, nonpapillary, and/or do not aceto-whiten should be biopsied. Biopsy is also recommended for aceto-whitened lesions that fail to respond to first-line treatment. Women with external genital warts or contacts thereof should have a Pap smear. Colposcopy is indicated for women with vulvar warts or those with atypical cervical cytology. Women at high risk for sexually transmitted diseases (STDs) should receive yearly Pap smears. Patients with condylomata located at the urethral meatus or perianal area should receive urethroscopic or proctoscopic examination, respectively. A diagnostic algorithm is provided in Figure 5.6.

Does the increased rate of detection of HPV infection and the ability to identify high- versus low-risk genotypes (see below) afforded by DNA hybridization techniques justify their use in a diagnostic schema? Until the natural history of subclinical and latent infection is known, routine use of these techniques cannot be recommended.

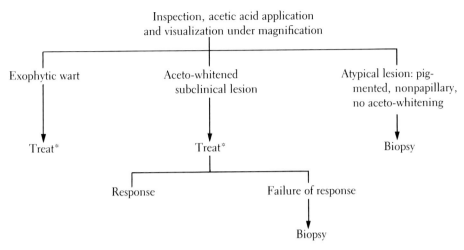

Figure 5.6   Diagnostic algorithm for patients with external anogenital warts and their contacts.

HUMAN PAPILLOMAVIRUS INFECTION: TREATMENT

Treatment of human papillomavirus infection is undertaken for cosmetic reasons, symptomatic improvement, reduction of viral transmission, and to prevent the development of neoplasia. Currently, there are no data to prove that treatment affects either transmission or the natural history of HPV infection. Treatment modalities are, for the most part, directed at macroscopically visible genital warts or areas of the epithelium in which HPV infection is detected histologically. Currently available therapeutic regimens do not eliminate the virus from the host. In addition, even if subclinical or latent infection were to be detected, management would be limited by the destructive nature of most treatment modalities; widespread destructive treatment of overtly normal-appearing tissue is unreasonable. Lastly, as with diagnostic approaches, the clinical study of the treatment of HPV infection has been hampered by a lack of knowledge of the natural history of the infection (2). Table 5.1 lists the currently available therapeutic regimens for HPV infection.

Cytotoxic agents

Podophyllin resin, an antimitotic agent, has been used as a first-line therapy for many years because of its convenience and low cost. A 10% to 25% solution of podophyllin in alcohol or tincture of benzoin is applied directly onto externally located genital warts and washed off after four to six hours. Within a few hours of application, the lesions blanch; sloughing occurs within two to four days (32). Repeated applications may be performed once or twice a week for approximately one month. Apparent cure rates with podophyllin

Table 5.1   HPV infection
treatment modalities

Cytotoxic agents
Podophyllin resin
Podophyllotoxin (Podofilox)
5-Fluorouracil

Ablative therapy
Biochloroacetic acid
Trichloroacetic acid
Cryotherapy
Surgical excision
Electrocautery
Electrodesiccation
Carbon dioxide laser therapy
Loop electro excisional procedure (LEEP)

Interferon
Intralesional interferon
Systemic interferon

---

are variable and have ranged in clinical trials from 22% to 90% (33–40), but recurrence rates are high, ranging from 11% to 74% (33–39). Podophyllin has disadvantages which include its variable potency and stability and lack of efficacy in the management of highly keratinized, old, or large warts (32). In addition, podophyllin may cause local toxicity, for example, erythema and tenderness, itching, burning and swelling; occasionally, superficial erosions (41), infection, and an allergic contact dermatitis (42) may occur. Podophyllin is systemically absorbed and, when used in large volumes, has resulted in toxicity, including neuropathy, hepatotoxicity, granulocytopenia, thrombocytopenia, coma, and occasionally death (43,44). Therefore, it is recommended that no more than 0.5 mL of 25% podophyllin be administered at each treatment session. Podophyllin is contraindicated during pregnancy where its use has resulted in fetal demise (45) and teratogenicity (46). In addition, podophyllin has been noted to have an oncogenic potential (47,48). Last, podophyllin should not be used in the treatment of warts located internally, for example, on the cervix, vagina, or in the urethra.

Podophyllotoxin (Podofilox) is a purified preparation of the major biologically active lignin present in podophyllin resin. Because of the purity and lower concentration of active drug, local adverse effects are reduced, and systemic absorption and toxicity are negligible. This preparation has been approved for patient self-application and provides a more convenient method of therapy. Podofilox is applied to warts twice a day for three days, followed by a four-day rest period. This treatment cycle may be repeated for two to four weeks. Clinical trials of podophyllotoxin (0.5% solution) have demonstrated complete response rates ranging from 45% to 100% and recurrence rates of 21% to 40% (37,49–51). Podophyllotoxin is contraindicated in pregnancy.

5-Fluorouracil (5-FU), an antimetabolite, has been used as a topical agent for treatment of both external and internal genital warts, including urethral condylomata.

Although open studies have revealed complete response rates of up to 95% (41), local side effects, including meatitis, vaginal discharge, vulvitis, and ulcerative balanitis, often make its use unacceptable. 5-FU has not been approved for treatment of genital warts in the United States.

Ablative therapy

Ablative methods of therapy include topical application of bi- or trichloroacetic acid (TCA) cryotherapy, surgical excision, electrocautery/electrodesiccation, carbon dioxide laser therapy, and the loop electro excisional procedure (LEEP). Bi- or tricholoracetic acids are caustic agents that, upon application, result in tissue destruction. A 50% to 85% solution is applied to the wart, with care taken to avoid normal tissue. Treatment is repeated on a weekly or biweekly basis but is unlikely to be successful if there is no response by three weeks (52). In contrast to podophyllin, TCA does not need to be washed off. Clinical trial data are limited, but, in one study, trichloracetic acid proved comparable to cryotherapy in efficacy, recurrence rates, and adverse effects (53). Adverse effects are local pain and irritation; some patients complain of an intense, albeit temporary, stinging sensation upon application. TCA may be advantageous because it can be used for pregnant women and in the treatment of vaginal or cervical warts.

The Centers for Disease Control (CDC) currently recommend cryotherapy as first-line management for anogenital condylomata, including vaginal, urethral meatal, and anal warts (54). Nitrous oxide or carbon dioxide, applied with a cryoprobe apparatus, has equal efficacy and is useful in the treatment of cervical intraepithelial neoplasia and cervical condylomata. Liquid nitrogen can be applied as a spray or swabbed onto the lesion, usually on a weekly basis. Each individual lesion is frozen down to its base, while also destroying a small area of the adjacent epithelium (32). However, unlike laser therapy (see below), the depth of destruction of tissue cannot be controlled, and cervical lesions extending into the endocervical canal cannot be reached. Clinical trials have revealed complete response rates for cryotherapy of 63% to 88%, with recurrence rates of 21% to 39% (5,34,36,53,55–57). Electrocautery, electrodesiccation, or surgical excision of warts is expensive and requires local anesthesia, operator skill, and longer healing periods. These methods eradicate the lesions 90% of the time, but recurrence rates range from 22% to 29% (35,36). In a randomized clinical trial, electrodesiccation was significantly more efficacious than cryotherapy or podophyllin in the treatment of external genital warts (36). Recurrence rates were similar for all three treatment modalities.

Carbon dioxide (CO_2) laser vaporization is used to treat warts that are refractory to other treatments or warts that are located internally in the anogenital area. Laser vaporization has also been used for the treatment of extensive disease because it provides precise definition of the treatment area and results in minimal damage to adjacent tissues (58–60). Clinical trials of CO_2 laser therapy in the treatment of genital warts have, for the most part, been conducted as open studies. Complete response rates following one treatment session have ranged from 27% to 94% with recurrence rates of 3% to 95% (5,58,61–67). However, there are disadvantages of CO_2 laser therapy; these include: (a) the need for operator experience, (b) healing times that are approximately three to six weeks in duration, (c) the need for local or general anesthesia, depending on wart size,

(d) resultant scarring, occurring in up to 28% of laser treatments (65), (e) expense, and (f) rare infectious complications (66). In addition, there are reports that suggest a potential for viral transmission during vaporization because of dispersion of HPV (68,69). Vaginal and vulvar adenosis following laser therapy has also been reported (70).

A newer ablative method, currently applied to the treatment of cervical lesions, is the loop electro excisional procedure. This consists of thin wire loops of various sizes coupled to an electrosurgical generator, which can be adjusted to employ a blend of cutting and coagulation current. The advantage of this procedure is that, when used with a colposcope, a cervical abnormality can be detected and treated at the same time (71). Intracervical local anesthesia is required.

Interferon therapy

Interferon may be administered topically, intralesionally, or systemically for the treatment of genital warts. Only intralesional interferon alpha has been approved for use with a recommended dose of 10^6 U injected/lesion (up to 5×10^6 U/treatment session) three times per week for three weeks. Topical interferon was proven ineffective in recent placebo-controlled trials (72–74) and thus is not recommended.

Randomized placebo-controlled trials have shown that intralesional interferon alpha is significantly more effective than placebo in the treatment of (refractory or recurrent) genital warts (Table 5.2). Complete response rates for interferon have ranged from 19% to 66% with recurrence rates of 0 to 33% (75–80). In one study (76), there was no significant difference in efficacy between three different recombinant interferon preparations: alpha 2b, alpha n1, and beta, administered in the same dosing regimen. One study found an increased response with 10^6 versus 10^5 U interferon alpha per injection (78).

Systemic interferon, administered subcutaneously or intramuscularly, has shown variable efficacy in the treatment of recurrent or refractory warts. Complete response rates for interferon alpha administered systemically and used in varying doses and regimens have ranged from 0% to 71% (81–86). However, two recent, large, randomized, placebo-controlled trials of interferon alpha (87,88) failed to show a significant difference in complete response rates of treated versus control groups. The only randomized, controlled study of systemic interferon beta (89) documented complete response rates of 82% (9/11) and 18% (2/11) for treated and control groups, respectively. Relapse rates among complete responders ranged from 0% to 23% in these studies.

In summary, intralesional interferon has efficacy in the treatment of recurrent or refractory genital warts. However, recurrence rates are high. The optimal dosing regimen and duration of treatment are not known. The efficacy of systemic interferon in the treatment of refractory or recurrent genital warts is questionable. Further studies may be required to determine if alterations in dosing regimens and treatment duration might improve efficacy rates. Problems with the use of interferon include: (a) expense, (b) difficulty of administration, and (c) frequent adverse effects, such as influenzalike symptoms, and reversible laboratory abnormalities, including leukopenia, thrombocytopenia, and abnormal liver and renal function tests. Similar to other therapeutic regimens, interferon does not eradicate the virus, even in patients who experience a complete remission (87,90).

Table 5.2 Randomized, controlled clinical trials of intralesional interferon

Reference	Type of interferon (IFN)	Regimen	Clearance*		Recurrence†
75	α-Recombinant (Schering)	Up to five warts injected with 10^6 U/lesion 3×/wk for 3 wks	IFN Placebo	7/16 (44) 3/21 (14)	0/7 0/3
76	a. α-Recombinant (Schering) b. α-Lymphoblastoid (Burroughs-Wellcome) c. β-Human fibroblast (Roswell Park, Buffalo, N.Y.)	One wart injected with 10^6 U 3×/wk for 4 wks	IFN Placebo	27/57 (47) 4/18 (22)	9/27 (33) 0/4 (0)
77	α-Human leukocyte (Ultrapure)	All warts injected with 2.5 to 5 × 10^5 U/mm^2 2×/wk for 8 wks (<8 wks if wart already cleared); maximal interferon/session, 2.5 × 10^6 U	IFN Placebo	41/66 (62) 14/66 (21)	9/36 (25) 3/13 (23)
78	α-Recombinant (Intron-A; Schering, Kenilworth, NJ)	One wart injected with 10^5 or 10^6 U 3×/wk for 3 wks	IFN (10^6 U) IFN (10^5 U) Placebo	16/30 (53) 6/32 (19) 4/29 (14)	— —
79	α-Recombinant (Intron-A)	One to three warts injected with 10^6 U 3×/wk for 3 wks	IFN Placebo	45/125 (36) 22/132 (17)	5/24 (21) —

80	α-Recombinant (Intron-A)	One to three warts injected with 10^6 U 3×/wk for 3 wks	IFN
			  HIV−
			  HIV+
			Placebo
			  HIV−
			  HIV+
				
				11/21 (52)
				0/8 (0)
				
				6/19 (32)
				1/5 (20)
					—
					—
					
					—
					—

*Results are expressed as number with complete clearance on gross examination/number treated (percentage with complete clearance).

†Results are expressed as number with recurrence evident on gross examination/number with complete clearance after treatment (percentage with recurrence).

SOURCE Reprinted with modification from Kraus SJ, Stone KM. Management of genital infection caused by human papillomavirus. *Rev Infec Dis* 1990;12 (Suppl 6): S620–S632.

Combination therapy

Combinations of treatment have been attempted to improve efficacy and diminish recurrence rates with variable results. Adjuvant 5-FU therapy following laser vaporization of subclinical warts in men failed to improve recurrence rates in one randomized trial (91), but, in a second open study (92), recurrence rates were low (6%) with this combination. The addition of systemic interferon therapy following laser vaporization significantly improved the complete response rate in another study (93). In a retrospective study, a reduced recurrence rate among patients treated with a combination of laser therapy and intralesional interferon was found, as compared with laser therapy alone (94). The addition of systemic interferon to podophyllin therapy has produced inconsistent results (85,95). There was neither improvement in complete response rates nor decrease in recurrence rates with the addition of systemic interferon to cryotherapy (96).

In summary and unfortunately, an ideal treatment for HPV is not currently available. Current treatment modalities are destructive in nature, produce local discomfort, and sometimes have systemic toxicity. Often, weekly visits to a physician are required, making management inconvenient. In addition, recurrence rates are high with all treatment modalities. The cost of therapy varies by the method used; intralesional interferon and laser therapy are the most expensive. There are numerous ways of managing the treatment of genital warts; one algorithm for the management of external anogenital warts is provided in Figure 5.7.

Vaginal warts are best managed with laser therapy. An algorithm for the management of cervical HPV-related infection is provided in Figure 5.8. Of note, there is

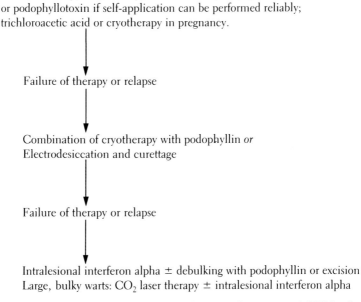

First-line therapy: Cryotherapy. Alternatives: podophyllin if mucosal lesions or podophyllotoxin if self-application can be performed reliably; trichloroacetic acid or cryotherapy in pregnancy.

Failure of therapy or relapse

Combination of cryotherapy with podophyllin *or* Electrodesiccation and curettage

Failure of therapy or relapse

Intralesional interferon alpha ± debulking with podophyllin or excision
Large, bulky warts: CO_2 laser therapy ± intralesional interferon alpha

Figure 5.7   Algorithm for the treatment of external anogenital HPV infection.

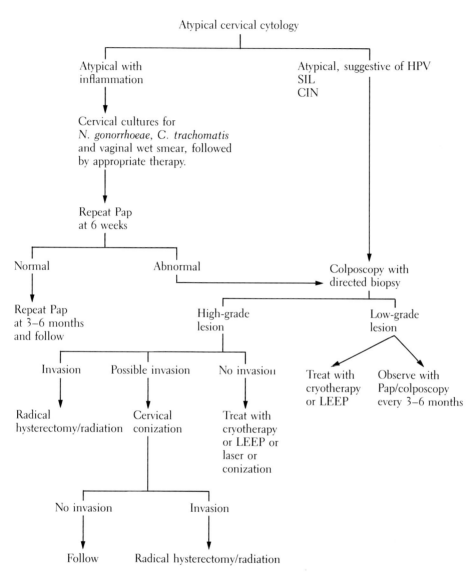

Figure 5.8   Algorithm for the management of HPV-related cervical infection/ atypical cervical cytology. SIL: Squamous intraepithelial lesion, Bethesda system for reporting cervical/vaginal cytologies (97). SIL, low grade, corresponds to HPV infection or CIN 1. SIL, high grade, corresponds to CIN 2 or CIN 3, i.e., moderate or severe dysplasia or carcinoma in situ.

controversy regarding the management of low-grade cervical HPV-related lesions. Some experts favor immediate treatment after proper workup, while others suggest careful observation. Proponents of the former approach cite the: (a) high cure rate for low-grade HPV/CIN lesions, (b) alleviation of anxiety in patients who have abnormal Pap smears, (c) questionable sensitivity of Pap smears as a tool for following patients, (d) often unacceptably low rates of patient compliance with follow-up examinations, and (e) the fact that a small percentage of patients with low-risk lesions will progress to advanced disease. Advocates for observation point out that: (a) low-grade lesions are at low risk for malignant progression; (b) spontaneous regression rates favor initial observation; (c) a high proportion of patients with cervical lesions also have vulvar and vaginal lesions, making eradication extremely difficult; and (d) the cost of treatment is high.

RELATIONSHIP TO ANOGENITAL NEOPLASIA

The biologic evidence for a role of HPV in carcinogenesis is presented in Table 5.3 (98). In animals, papillomaviruses have been associated with tumor development (4,98). In humans, nongenital papillomavirus infection has been associated with the development of skin cancer in patients with epidermodysplasia verruciformis (4). Transfected HPV 16 or 18 DNA can immortalize human cell lines (107,108). In addition, in genital cancers, HPV DNA is integrated into the host cell genome and is transcriptionally active. In benign lesions, it is generally located episomally (3,102,109–111). Integration of HPV DNA may occur near cellular proto-oncogenes, such as c-*myc* (112), and its integration in the HPV genome may result in deregulated expression of the viral E6 and E7 transforming genes (103,104,113–115). These transforming genes have been shown to bind retinoblastoma anti-oncogene product and the p53 tumor-suppressing gene product (105,106). It is believed that, as a result of this binding, the retinoblastoma anti-oncogene product is inactivated, and p53 undergoes rapid degradation (116).

With the application of PCR to HPV diagnostics, HPV DNA has been found in nearly all cervical tumor specimens (98,117). Using the various DNA hybridization

Table 5.3 Biological evidence in support of a carcinogenic role for HPVs

Nature of evidence	*Reference*
PVs associated with tumors in other species	99
HPV found in early and advanced lesions of the same tumor	100
Transcriptionally active viral genome frequently found in tumors	101
Viral DNA integrated in invasive tumors and episomal in premalignant lesions	102
Malignant transformation upon transfection of viral DNA into cultured cells	103
Cooperation between HPV and oncogenes in transformation	104
HPV E7 protein binds to the retinoblastoma anti-oncogene product	105
HPV E6 protein binds to the p53 tumor-suppressing gene product	106

SOURCE Reprinted by permission of University of Chicago Press from: Franco E.L. Viral etiology of cervical cancer: A critique of the evidence. University of Chicago Press, 1991 (98).

techniques, HPV DNA may be detected in 15% to 92% of cervical cancers (118). HPV DNA has also been detected in metastatic lesions from disseminated cervical cancer, in a majority of neoplastic lesions of the vulva and penis (4), and in neoplastic lesions of the anus (119–121). The most common genotypes associated with neoplasia are 16 and 18; less common types are 31, 33, and 35. Although types 6 and 11 are the most common types to infect the anogenital region, they are usually found only in condylomata and CIN 1.

Epidemiologic studies support the idea that a sexually transmitted pathogen may be important in the pathogenesis of cervical carcinoma. A consistent epidemiologic finding has been the association of enhanced risk of cervical cancer with sexual behavior, specifically, age at first intercourse and lifetime number of sexual partners (98). Associations have also been made between the risk for cervical cancer and the sexual behavior of partners (122,123), including an association of cervical and penile carcinoma in partners (98,124–127).

Although HPV DNA is detected in anogenital tumors, certain epidemiologic data suggest that HPV infection alone is not sufficient to result in carcinoma (98). Supporting evidence include the following: (a) PCR may detect high rates of cervical infection with HPV types 16 or 18 in women with no cervical cytologic abnormalities (up to 70%) (98); (b) despite increasing overall rates of HPV infection, mortality and morbidity rates due to in situ and invasive cervical cancer have steadily declined (98). Furthermore, some studies have failed to document a parallel between rates of HPV infection and an increased risk of cervical cancer in specific geographic areas (128,129). Finally, a case control study (130) has found sexual behavior to be an independent risk factor for cervical cancer, even after adjustment for HPV infection.

These findings and the observation that most patients infected with a high-risk HPV type do not develop cancer suggest the importance of additional cofactors for the development of carcinoma in HPV-infected patients. Suggested possible cofactors have included other infections, smoking, oral contraceptive use, dietary deficiency, immunodeficiency (3,98), and sex steroid receptivity (131,132).

Several prospective studies of women with cervical HPV infection have documented progression to CIN in (on average) 11%, with follow-up periods varying from 12 months to six years (133–136). However, another study noted progression to CIN over an average of 11 months (range four to 20 months) in 37% of women with cervical HPV infection (137). Progression rates from CIN 1 to CIN 3 over a maximum 30-month follow-up period were noted to vary by genotype in another study with rates of 56% and 20% for HPV 16 and HPV 6-associated lesions, respectively (138). Of note, rates of spontaneous regression of lesions are also variable, occurring in 7% to 47% (136–138), and may also be related to genotype (138).

Interpretation of the results of these studies are limited for several reasons (3). First, given the multicentric nature of HPV infection, it is possible that initial tissue biopsy specimens may fail to represent the most advanced lesion present. Second, the initial and follow-up biopsies may alter the natural history of the infection. Studies that use only cytologic examination often suffer from a lack of precision of a cytologic diagnosis of CIN and from the potential lack of detection of a more advanced, underlying histologic abnormality. Therefore, actual progression rates are uncertain.

TRANSMISSION

The transmission of HPV has been evaluated by studying the prevalence of clinical and subclinical HPV infection in partners of individuals with HPV-related lesions. Thus, actual transmission rates are not known. The prevalence rates vary by the detection methods used: for example, whether acetic acid application followed by examination under magnification was performed and if DNA hybridization techniques were used. Also, prevalence rates may be influenced by the type of HPV infection in the index case (subclinical versus clinical) and the genotype of the infecting virus. According to several studies, the prevalence of HPV-related lesions, including subclinical disease, in male partners of women with cervical HPV infection, range from 53% to 88% (12–14,124,139). Male partners of women with flat cervical condylomata versus CIN have a prevalence of 41% and 5%, respectively, of HPV-related lesions (124). In this study, a correlation between the presence of CIN in women and penile intraepithelial neoplasia (PIN) was also documented in the male partners.

HPV infection can be vertically transmitted, presumably from contact with vaginal secretions during delivery. Cases of HPV transmission following cesarean delivery (140) and the finding of HPV DNA in amniotic fluid (141) suggest the possibility of in utero transmission. The risk of transmission to the fetus is thought to be low, but actual rates are not known. Juvenile laryngeal papillomatosis (JLP) and/or external anogenital and conjunctival warts may occur as a result of HPV transmission during pregnancy. The risk of JLP has been estimated to be 1/1,500 pregnancies with genital condylomata (141) or lower (142). HPV DNA has been detected in the nasopharyngeal aspirate of 48% (11/23) of neonates born to mothers with evidence of cervical HPV infection (143), but this may result from contamination rather than from infection. Because of the low risk of transmission, elective cesarean section is not indicated for pregnant women with anogenital warts. However, cesarean section is the favored route of delivery if large, bulky warts present a mechanical obstruction to vaginal delivery.

PREVENTION

Sex partners should be referred for examination and treatment of warts. Treatment failure may result from latent infection, but reinfection may also occur from continued sexual contact with infected partners. Patients with genital warts should be counseled regarding the sexually transmitted nature of this infection. Although there are no clinical trials to support the use of condoms and/or nonoxynol 9 in the prevention of HPV transmission, use of these agents, particularly in combination, is advocated (144). Patients who are receiving treatment for genital warts should abstain from sex until the lesions resolve. Condoms should be used thereafter with uninfected partners, i.e., new or recent partners, to prevent transmission to or from the penis. However, condoms are unlikely to be of benefit for partners in a long-term monogamous relationship because of the high likelihood that both are infected.

ACKNOWLEDGMENT

We gratefully acknowledge the expert guidance given by Elliot J. Androphy, M.D., Amal K. Kurban, M.D., and J.C. O'Keane, M.D. in preparing this chapter. We also thank Dipanita Gupta, B.S., for her excellent technical assistance.

REFERENCES

1 **Hatch KD.** Vulvovaginal human papilloma-virus infections: Clinical implications and management. *Am J Obstet Gynecol* 1991;165:183–188.

2 **Reichman RC, Strike DG.** Pathogenesis and treatment of human genital papillomavirus infections: a review. *Antiviral Research* 1989;11:109–118.

3 **Koutsky LA, Wolner-Hanssen P.** Genital papil-lomavirus infections: Current knowledge and future prospects. *Obstetrics and Gynecology Clinics of North America* 1989;16(3):541–563.

4 **Douglas JM Jr, Werness BA.** Genital human papillomavirus infections. *Clinics in Labora-tory Medicine* 1989;9(3):421–444.

5 **Ferencxy A, Mitao M, Nagai N, Silverstein SJ, Crum CP.** Latent papillomavirus and recur-ring genital warts. *N Engl J Med* 1985;313:784–788.

6 **Reichman RC, Bonnez W.** Papillomaviruses. In: Mandell GL, Douglas RG Jr, Bennett JE, eds. *Principles and Practice of Infectious Dis-eases. Third ed.* New York: Churchill Living-stone Inc, 1990;1191–1200.

7 **Campion MJ.** Clinical manifestations and natural history of genital human papilloma-virus infection. *Dermatologic Clinics* 1991;9(2):235–249.

8 **Oriel D.** Genital human papillomavirus infec-tion. In: Holmes KK, Mardh P, Sparling PF, Wiesner PJ, et al., eds. *Sexually Transmitted Diseases. Second ed.* New York: McGraw-Hill Inc, 1990:433–441.

9 **Larsen J, Petersen CS, Weismann K.** Pro-longed application of acetic acid for detection of flat vulval warts. *Danish Med Bull* 1990;37:286–287.

10 **Coppleson M.** Colposcopic features of papillo-maviral infection and premalignancy in the female lower genital tract. *Dermatologic Clin-ics* 1991;9(2):251–266.

11 **Comite SL, Castadot MJ.** Colposcopic evalua-tion of men with genital warts. *J Am Acad Dermatol* 1988;18:1274–1278.

12 **Sedlacek TV, Cunnane M, Carpiniello V.** Colposcopy in the diagnosis of penile condy-loma. *Am J Obstet Gynecol* 1986;154:494–496.

13 **Hippelainen M, Yliskoski M, Saarikoski S, Syrjanen S, Syrjanen K.** Genital human papillo-mavirus lesions of the male sexual partners: the diagnostic accuracy of peniscopy. *Genitourin Med* 1991;67:291–296.

14 **Schultz RE, Skelton HG.** Value of acetic acid screening for flat genital condylomata in men. *J of Urol* 1988;139:777–779.

15 **Sonnex C, Scholefield JH, Kocjan G, et al.** Anal human papillomavirus infection: a com-parative study of cytology, colposcopy and DNA hybridisation as methods of detection. *Genitourin Med* 1991;67:21–25.

16 **Tawa K, Forsythe A, Cove JK, Saltz A, Peters HW, Watring WG.** Comparison of Papani-colaou-smear and the cervigram: Sensitivity, specificity and cost analysis. *Obstet Gynecol* 1988;71:229–235.

17 **Gunderson J, Schauberger C, Rowe N.** The Papanicolaou smear and the cervicogram: A pre-liminary report. *J Reprod Med* 1988;33:46–48.

18 **Lorincz AT.** Human papillomavirus detection tests. In: Holmes KK, Mardh P, Sparling PF, Wiesner PJ, et al, eds. *Sexually Transmitted Diseases. Second ed.* New York: McGraw-Hill, Inc, 1990:953–959.

19 **Petersen CS, Lindeberg H, Thomsen HK.** Human papillomavirus types in cervical biopsy specimens from Pap-smear-negative women with external genital warts. *Acta Obstet Gynecol Scand* 1991;70:69–71.

20 **Nuovo GJ.** Human papillomavirus DNA in genital tract lesions histologically negative for condylomata. Analysis by *in situ*, Southern blot hybridization and the polymerase chain reaction. *Am J Surg Path* 1990;14(7):643–651.

21 **Lorincz AT, Temple GF, Kurman RJ, Jenson AB, Lancaster WD.** Oncogenic association of specific human papillomavirus types with cervi-cal neoplasia. *J Natl Cancer Inst* 1987;79:671–677.

22 Nuovo GJ. Correlation of histology with human papillomavirus DNA detection in the female genital tract. *Gynecol Oncol* 1988;31:176–181.

23 Nuovo GJ, O'Connell M, Blanco JB, Levine RU, Silverstein SJ. Correlation of histology and human papillomavirus DNA detection in condyloma acuminatum and condyloma-like vulvar lesions. *Am J Surg Pathol* 1989;13:700–706.

24 Reid R, Greenberg M, Jenson AB, et al. Sexually transmitted papillomaviral infections I. The anatomic distribution and pathologic grade of neoplastic lesions associated with different viral types. *Am J Obstet Gynecol* 1987;156:212–222.

25 Garuti G, Boselli F, Genazzani AR, Silvestri S, Ratti G. Detection and typing of human papillomavirus in histologic specimens by *in situ* hybridization with biotinylated DNA probes. *Am J Clin Pathol* 1989;92:604–612.

26 Meyer MP, Markiw CA, Matuscak RR, Saker A, McIntyre-Seltman K, Amortegui AJ. Detection of human papillomavirus DNA in genital lesions by using a modified commercially available *in situ* hybridization assay. *J Clin Micro* 1991;29(7):1308–1311.

27 Skyldberg B, Kalantari M, Karki M, Johansson B, Hagmar B, Walaas L. Detection of human papillomavirus infection in tissue blocks by *in situ* hybridization as compared with a polymerase chain reaction procedure. *Hum Pathol* 1991;22:578–582.

28 Caussy D, Orr W, Daya AD, Roth P, Reeves W, Rawls W. Evaluation of methods for detecting human papillomavirus deoxyribonucleotide sequences in clinical specimens. *J Clin Micro* 1988;26:236–243.

29 Schadendorf D, Tiedemann KH, Haas N, Czarnetzki BM. Detection of human papillomaviruses in paraffin-embedded condylomata acuminata—Comparison of immunohistochemistry, in situ hybridization, and polymerase chain reaction. *J Invest Dermatol* 1991;97:549–554.

30 Brown DR, Bryan J, Rodriguez M, Rose RC, Strike DG. Detection of human papillomavirus types 6 and 11 E4 gene products in condylomata acuminatum. *J Med Vir* 1991;34:20–28.

31 Lacey CJN, Wells M, Macdermott RIJ, Gibson PE. Human papillomavirus type 16 infection of the cervix: a comparison of differing DNA detection modes and the use of monoclonal antibodies against the major capsid protein. *Genitourin Med* 1991;67:87–91.

32 Kaufman RH, Friedrich EG Jr., Gardner HL. *Benign Diseases of the Vulva and the Vagina. Third ed.* London: Yearbook Press, 1989:106–158.

33 Simmons PD. Podophyllin 10% and 25% in the treatment of anogenital warts: a comparative double-blind study. *Br J Vener Dis* 1981;57:208–209.

34 Bashi SA. Cryotherapy versus podophyllin in the treatment of genital warts. *Int J Dermatol* 1985;24:535–536.

35 Jensen SL. Comparison of podophyllin application with simple surgical excision in clearance and recurrence of perianal condylomata acuminata. *Lancet* 1985;2:1146–1148.

36 Stone K, Becker T, Hadgu LA, Kraus S. Treatment of external genital warts: a randomized clinical trial comparing podophyllin, cryotherapy, and electrodesiccation. *Genitourin Med* 1990:66:16–19.

37 Lassus A, Haukka K, Forsstromm S. Podophyllotoxin for treatment of genital warts in males: a comparison with conventional podophyllin therapy. *European J Sex Trans Dis* 1984;2:31–33.

38 von Krogh G. Topical treatment of penile condylomata acuminata with podophyllin, podophyllotoxin and colchicine. *Act Derm Venereol (Stockh)* 1978;58:163–168.

39 Gabriel G, Thin RNT. Treatment of anogenital warts: comparison of trichloroacetic acid and podophyllin versus podophyllin alone. *Br J Vener Dis* 1983;59:124–126.

40 Khawaja HT. Treatment of condyloma acuminatum. *Lancet* 1986;1:208–209.

41 Kraus SJ, Stone KM. Management of genital infection caused by human papillomavirus. *Rev Infect Dis* 1990;12(Suppl 6):S620–S632.

42 Marcus J, Camisa C. Podophyllin therapy for condyloma acuminatum. *Int J Derm* 1990;29(10):693–698.

43 Slater GE, Rumack BH, Peterson RG. Podophyllin poisoning: Systemic toxicity following cutaneous application. *Obstet Gynecol* 1978;52:94–99.

44 Ward JW, Clifford WS, Monaco AR, Bickerstaff HJ. Fatal systemic poisoning following podophyllin treatment of condyloma acuminatum. *South Med J* 1954;47:1204–1206.

45 Chamberlain MJ, Reynolds AL, Yeoman WB. Toxic effect of podophyllin in pregnancy. *Br Med J* 1972;3:391–392.

46 Thiersch JB. Effect of podophyllin (P) and podophyllotoxine (PT) on the rat litter in utero. *Proc Soc Exp Biol Med* 1963;113:124–127.

47 Gueson ET, Liu CT, Emich JP Jr. Dysplasia following podophyllin treatment of vulvar condylomata acuminata. *J Reprod Med* 1971;6:159–161.

48 Kaminetzky HA, Swerdlow M. Podophyllin and the mouse cervix: Assessment of carcinogenic potential. *Am J Obstet Gynecol* 1965;93: 486–490.

49 Beutner KR, Conant MA, Friedman-Kien AE, et al. Patient-applied podofilox for treatment of genital warts. *Lancet* 1989;1:831–834.

50 Greenberg MD, Rutledge LH, Reid R, Berman NR, Precop SL, Elswick RK Jr. A double-blind, randomized trial of 0.5% podofilox and placebo for the treatment of genital warts in women. *Obstet Gynecol* 1991;77:735–739.

51 Baker DA, Douglas JM Jr, Buntin DM, Micha JP, Beutner KR, Patsner B. Topical podofilox for the treatment of condylomata acuminata in women. *Obstet Gynecol* 1990;76:656–659.

52 Friedrich EG Jr. *Vulvar Disease. Second ed.* Philadelphia: W.B. Saunders Co., 189–215.

53 Godley MJ, Bradbeer CS, Gellan M, Thin RNT. Cryotherapy compared with trichloroacetic acid in treating genital warts. *Genitourin Med* 1987;63:390–392.

54 Centers for Disease Control. STD treatment guidelines. *MMWR* 1989;38:18–21.

55 Balsdon MJ. Cryosurgery of genital warts. *Br J Vener Dis* 1978;54:352–353.

56 Ghosh AK. Cryosurgery of genital warts in cases in which podophyllin treatment failed or was contraindicated. *Br J Vener Dis* 1977;53:49–53.

57 Simmons PD, Langlet F, Thin RNT. Cryotherapy versus electrocautery in the treatment of genital warts. *Br J Vener Dis* 1981;57:273–274.

58 Reid R. Superficial laser vulvectomy. I. The efficacy of extended superficial ablation of refractory and very extensive condylomas. *Am J Obstet Gynecol* 1985;151:1047–1052.

59 Reid R, Elson L, Absten G. A practical guide to laser safety. *Colposcopy Gynecol Laser Surg* 1986;2:121–132.

60 Reid R. Physical and surgical principles governing expertise with carbon dioxide laser. *Obstet Gynecol Clin North Am* 1987;14:513–535.

61 Bellina JH. The use of the carbon dioxide laser in the management of condyloma acuminatum with eight-year follow-up. *Am J Obstet Gynecol* 1983;147:375–378.

62 Kryger-Baggesen N, Larsen JF, Pedersen PH. CO2-Laser treatment of condylomata acuminata. *Acta Obstet Gynecol Scand* 1984;63: 341–343.

63 Baggish MS. Improved laser techniques for the elimination of genital and extragenital warts. *Am J Obstet Gynecol* 1985;153:545–550.

64 Krebs H-B, Wheelock JB. The CO2 laser for recurrent and therapy-resistant condylomata acuminata. *J Reprod Med* 1985;30:489–492.

65 Duus BR, Philipsen T, Christensen JD, Lundvall F, Sondergaard J. Refractory condylomata acuminata: a controlled clinical trial of carbon dioxide laser versus conventional surgical treatment. *Genitourin Med* 1985;61:59–61.

66 Bar-Am A, Shilon M, Peyser MR, Ophir J, Brenner S. Treatment of male genital condylomatous lesions by carbon dioxide laser after failure of previous nonlaser methods. *J Am Acad Dermatol* 1991;24:87–89.

67 Larsen J, Petersen CS. The patient with refractory genital warts in the STD-clinic. Treatment failure with CO2-laser. *Dan Med Bull* 1990;37:194–195.

68 Andre P, Orth G, Evenou P, Guillaume JC, Avril MF. Risk of papillomavirus infection in carbon dioxide laser treatment of genital lesions. *J Am Acad Dermatol* 1990;22:131–132.

69 Ferenczy A, Bergeron C, Richart RM. Carbon dioxide laser energy disperses human papillomavirus deoxyribonucleic acid onto treatment fields. *Am J Obstet Gynecol* 1990;163: 1271–1274.

70 Sedlacek TV, Riva JM, Magen AB, Mangan CE, Cunnane MF. Vaginal and vulvar adenosis. An unsuspected side effect of CO2 laser vaporization. *J Repro Med* 1990;35:995–1001.

71 Wright T Jr., Gagnon S, Ferenczy A, Richart R. Excising CIN lesions by loop electrosurgical procedure. *Contemp Obstet Gynecol* 1991;36: 56–74.

72 Keay S, Teng N, Eisenberg M, Story B, Sellers PW, Merigan TC. Topical interferon for treating condyloma acuminata in women. *J Infect Dis* 1988;158:934–939.

73 Vesterinen E, Meyer B, Purola E, Cantell K. Treatment of vaginal flat condyloma with interferon cream. *Lancet* 1984;1:157.

74 Vesterinen E, Meyer B, Cantell K, Purola E. Topical treatment of flat vaginal condyloma with human leukocyte interferon. *Obstet Gynecol* 1984;64:535–538.

75 Welander CE, Homesley HD, Smiles KA, Peets EA. Intralesional interferon alfa-2b for the treatment of genital warts. *Am J Obstet Gynecol* 1990;162:348–354.

76 Reichman RC, Oakes D, Bonnez W, et al. Treatment of condyloma acuminatum with three different interferons administered intralesionally. *Ann Intern Med* 1988;108:675–679.

77 Friedman-Kien AE, Eron LJ, Conant M, et al. Natural interferon alfa for treatment of condylomata acuminata. *JAMA* 1988;259:533–538.

78 Vance JC, Bart BJ, Hansen RC, et al. Intralesional recombinant alpha-2 interferon for the treatment of patients with condyloma

acuminatum or verruca plantaris. *Arch Dermatol* 1986;122:272–277.

79 Eron LJ, Judson F, Tucker LS, et al. Interferon therapy for condylomata acuminata. *N Engl J Med* 1986;315:1059–1064.

80 Douglas JM Jr., Roger M, Judson FN. The effect of asymptomatic infection with HTLV-III on the response of anogenital warts to intralesional treatment with recombinant alpha 2 interferon. *J Infect Dis* 1986;154:331–334.

81 Gross G, Ikenberg H, Roussaki A, Drees N, Schopf E. Systemic treatment of condylomata acuminata with recombinant interferon-alpha-2-A: low-dose superior to the high dose regimen. *Chemotherapy* 1986;32:537–541.

82 Gross G, Ikenberg H, Roussaki A, Kunze B, Drees N. Does the papillomavirus DNA persist in the epithelium after successful treatment of genital warts with subcutaneous injections of recombinant interferon alpha [abstract]? *J Invest Dermatol* 1988;90:242.

83 Gall SA, Hughes CE, Trofatter K. Interferon for the therapy of condyloma acuminatum. *Am J Obstet Gynecol* 1985;153:157–163.

84 Gall SA, Hughes CE, Mounts P, Segriti A, Weck PK, Whisnant JK. Efficacy of human lymphoblastoid interferon in the therapy of resistant condyloma acuminata. *Obstet Gynecol* 1986;67:643–651.

85 Weck PK, Buddin DA, Whisnant JK. Interferons in the treatment of genital human papillomavirus infections. *Am J Med* 1988; 85(Suppl 2A):159–164.

86 Paavonen J. Subcutaneous interferon alpha in the treatment of refractory condylomata. *Sex Trans Dis* 1990 (17): 152–153.

87 Reichman RC, Oakes D, Bonnez W, et al. Treatment of condyloma acuminatum with three different interferon-alpha preparations administered parenterally: A double-blind, placebo-controlled trial. *J Infect Dis* 1990;162:1270–1276.

88 Condylomata International Collaborative Study Group. Recurrent condylomata acuminata treated with recombinant interferon alfa-2a. A multicenter double-blind placebo-controlled clinical trial. *JAMA* 1991;265:2684–2687.

89 Schonfeld A, Schattner A, Crespi M, et al. Intramuscular human interferon-beta injections in treatment of condylomata acuminata. *Lancet* 1984;1:1038–1042.

90 Macnab JCM, Walkinshaw SA, Cordiner JW, Clements JB. Human papillomavirus in clinically and histologically normal tissue of patients with genital cancer. *N Engl J Med* 1986;315:1052–1058.

91 Carpiniello VL, Malloy TR, Sedlacek TV, Zderic SA. Results of carbon dioxide laser therapy and topical 5-fluorouracil treatment for subclinical condyloma found by magnified penile surface scanning. *J Urol* 1988;140: 53–54.

92 Bergman A, Nalick R. Genital human papillomavirus infection in men. Diagnosis and treatment with a laser and 5-fluorouracil. *J Repro Med* 1991;36:363–366.

93 Petersen CS, Bjerring P, Larsen J, et al. Systemic interferon alpha-2b increases the cure rate in laser treated patients with multiple persistent genital warts: a placebo-controlled study. *Genitourin Med* 1991;67:99–102.

94 Vance JC, Davis D. Interferon alpha-2b injections used as an adjuvant therapy to carbon dioxide laser vaporization of recalcitrant ano-genital condylomata acuminata. *J Invest Dermatol* 1990;95:146S–148S.

95 Douglas JM, Eron LJ, Judson FN, et al. A randomized trial of combination therapy with intralesional interferon alpha 2b and podophyllin versus podophyllin alone for the therapy of anogenital warts. *J Infect Dis* 1990;162:52–59.

96 Handley JM, Horner T, Maw RD, Lawther H, Dinsmore WW. Subcutaneous interferon alpha 2a combined with cryotherapy vs cryotherapy alone in the treatment of primary anogenital warts: a randomised, observer-blind, placebo-controlled study. *Genitourin Med* 1991;67:297–302.

97 National Cancer Workshop. The 1988 Bethesda system for reporting cervical/vaginal cytologic diagnosis. *Acta Cytol* 1989;33: 567–574.

98 Franco EL. Viral etiology of cervical cancer: A critique of the evidence. *Rev Infect Dis* 1991;13:1195–1206.

99 Campo MLS, Moar MH, Jarrett WFH, Laird HM. A new papillomavirus associated with alimentary cancer in cattle. *Nature* 1980;286: 180–182.

100 Schneider A, Olterdorf T, Schneider V, Gissmann L. Distribution pattern of human papilloma virus 16 genome in cervical neoplasia by molecular *in situ* hybridization of tissue sections. *Int J Cancer* 1987;39:717–721.

101 Schwartz E, Freese UK, Gissmann L, et al. Structure and transcription of human papillomavirus sequences in cervical carcinoma cells. *Nature* 1985;314:111–114.

102 McCance DJ. Human papillomavirus (HPV) infections in the aetiology of cervical cancer. *Cancer Surv* 1988;7:499–506.

103 Bedell MA, Jones KH, Laimins LA. The E6-E7 region of human papillomavirus type 18 is

sufficient for transformation of NIH 3T3 and rat-1 cells. *J Virol* 1987;61:3635–3640.

104 Matlashewski G, Schneider J, Banks L, Jones N, Murray A, Crawford L. Human papillomavirus type 16 DNA cooperates with activated *ras* in transforming primary cells. *EMBO J* 1987;6:1741–1746.

105 Dyson N, Howley PM, Munger K, Harlow E. The human papilloma virus-16 E7 oncoprotein is able to bind to the retinoblastoma gene product. *Science* 1989;243:934–937.

106 Werness BA, Levine AJ, Howley PM. Association of human papillomavirus types 16 and 18 E6 proteins with p53. *Science* 1990; 248:76–79.

107 Durst M, Dzarlieva-Pertrusevzka P, Boukamp P, et al. Molecular and cytologic analysis of immortalized human primary keratinocytes obtained after transfection with human papilloma virus type 16 DNA. *Oncogene* 1987;1:251–256.

108 Kaur P, McDougall JK. Characterization of primary human keratinocytes transformed by human papillomavirus type 18. *J Virol* 1988; 62:1917–1924.

109 Lehn H, Villa LL, Mariziona F, Hilgarth M, Hillemans HG, Sauer G. Physical state and biological activity of human papillomavirus genomes in precancerous lesions of the female genital tract *J Gen Virol* 1988;69:187–196.

110 Yee C, Krishnan-Hewlett I, Baker CC, Schlegel R, Howley PM. Presence and expression of human papillomavirus sequence in human cervical carcinoma cell lines. *Am J Pathol* 1985;119:361–366.

111 Howley PM, Schlegel R. The human papillomaviruses. *Am J Med* 1988;85(Suppl2A): 155–158.

112 Durst M, Croce CM, Gissmann L, Schwarz E, Huebner K. Papillomavirus sequences integrate near cellular oncogenes in some cervical carcinomas. *Proc Natl Acad Sci USA* 1987;84:1070–1074.

113 Schneider-Gadicke A, Schwarz E. Different human cervical carcinoma cell lines show similar transcription patterns of human papillomavirus type 18 early genes. *EMBO J* 1986;5:2285–2292.

114 Smotkin D, Wettstein FO. Transcription of human papillomavirus type 16 early genes in a cervical cancer and a cancer-derived cell line and identification of the E7 protein. *Proc Natl Acad Sci USA* 1986;83:4680–4684.

115 Takebe N, Tsunokawa Y, Nozawa S, et al. Conservation of E6 and E7 regions of human papillomavirus types 16 and 18 present in

cervical cancers. *Biochem Biophys Res Commun* 1987;143:837–844.

116 Howley PM. Molecular mechanisms of human papillomavirus-associated carcinogenesis. Symposium: Sexually transmitted diseases, 31st Interscience Conference on Antimicrobial Agents and Chemotherapy, Chicago, IL, 1991.

117 Resnick RM, Cornelissen MT, Wright DK, et al. Detection and typing of human papillomavirus in archival cervical cancer specimens by DNA amplification with consensus primers. *J Natl Cancer Inst* 1990;82:1477–1484.

118 Munoz N, Bosch X, Kaldor JM. Does human papillomavirus cause cervical cancer? The state of epidemiological evidence. *Br J Cancer* 1988;57:1–5.

119 Taxy JB, Gupta PK, Gupta JW, Shah KV. Anal cancer. Microscopic condyloma and tissue demonstration of human papillomavirus capsid antigen and viral DNA. *Arch Pathol Lab Med* 1989;113:1127–1131.

120 Oriel JD. Human papillomaviruses and anal cancer. *Genitourin Med* 1989;65:213–215.

121 Duggan MA, Boras VF, Inoue M, McGregor SE, Robertson DI. Human papillomavirus DNA determination of anal condylomata, dysplasias, and squamous carcinomas with *in situ* hybridization. *Am J Clin Pathol* 1989;92: 16–21.

122 Buckley JD, Doll R, Harris RWC, Vessey MP, Williams PT. Case-control study of the husbands of women with dysplasia or carcinoma of the cervix uteri. *Lancet* 1981;2: 1010–1014.

123 Zunzunegui MV, King MC, Coria CF, Charlet J. Male influences on cervical cancer risk. *Am J Epidemiol* 1986;123:302–307.

124 Barrasso R, De Brux J, Croissant O, Orth G. High prevalence of papillomavirus-associated penile intraepithelial neoplasia in sexual partners of women with cervical intraepithelial neoplasia. *N Eng J Med* 1987;317: 916–923.

125 Martinez I. Relationship of squamous cell carcinoma of the cervix uteri to squamous cell carcinoma of the penis among Puerto Rican women married to men with penile carcinoma. *Cancer* 1969;24:777–780.

126 Graham S, Priore R, Graham M, Browne R, Burnett W, West D. Genital cancer in wives of penile cancer patients. *Cancer* 1979;44: 1870–1874.

127 Smith PG, Kinlen LJ, White GC, Adelstein AM, Fox AJ. Mortality of wives of men dying with cancer of the penis. *Br J Cancer* 1980;41:422–428.

128 Kjaer SK, DeVilliers E-M, Haugaard BJ, et al. Human papillomavirus, herpes simplex virus and cervical cancer incidence in Greenland and Denmark. A population-based cross-sectional study. *Int J Cancer* 1988;41: 518–524.

129 Acs J, Hildesheim A, Reeves WC, et al. Regional distribution of human papillomavirus DNA and other risk factors for invasive cervical cancer in Panama. *Cancer Res* 1989; 495:5725–5729.

130 Reeves WC, Brinton LA, Garcia M, et al. Human papillomavirus infection and cervical cancer in Latin America. *N Engl J Med* 1989;320:1437–1441.

131 Monsonego J, Magdelenat H, Catalan F, Coscas Y, Zerat L, Sastre X. Estrogen and progesterone receptors in cervical human papillomavirus related lesions. *Int J Cancer* 1991;48:533–539.

132 Konishi I, Fujii S, Nonogaki H, Nanbu Y, Iwai T, Mori T. Immunohistochemical analysis of estrogen receptors, progesterone receptors, Ki-67 antigen, and human papillomavirus DNA in normal and neoplastic epithelium of the uterine cervix. *Cancer* 1991;68:1340–1350.

133 Syrjanen IK, Mantyjarvi R, Vayrynan M, et al. Assessing the biological potential of human papillomavirus infections in cervical carcinogenesis. In: Steinberg BV, Brandsma JL, Taichman LB, eds. *Cancer Cells. 5. Papillomaviruses.* Cold Spring Harbor, NY: Cold Spring Harbor Laboratory, 1987: p 281.

134 de Brux J, Orth G, Croissant O, et al. Lesions condylomateuses du col uterin: Evolution chex 2,466 patientes. *Bull Cancer (Paris)* 1983;70:410–422.

135 Mitchell H, Drake M, Medley G. Prospective evaluation of risk of cervical cancer after cytological evidence of human papillomavirus infection. *Lancet* 1986;1:573–575.

136 Evans AS, Monaghan JM. Spontaneous resolution of cervical warty dysplasia: The relevance of clinical and nuclear DNA features: A prospective study. *Br J Obstet Gynaecol* 1985; 92:165–169.

137 Nash JD, Burke TW, Hoskins WJ. Biologic course of cervical human papillomavirus infection. *Obstet Gynecol* 1987;69:160–162.

138 Campion MJ, McCance DJ, Cuzick J, et al. Progressive potential of mild cervical atypia: prospective cytological, colposcopic, and virological study. *Lancet* 1986;2:237–240.

139 Levine RU, Crum CP, Herman E, Silvers D, Ferenczy A, Richart RM. Cervical papillomaviruses and intraepithelial neoplasia: a study of male sexual partners. *Obstet Gynecol* 1984;64: 16–20.

140 Holinger PH, Shield JA, Maurizi DG. Laryngeal papilloma: Review of etiology and therapy. *Laryngoscope* 1968;782:1462–1474.

141 Ferenczy A. HPV-associated lesions in pregnancy and their clinical implications. *Clin Obstet and Gynecol* 1989;32:191–199.

142 Patsner B, Baker DA, Orr JW Jr. Human papillomavirus genital tract infections during pregnancy. *Clin Obstet and Gynecol* 1990;33: 258–267.

143 Sedlacek TV, Lindheim S, Eder C, et al. Mechanism for human papillomavirus transmission at birth. *Am J Obstet Gynecol* 1989;161:55–59.

144 Eron LJ. Update: Prevention and therapy of genital warts. *Comprehen Ther* 1988;14:7–11.

Varicella in a susceptible pregnant woman

DENNIS A. CLEMENTS
SAMUEL L. KATZ

INTRODUCTION

Varicella epidemiology

Varicella is a disease of childhood. It is estimated that 90% to 95% (1,2) of the United States population has acquired the infection by 20 years of age. Morbidity and mortality from the disease are high in the first year of life and, after 20 years of age, primarily due to pneumonia. During the postinfant to adult years, the disease is characteristically mild, so much so that some parents purposefully expose their children to varicella-infected children "to get the disease over with."

Varicella in neonates, adults, and immunocompromised hosts, however, has much greater morbidity and mortality. Susceptible pregnant women, their fetuses, and newborn infants are special cases that will be examined in this chapter.

Brief clinical description

Varicella infection is usually manifested by a characteristic constellation of symptoms (3,4). There is a mild prodrome with flulike symptoms in adults (coryza and cough) or frequently no symptoms in children. Then there is the onset of a characteristic rash that begins centrally and spreads outwardly to the extremities. The rash consists of small red macules evolving to papules that then develop central clear vesicles. This typically occurs over a few days. Occasionally, there is only a minimal rash which remains unchanged, or, after a few days, it may spread over the body. The rash occurs most commonly in sun-exposed or traumatized areas where there is increased blood flow. The rash can be sparse or cover the entire body. The rash is customarily pruritic during the healing phase except in the youngest children. Secondary infection of the viral pustules, particularly with β-hemolytic group A *Streptococcus pyogenes* or *Staphylococcus aureus*, is common, particularly in children.

123

Complications: CDC data on rates, hospitalizations, deaths

There are an estimated 3.5 million cases of varicella each year in the United States, which is equivalent in size to the annual birth cohort (1). Children between the ages of one and 14 years account for 90% of cases, and only 2% of cases occur in adults. The incidence of varicella encephalitis is decreasing in children, but not in adults (1). There are approximately 75 deaths per year due to varicella, almost 50% of which occur in adults (>20 years of age). Additionally, adults have been found to be ten times more likely to be hospitalized and three to four times more likely to visit a physician than are children (2).

ASCERTAINMENT OF SUSCEPTIBILITY

History

A history of varicella is usually sufficient to document past disease. Unlike other exanthematous diseases, the rash of varicella is sufficiently characteristic that a history of disease is usually accurate. A negative history, however, is less likely to be so. Serologic surveys suggest that approximately 75% of people with a negative history of disease do in fact have varicella antibody (3). Adults with childhood histories of varicella in siblings and other family members are likely to be immune. It is not uncommon for one child to have undergone such mild disease that the lesions were unrecognized or dismissed as insect bites until two weeks later, when siblings developed typical varicella lesions (or vice versa). However, for patients with a negative history of varicella, serological tests are available to assess immunity (4,5).

Serology

Serologic tests to confirm varicella immunity include complement fixation (CF), radioimmunoassay (RIA), enzyme-linked immunosorbent assay (ELISA), and fluorescent antimembrane antibody assay (FAMA). Although the latter is the most sensitive of the tests, it is frequently unavailable. The ELISA test is becoming the most readily available serologic test, and a recent report confirms its high sensitivity and specificity (6). It is slightly less sensitive than FAMA so that a few patients classified as negative may actually have a small but detectable antibody level. It is, however, very specific and, most importantly, gives few, if any, false positives (7). RIA is less commonly available but has similar specificity and sensitivity to the ELISA assay. The CF test is unreliable and should not be used.

PATHOGENESIS

Respiratory spread

Varicella-zoster virus (VZV) is a DNA double-stranded Herpes family virus related to herpes simplex viruses 1 and 2 (HSV), cytomegalovirus (CMV), human herpes virus 6

(HHV 6) and Epstein-Barr virus (EBV). All the members of this family have the ability to cause significant morbidity during primary infection and then become latent. When subsequent reactivation occurs, it is often asymptomatic except for VZV which causes painful shingles and HSV which may cause recurrent local genital or orofacial lesions.

Varicella is thought to spread primarily by airborne droplets to the conjunctivae and upper respiratory tract of susceptible individuals (4,8). The concept of airborne spread has recently been strengthened because of documentation of disease transmission without contacts being in the same room at the same time (9). The dose of the viral inoculum is thought to influence the severity of the disease. Intense exposures, such as those within households, provide repeated doses of virus in confined spaces and thereby the largest inoculum with usually the most severe disease. It is assumed that more virus is able to replicate before activation of host defenses adequate to limit infection.

Primary and secondary viremia; viral persistence and latency

Animal studies suggest that VZV then replicates in the cervical and regional lymph nodes before disseminating to the reticuloendothelial system during a primary viremia (10). After a period of replication, usually 14 (7–21) days, a secondary viremia occurs which produces the characteristic flulike symptoms in adults. During this period, the host is contagious, presumably through aerosolized respiratory droplets. Concurrently, the characteristic macular/papular, then vesicular, rash appears over five to seven days, crusts, and scabs over. It begins centrally on the trunk and face and then spreads to the extremities. During the secondary viremia, adults often have significant constitutional symptoms of fever, myalgias, and associated clinical syndromes of pneumonia or hepatitis. The virus then becomes latent in sensory dorsal root ganglia, probably by ascending from the dermatomes where skin lesions were most concentrated. Later, VZV may reactivate, and painful clusters of vesicular lesions known as zoster appear in the same dermatomal patterns.

Complications

The most significant complications of primary varicella infection in adults are pneumonia, hepatitis, and death (1). In children, bacterial secondary infection of the skin lesions, pneumonia, and encephalitis are the most common complications (1). Whereas children over age one have a 1% incidence of pneumonia, adults have a much higher incidence (up to 20%). It is still debatable whether pregnant women have an increased incidence of pneumonia above that seen in other adults, but it is not thought to be less.

Immunocompromised patients

Immunocompromised patients have a much higher incidence of complications than do normal children and adults. It is assumed that a defect in cell-mediated immunity is primarily responsible for this effect. Untreated primary infections in this group permit widespread dissemination and can result in a 7% mortality rate. Those patients with pneumonia (40%) may have a 25% mortality rate (12).

Vertical transmission

About 25% of infants born to mothers who had primary varicella infection during pregnancy have serologic evidence of intrauterine infection (13). Infection in the first trimester is most likely to have adverse sequelae on the fetus, but this risk is small, and most of these infections are asymptomatic (13–15). There is no evidence that maternal reactivation of VZV (zoster) leads to fetal infection. Vertical transmission of VZV is most dangerous within a few days of delivery, and approximately 25% of infants born to mothers with active varicella at the time of birth acquire overt infection (13).

VARICELLA INFECTION DURING PREGNANCY

Increased morbidity and mortality of adults

There is evidence that primary VZV infections in adults have increased morbidity and mortality compared with that seen in children (1). This is not dissimilar to what is noted with other viral infections such as poliomyelitis, hepatitis A, measles, and mumps. Although only 2% of varicella infections each year occur in adults, 25% to 50% of the reported mortality is in adults, primarily due to varicella pneumonia (1). Adults are also more likely to have visceral involvement significant enough to require medical attention.

Suggested increased morbidity and mortality of pregnant women

Although varicella infection during pregnancy is estimated to occur in only five to 10 of 10,000 pregnancies (16–18), anecdotally, there seems to be an increased incidence of complications due to primary infections in these women. Paryani and Arvin reported in 1986 (13) that, of the 43 women they followed, pneumonia occurred in 9%, premature labor in 10%, premature delivery in 5%, and maternal death in 2%. The rates of pneumonia and death are between those expected for normal and immunocompromised hosts, which may reflect the physiologic immunosuppression of pregnancy.

It appears that varicella acquired during the latter part of pregnancy, compared to that acquired earlier, has increased morbidity, for there is a greater incidence of both pneumonia and hospitalization in this group (19–21). This may be the result of the heightened immunosuppressive state of the mother or a possible bias from the likelihood of admission because of heightened concern by the patient and/or her physician.

Before the availability of specific antiviral therapy, mortality from varicella pneumonia was as high as 41% (19). Recent studies have documented lessened mortality, probably due to improved supportive care.

Effects on embryo, fetus, and newborn

Approximately 25% of infants exposed to maternal varicella infections in utero acquire infection (13). This is supported by serologic studies. There are four clinical manifestations of disease (22). If exposed in the first 13 to 20 weeks of gestation, congenital varicella syndrome occurs in about 1% to 5% of such pregnancies (13–15,23–26). There seem to be few effects on the fetus if exposure occurs between 20 weeks' gestation and three weeks prior to delivery, but many of these infants later manifest zoster as their first overt VZV disease soon after birth (27). Infection occurring in the interval between 21 and five days prior to delivery can lead to a mild postnatal varicella infection of the infant because of attenuation of the disease by passively acquired maternal antibody. Exposure a few days before or after delivery is the most dangerous time for the infant and can lead to severe neonatal infection (3,12,28).

Several investigations have looked at the effects of primary maternal VZV infection on the fetus. Case reports and retrospective studies have suggested (13–15,23–26) that a congenital varicella syndrome or varicella embryopathy exists. Distinguishing features include abnormalities of the skin, limbs, eye, and brain. When present, skin lesions conform to dermatomal patterns, and hypoplastic or paralyzed limbs are ipsilateral and distal to the cicatrizing skin lesions. Microcephaly and motor/sensory paralysis are common. Virus has been detected from at least one such infant (29).

In spite of these observations, prospective studies following pregnant women with primary VZV infection have not shown an increased incidence of congenital abnormalities overall (13,15,16,28). Thus, the incidence of the well-described syndrome must be very low. Those infants with abnormalities were primarily exposed to infection before 12 to 20 weeks of gestation.

Infants exposed during the last few weeks of pregnancy (but prior to five days before delivery) are often born with, or develop soon after delivery, a mild varicella skin infection. It is felt that this represents infection modified by passively acquired maternal antibody.

Infants exposed from five days before to two days after delivery manifest the most severe symptoms. It is assumed that they acquire a larger viral inoculum from the mother in the absence of any protective antibody. They frequently have involvement of the lungs, liver, and skin, and infants thus affected have a case mortality rate of up to 50% (4).

INTERVENTIONS

Varicella-zoster immune globulin (mother and/or infant)

There is evidence that varicella-zoster immune globulin (VZIG) modifies primary VZV infections, even in immunocompromised individuals, if given within 96 hours of exposure (30). It is presumed that this is the interval when virus is replicating in the regional respiratory lymph nodes and prior to the primary viremia. One European report (16) suggested that expression of the disease can be blocked frequently in pregnant women, but this has not been replicated in the United States. It may be important to remember that since there can be differences in the antibody content of immunoglobulin preparations among countries, results (when available) from the United States may not be identical. The recommended dose for seronegative pregnant women exposed to varicella is four to five vials of 2 to 2.5 cc of VZIG, each given intramuscularly in a separate site within 96 (preferably 48) hours of exposure.

For infants, the period of greatest vulnerability is when the mother manifests disease between five days prior to and two days after delivery. If the mother becomes ill more than five days prior to delivery, sufficient placental transfer of VZV-specific IgG occurs to protect (at least partially) the infant. If the mother manifests the disease more than two days after delivery, then the secondary viremia did not occur prenatally, and the child's exposure will be postnatally due to maternal respiratory spread. This inoculum is likely to be considerably less than that from placental transfer of virus prior to birth. Infants whose mothers manifest disease within this narrow six-day peripartum period should receive one vial of VZIG as soon after birth as possible (31). There is evidence that VZIG may attenuate the disease in some infants; nevertheless, there are case reports of death in spite of VZIG and acyclovir therapy (32,33).

Acyclovir (mother and/or infant)

Although acyclovir (ACV) is readily detectable in cord blood and neonatal urine after delivery, there is no evidence that treating pregnant women with ACV affects the course of fetal infection or produces fetal embryopathy; thus, treatment of women with ACV should be predicated on the extent of maternal disease. There is evidence in nonpregnant adults that treatment with ACV yields significant improvement in respiratory status after starting the drug (34). Because varicella pneumonia in pregnant women can have a reported mortality rate as high as 41% (19) (this is likely an overestimation), ACV should be used in any varicella-susceptible mother exposed to varicella if respiratory symptoms develop 10 days after exposure. The recommended dose is 10 to 15 mg/kg (500 mg/m^2) IV every eight hours for seven days.

Vaccine (investigative studies)

A vaccine to provide protection against varicella has been used since 1974 in Japan and more recently in several European countries. In the United States, Varivax®, derived from the same Oka Japanese strain and produced by Merck Research Laboratories, is currently under investigation in children, adolescents, and adults. To date, it has been administered to approximately 10,000 healthy adults and children in the United States.

Presently, Varivax® is undergoing consistency lot trials prior to licensure. It has been shown to produce seroconversion in up to 95% of immunized children and adults (35) and has been reported to be safe and effective in preventing varicella (36). A portion of recipients have had modified varicella disease when later exposed to natural VZV, but this is characteristically benign. Seronegative adults may require two injections of vaccine for seroconversion.

If this product is licensed, it would be appropriate for nonimmune women of childbearing age to be immunized prior to pregnancy. To date, in clinical trials of women of childbearing age, no subject received an initial vaccination while pregnant. A few study participants have inadvertently become pregnant within a few weeks of receipt of the vaccine, but there have been no apparent adverse effects to either the fetus or the mother in these cases (personal communication, Merck Research Laboratories).

CONCLUSIONS

At present, VZIG and ACV are the only available interventions for varicella-exposed, nonimmune, pregnant women. In the near future, a vaccine may be available that, if used prior to pregnancy, can provide immunity or at least partial protection against disease.

When the clinician is faced with the problem of varicella exposure to an allegedly susceptible pregnant woman, the appropriate steps are:

1   Determine varicella susceptibility as soon as possible by a reliable serologic test, remembering that VZIG should be given within 96 hours, but preferably 48 hours.

2   Administer VZIG as soon as possible if needed or if the results of the serologic test will be delayed.

3   Be prepared to intervene with ACV if maternal illness develops with any severity.

4   Reassure the mother about the infrequency of fetal problems, particularly after the first trimester, but make her aware that zoster may be her child's first manifestation of VZV infection.

5   For maternal infection manifested from five days before delivery to two days after delivery, give VZIG to the mother *and* infant (after birth) and use ACV for the child if any symptoms occur and for the mother if necessary.

REFERENCES

1   **Preblud SR.** Varicella: Complications and costs. *Pediatrics* 1986;78(suppl):728–735.

2   **Guess HA, Broughton MD, Melton LJ, Kurland TL.** Population-based studies of varicella complications. *Pediatrics* 1986;78(suppl): 723–737.

3   **Gershon AA.** Chickenpox, measles and mumps. In: Remington JS, Klein JO, eds. *Infectious Diseases of the Fetus and Newborn Infant.* 2d ed. Philadelphia: Saunders, 1990;395–445.

4   **Straus SE, Ostrove JM, Inchauspe G, et al.** NIH conference. Varicella-zoster virus infections. Biology, natural history, treatment, and prevention. *Ann Intern Med* 1988;108: 221–237.

5   **Shehab ZM, Brunell PA.** Susceptibility of hospital personnel to varicella-zoster virus. *J Infect Dis* 1984;150:786.

6   **Enders G.** Management of varicella-zoster contact and infection in pregnancy using a standardized varicella-zoster ELISA test. *Postgrad Med J* 1985;61(S4):23–30.

7   **Steinberg SP, Gershon AA.** Measurement of antibodies to varicella-zoster virus by using a latex agglutination test. *J Clin Microbiol* 1991; 29:1527–1529.

8   **Le CT, Lipson M.** Difficulty in determining varicella-zoster immune status in pregnant women. *Pediatr Infect Dis J* 1989;8:650–651.

9   **Brunell PA.** Transmission of chickenpox in a school setting prior to the observed exanthem. *Am J Dis Child* 1989;143:1451–1452.

10 **Gustafson TL, Lavely GB, Brawner ER, Hutcheson RH, Wright PF, Schaffner W.** An outbreak of airborne nosocomial varicella. *Pediatrics* 1982;70:550–556.

11 **Plotkin SA.** Clinical and pathogenetic aspects of varicella-zoster. *Postgrad Med J* 1985;61 (suppl 4): 7–14.

12 **Feldman S.** Varicella Zoster infections of the fetus, neonate and immunocompromised child. *Adv Pediatr Infect Dis* 1986;99–115.

13 **Paryani SG, Arvin AM.** Intrauterine infection with varicella-zoster virus after maternal varicella. *N Engl J Med* 1986;314:1542–1546.

14 **Siegel M, Fuerst HT, Peress NSA.** Comparative fetal mortality in maternal virus diseases: a prospective study on rubella, measles, mumps, chickenpox and hepatitis. *N Engl J Med* 1966;274:768–771.

15 **Siegel M.** Congenital malformations following chickenpox, measles, mumps, and hepatitis. Results of a cohort study. *JAMA* 1973;226:1521–1524.

16 **Enders G.** Varicella-zoster virus infection in pregnancy. *Prog Med Virol* 1984;29:166–196.

17 **Fox GN, Strangarity JW.** Varicella-zoster virus infections in pregnancy. *Am Fam Physician* 1989;39:89–99.

18 **Stagno S, Whitley RJ.** Herpesvirus infections of pregnancy. 11. Herpes simplex virus and varicella-zoster virus infections. *N Engl J Med* 1985;313:1327–1330.

19 **Harris RD, Rhoades EF.** Varicella pneumonia complicating pregnancy: Report of a case and a review of the literature. *Obstet Gynecol* 1965;25:734–740.

20 **Smego RA, Asperilla MO.** Use of acyclovir for varicella pneumonia during pregnancy. *Obstet Gynecol* 1991;78:1112–1116.

21 **Broussard RC, Payne DK, George RB.** Treatment with acyclovir of varicella pneumonia in pregnancy. *Chest* 1991;99:1045–1047.

22 **Prober CG, Gershon AA, Grose C, McCracken GH, Nelson JD.** Consensus: Varicella-zoster infections in pregnancy and the perinatal period. *Pediatr Infect Dis J* 1990;9:865–869.

23 **LaForet EG, Lynch C.** Multiple congenital defects following maternal varicella. *N Engl J Med* 1947;236:534–537.

24 **Alkalay AL, Pomerance JJ, Rimoin DL.** Fetal varicella syndrome. *J Pediatr* 1987;111:320–323.

25 **Hammad E, Helin I, Pacsa A.** Early pregnancy varicella and associated congenital anomalies. *Acta Paediatr Scand* 1989;78:963–964.

26 **Lambert SR, Taylor D, Kriss A, Holzel H, Heard S.** Ocular manifestations of the congenital varicella syndrome. *Arch Opthalmol* 1989;107:52–56.

27 **Brunell PA, Kotchmar GS.** Zoster in infancy, the failure to maintain virus latency following intrauterine infection. *J Pediatr* 1981;98:71–73.

28 **Sterner G, Forsgren M, Enocksson E, Gandien M, Granström G.** Varicella-zoster infections in late pregnancy. *Scand J Infect Dis* 1990;71(suppl):30–35.

29 **Scharf A, Scherr O, Enders G, Helftenbein E.** Virus detection in the fetal tissue of a premature delivery with a congenital varicella syndrome. A case report. *J Perinat Med* 1990;18:317–322.

30 **Orenstein WA, Heymann DL, Ellis RJ, et al.** Prophylaxis of varicella in high-risk children: Dose-response effect of zoster immune globulin. *J Pediatr* 1981;98:368.

31 **Miller E, Cradock-Watson JE, Ridehalgh MKS.** Outcome in newborn babies given anti-varicella-zoster immunoglobulin after perinatal maternal infection with varicella-zoster virus. *Lancet* 1989;8:371–373.

32 **King SM, Gorenesk M, Ford-Jones EL, Read SE.** Fatal varicella-zoster infection in a newborn treated with varicella-zoster immunoglobulin. *Pediatr Infect Dis J* 1986;5:588–589.

33 **Bakshi SS, Miller TC, Kaplan M, Hammerschlag MR, Prince A, Gershon AA.** Failure of varicella-zoster immunoglobulin in modification of severe congenital varicella. *Pediatr Infect Dis* 1986;5:699–702.

34 **Haake DA, Zakowski PC, Haake DL, Bryson YJ.** Early treatment with acyclovir for varicella pneumonia in otherwise healthy adults: Retrospective controlled study and review. *Rev Infect Dis* 1990;12:788–798.

35 **Hardy IRB, Gershon AA.** Prospects for use of a varicella vaccine in adults. *Infect Dis Clin North Am* 1990;4(1):159–173.

36 **Gershon AA.** Live attenuated vaccine. *Annu Rev Med* 1987;38:41–50.

Evaluation and treatment of patients with prior reactions to β-lactam antibiotics

MICHAEL E. WEISS

CLASSIFICATION OF β-LACTAM REACTIONS

Since the introduction of penicillin by Fleming in the mid-1940s, the number of β-lactam antibiotics developed has grown dramatically. Currently, there are 46 β-lactam antibiotics licensed for use in the United States. Other than allergy, these drugs have remarkably low toxicity when used in moderate doses. In fact, the principal toxicity of β-lactam antibiotics is allergic reactions. The first case of anaphylaxis due to penicillin was reported in 1946 (1), and the first reported death due to an allergic reaction was in 1949 (2). Allergic reactions occur at a frequency of between 0.7% and 4% of penicillin treatment courses (3). Studies have indicated that as much as half of all allergic drug reactions occurring in hospitalized patients are attributed to β-lactam antibiotics (4). A wide range of different allergic reactions has been caused by β-lactam antibiotics. It is possible to classify allergic reactions to β-lactam antibiotics using the Gell and Coombs immunopathologic classification system (5) or Levine's classification system, which is based on time of onset of the reaction (6), or by classifying the reaction based on the predominate clinical manifestation.

Gell and Coombs classified four different types of immunopathologic reactions, all of which have been seen with β-lactam antibiotics (Table 7.1).

Type I: immediate hypersensitivity

These reactions result from the interaction of β-lactam antigens with preformed β-lactam-specific IgE antibodies that are bound to tissue mast cells and/or circulating basophils via high-affinity IgE receptors. Cross-linking two or more IgE receptors by β-lactam antigens leads to the release of both preformed mediators (histamine, proteases, and chemotactic factors) and newly generated mediators (prostaglandins, leukotrienes, and platelet activating factor) which are stimulated by the metabolism of arachidonic acid (7). Release of these mediators can lead to urticaria, laryngeal edema, and bronchospasm, with or without cardiovascular collapse. Anaphylactic reactions have been

131

Table 7.1 Classification of immunopathologic reactions according to the scheme of Gell and Coombs

Type of reactions	Description	Antibody	Cells	Other	Clinical reactions
I	Anaphylactic (reagenic); immediate hypersensitivity	IgE	Basophils, mast cells		Anaphylaxis, urticaria
II	Cytotoxic or cytolytic	IgG, IgM	Any cell with isoantigen	C', RES*	Hemolytic anemia cytopenias; nephritis
III	Immune complex disease	Soluble immune complexes (Ag-Ab)*	None directly	C'	Serum sickness; drug fever
IV	"Delayed" or cell-mediated hyper-sensitivity	None known	Sensitized T lymphocytes		Contact dermatitis
V	Idiopathic		?* ? ? ?	? ? ? ?	Maculopapular eruptions; eosinophilia; Stevens-Johnson syndrome; exfoliative dermatitis

*C' = complement, RES = reticuloendothelial system; Ag-Ab = antigen-antibody; ? = immunopathologic mechanism is in doubt.
SOURCE Modified from Weiss and Adkinson (27) with permission.

noted to occur in 0.004% to 0.015% of penicillin treatment courses (8). Fatality from β-lactam anaphylaxis has been reported to occur once in every 50,000 to 100,000 treatment courses (8). The use of β-adrenergic antagonists may increase the risk of death if anaphylaxis occurs, as treatment of an anaphylactic reaction is made more difficult (9). IgE type I acute allergic reactions cause the greatest clinical concern because of the risk of life-threatening anaphylaxis.

Type II: cytotoxic antibodies (usually IgG and/or IgM)

These reactions result when β-lactam-specific IgG or IgM antibodies become attached to circulating blood cells or renal interstitial cells that have β-lactam antigens bound to their cell surface. This antigen-antibody interaction activates the complement system, resulting in cell lysis. Type II reactions may also be complement independent. IgG or IgM antibody may bind to β-lactam antigens on cell membranes, resulting in neutrophil or macrophage attachment and activation via IgG or IgM Fc receptors. This opsonization can result in injury to the antigen-laden cell. Examples include hemolytic anemia, leukopenia, thrombocytopenia, or drug-induced nephritis. Long-term, high-dose β-lactam treatment is usually required for this form of allergic reaction to occur.

Type III: immune complexes (arthus reaction)

β-lactam-specific IgG or IgM antibodies may form circulating complexes with β-lactam antigens. These circulating complexes can fix complement and then lodge in tissue sites, causing serum-sicknesslike reactions and possibly drug fever. In children, serum sickness is 15 times more likely to occur secondary to administration of cefaclor compared with amoxicillin (10). These reactions typically occur seven to 14 days after the initiation of β-lactam therapy. The syndrome can occur even after the termination of therapy.

Type IV: cell-mediated hypersensitivity

These reactions are not mediated by an antibody, but rather by T lymphocytes. A T lymphocyte recognizes the β-lactam antigen through an antigen-specific T-cell receptor. This triggers the T-cell to release cytokines, which orchestrate an immune response by recruiting and stimulating proliferation of other lymphocytes, and mononuclear cells, which ultimately cause tissue inflammation and injury. Contact dermatitis is a clinical manifestation of a type IV reaction. The high rate of penicillin-related contact dermatitis (5% to 10%) in the 1940s led to the discontinuation of its use as a topical antibiotic.

Idiopathic reactions

Some reactions to β-lactam antibiotics have an obscure pathogenesis and are not included in the Gell and Coombs classification system. These reactions include pruritus, maculopapular (morbilliform) exanthems, erythema multiforme, erythema nodosum, photosensitivity reactions, fixed drug reactions, and exfoliative dermatitis. The very common maculopapular rash appears late in the treatment course in 2% to 3% of penicillin treatments. Ampicillin (amoxicillin)-induced rashes occur with much greater frequency (5.2% to 9.5% of treatment courses) in uncomplicated cases (4,11,12). When ampicillin or amoxicillin is given during infections with Epstein-Barr virus or cyto-megalovirus or to patients with acute lymphocytic leukemia, a much higher incidence of rash (69% to 100%) occurs (13). Other reactions caused by unknown mechanisms include the Stevens-Johnson syndrome, involving rash (usually erythema multiforme) plus involvement of two or more mucous membranes and Lyell's syndrome, also known as toxic epidermal necrolysis. Patients who have had Stevens-Johnson or Lyell's syndromes associated with β-lactam antibiotics should not receive that medication in the future. Attempting to desensitize individuals to β-lactam antibiotics that have caused these syndromes is also not recommended.

Levine classified reactions to penicillin according to their time of onset (6) (Table 7.2). Immediate reactions occur within the first hour after β-lactam administration, and they are almost always IgE-mediated (anaphylaxis and urticaria). Accelerated reactions occur one to 72 hours after initial treatment with β-lactams; they most commonly involve urticaria. Late reactions occur more than 72 hours after onset of therapy. Anaphylaxis does not occur later in the course of continuous β-lactam therapy; maculopapular reactions are most common, but types II to IV reactions also occur during this time frame. Allergic reactions may also be classified according to their predominate clinical manifestations as seen in Table 7.3.

Table 7.2   Classification of allergic reactions based on their time of onset

Reaction type	Onset	Clinical reactions
Immediate	0 to 1 h	Anaphylaxis Hypotension Laryngeal edema Urticaria/angioedema Wheezing
Accelerated	1 to 72 h	Urticaria/angioedema Laryngeal edema Wheezing
Late	>72 h	Morbilliform rash Interstitial nephritis Hemolytic anemia Neutropenia Thrombocytopenia Serum sickness Drug fever Stevens-Johnson syndrome Exfoliative dermatitis

SOURCE Adapted from Levine (6) with permission.

Table 7.3   Classification of allergic reactions according to their predominant clinical manifestations

Anaphylaxis	Laryngeal edema
	Hypotension
	Bronchospasm
Cutaneous reactions	Urticaria/angioedema
	Vasculitis
	Stevens-Johnson syndrome
	Exfoliative dermatitis
	Contact sensitivity
	Fixed drug eruption
	Toxic epidermal necrolysis
	Pruritus
	Maculopapular (morbilliform) rash
	Erythema multiforme
	Erythema nodosum
	Photosensitivity reactions
Destruction of formed elements of blood	Hemolytic anemia
	Neutropenia
	Thrombocytopenia
Renal reactions	Interstitial nephritis
	Glomerulonephritis
	Nephrotic syndrome
Serum sickness	
Drug fever	
Systemic vasculitis	
Lymphadenopathy	

IMMUNOCHEMISTRY OF β-LACTAM ANTIBIOTICS

Penicillins consist of a β-lactam ring, on which antimicrobial activity depends, and a five-membered thiazolidine ring (Figure 7.1). Since penicillin is a low-molecular-weight compound (molecular weight 356) it must first covalently combine with tissue macromolecules (presumably proteins) to produce multivalent hapten-protein complexes which are required both for the induction of an immune response and the later elicitation of an allergic reaction (Figure 7.2) (14). The most common form of haptenization by penicillin is in the penicylloyl configuration. Since the penicylloyl determinant is the most abundant derivative of penicillin in vivo, it has been labeled the "major determinant." While the formation of the penicylloyl group has been shown to occur spontaneously under physiologic conditions, recent evidence suggests that penicillin haptenization may be facilitated by serum molecules (15,16). This reaction occurs with the prototype benzylpenicillin and virtually all semisynthetic penicillins.

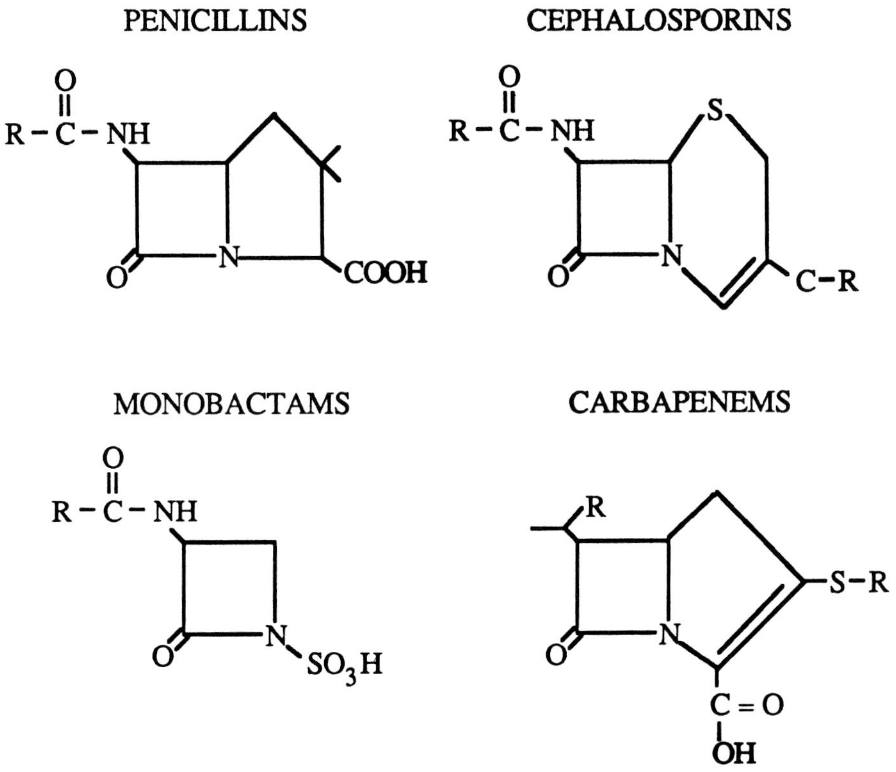

PENICILLINS   CEPHALOSPORINS

MONOBACTAMS   CARBAPENEMS

Figure 7.1 Structure of four classes of β-lactam antibiotics in use in the United States today. (From Weiss ME, Adkinson NF Jr. Immediate hypersensitivity to penicillin and related antibiotics. *Clin Allergy* 1988;18:515–540, with permission.)

Penicillin can also be degraded by other metabolic pathways to form additional antigenic determinants (17). These derivatives are formed in small quantities and stimulate a variable immune response; hence they have been termed the "minor determinants." The minor determinants of penicillin consist of benzylpenicillin, its alkaline hydrolysis product (benzylpenicilloate), and an acid hydrolysis product (benzylpenilloate), collectively called the "minor determinant mixture" (MDM). Therefore, for penicillin and other β-lactam antibiotics, IgE antibodies can be produced against a number of haptenic determinants labeled major and minor determinants. Anaphylactic reactions to penicillin are usually mediated by IgE antibodies directed against minor determinants, although some anaphylactic reactions have occurred in patients with only penicylloyl-specific IgE antibodies (6,17,18). Accelerated and late urticarial reactions are usually mediated by penicylloyl-specific IgE antibodies (major determinant) (6).

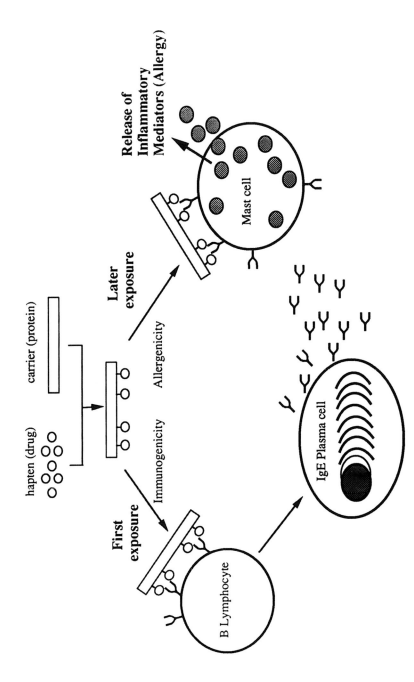

Figure 7.2 Illustration of drug hapten combining with carrier molecule to induce IgE antibody production against drug (sensitization). On subsequent exposure, drug combines with IgE antibody on mast cell surface, leading to anaphylactic reaction (immune response).

RISK FACTORS FOR β-LACTAM REACTIONS

Immune responses to β-lactam antibiotics occur in only a small percentage of exposed patients, and clinical expression of β-lactam allergy occurs in only a fraction of the patients demonstrating an immune response. The generation of a sustained immune response to a β-lactam antibiotic is probably controlled in part by the genetic makeup of that individual (19). The half-life of β-lactam IgE antibodies has been shown to range from as short as 10 days to an indeterminantly long interval (more than 1000 days) (20). Obviously, an individual whose β-lactam-specific IgE antibody response persists is at greater cumulative risk for allergic reactions to β-lactam antibiotics than one whose IgE antibody quickly disappears.

Parenteral administration of β-lactam antibiotics produces more allergic reactions than orally administered β-lactam antibiotics (21). However, recent evidence suggests that this may be more related to dose than route of administration. When higher oral doses are given, as in the treatment of gonorrhea, the incidence of allergic reactions is no different from that of intramuscular procaine penicillin at a comparable dose (22).

A history of atopy (allergic rhinitis, asthma, and/or atopic dermatitis) does not seem to be an independent risk factor for the development of β-lactam allergy (20,23), although atopic individuals seem to be predisposed to severe and fatal reactions to β-lactam antibiotics should anaphylaxis occur (8).

Individuals with a history of prior penicillin reactions have a four- to six-fold increased risk of subsequent reactions to β-lactam antibiotics compared with those without previous reaction histories (23). The risk is particularly pronounced if the previous reaction was anaphylaxis or urticaria (20). However, since most serious and fatal allergic reactions to β-lactam antibiotics occur in individuals who have never had a prior allergic reaction, a negative history of β-lactam allergy should not leave one with a false sense of security. Sensitization in these individuals probably occurred from their last therapeutic course of penicillin. A randomized, controlled trial of routine penicillin skin testing in history-negative patients was shown not to be cost effective, and, therefore, skin testing at this time is only recommended for patients with prior history of β-lactam allergy (24).

In general, the likelihood of sustaining IgE-specific β-lactam antibodies declines with increasing time from the previous reaction. Sullivan and collaborators reported that skin tests done within the first one or two months after an acute allergic reaction were positive 80% to 90% of the time. Thereafter, there was a time-dependent decline in the rate of positive skin tests to less than 20% by 10 years (25). Patients who have had serum-sicknesslike reactions to β-lactam antibiotics often persist with an intense antibody reaction and may remain at high risk for allergic reactions for many years.

DIAGNOSING β-LACTAM ALLERGY

An important question facing clinicians is how to assess patients who present with histories of prior β-lactam reactions, but who have a current clinical need for β-lactam antibiotics. Approximately 5% to 20% of patients give a history of prior allergy to β-lactam antibiotics. By current medical standards, all of these subjects would be denied therapy with β-lactam antibiotics for the rest of their lives unless further evaluation is undertaken. The most useful single piece of information in assessing an individual's risk for a type I, IgE-mediated reaction (anaphylaxis and urticaria) is the skin test response to major and minor penicillin determinants.

The major (penicylloyl) determinant of penicillin can be assessed by skin testing with penicylloyl-polylysine (PPL). This commercially available skin test reagent (PRE-PEN, Kremers-Uraban, Milwaukee, WI) contains multiple penicylloyl molecules synthetically coupled to a weakly immunogenic polylysine carrier. Unfortunately, minor determinants of penicillin are not commercially available in the United States at present. It is hoped that this will change in the near future. Skin testing should begin with an epicutaneous test for safety. If there is no induration (or systemic symptoms) after 15 minutes, intradermal injections are placed, raising 3- to 4-mm blebs. Testing should be done with PPL, MDM, a positive control (histamine), and a negative diluent control. The diameter of induration at 15 to 20 minutes is read; if it is greater than 5 mm, the test is considered positive (26). Antihistamines, tricyclic antidepressants, and adrenergic drugs, all of which may inhibit skin test results, should be discontinued at least 48 hours prior to skin testing. Antihistamines with long half-lives need to be discontinued for appropriate intervals.

Extensive worldwide experience has shown that patients with prior histories of penicillin reactions can be safely retreated with penicillin or related antibiotics if intradermal skin tests with PPL and a suitable minor determinant mixture are shown to be negative. When therapeutic doses of penicillin are given to patients with histories of penicillin allergy, but with negative skin tests to PPL and MDM, IgE-mediated reactions occur very rarely and are almost always mild and self-limited. Penicillin anaphylaxis has not been reported in skin-test-negative patients in the United States. When penicillin is given after negative skin tests, about 1% to 3% of patients will develop urticarial or other mild cutaneous reactions (27,28). If the major determinant penicillin is used alone as a skin test reagent, approximately 10% to 25% of all potential positive reactions would be missed (25). If one uses benzylpenicillin-G, diluted to a concentration of 10,000 units/mL (10^{-2} M) as the sole minor determinant, about 5% to 10% of skin-test-positive patients will be missed (25). Since readministration of β-lactam antibiotics may resensitize a patient, one needs to consider retesting the patient with a positive history of a penicillin reaction before each new course of β-lactam antibiotics.

Recently, Blanca and associates in Spain suggested that skin testing with major and minor determinants of benzylpenicillin may not protect all individuals with ampicillin/amoxicillin-specific allergy (29), Mendelson et al. studied 443 patients with a history of penicillin allergy who were skin-test-negative to PPL and a MDM of penicillin. The 443 patients tolerated a 10-day penicillin challenge, but, when given 10 days of amoxicillin, 18.7% developed cutaneous reactions (Mendelson, personal communication). Thus, amoxicillin/ampicillin seems to have a greater propensity for causing cutaneous allergic reactions. It has been postulated that the diamino acyl side chain contained in ampicillin/amoxicillin allows more readily for the formation of linear polymers of varying lengths, which may explain the higher cutaneous reaction rate seen with ampicillin/amoxicillin. Studies in the 1960s showed that patients with late-occurring maculopapular rashes from ampicillin could be retreated safely with the antibiotics without any increased risk for acute allergic reactions. Skin testing in these individuals with PPL and MDM is useful to rule out concomitant type I, IgE-mediated sensitivity.

A limited number of skin-test-positive patients have been treated with therapeutic doses of penicillin. The risk of an acute immediate or accelerated allergic reaction ranges from about 10% in history-negative to 50% to 70% in history-positive subjects (27). Patients with a history of exfoliative dermatitis or Stevens-Johnson or Lyell's syndromes, reactions that constitute absolute contraindications for penicillin administration, should not be evaluated by skin testing.

Type II reactions, such as hemolytic anemias, cytopenias, and interstitial nephritis, usually follow high-dose, long-term β-lactam therapy. Anecdotal experience suggests that short courses of β-lactam therapy in moderate doses can be tolerated by most, if not all, patients with these histories. Penicillin skin testing is important to rule out concomitant type I sensitivity but would not be predictive of type II or III reactions. If skin tests are negative in these patients and β-lactam antibiotics are strongly indicated, gradual dose escalation under careful medical observation can be prudently attempted. If cytopenia, hemolytic anemia, hematuria, or proteinuria develop, therapy should be promptly stopped and high-dose glucocorticoids administered. Most subjects can be retreated, however, without recurrence, especially if the prior history of reaction is remote.

Solid-phase immunoassays such as the radioallergosorbent test (RAST) have been developed to detect serum IgE antibodies directed against the penicylloyl determinant. At present, there is no in vitro RAST for minor determinant antibodies (26). Because it is more time-consuming, more expensive, less sensitive for detection of the major determinant IgE antibodies than skin testing, and presently unavailable for minor determinant antibody detection, the RAST and other in vitro analogs have limited clinical utility at this time.

β-LACTAM DESENSITIZATION

Effective, non-cross-reacting alternative antibiotics are usually available for patients with positive skin tests to penicillin. If alternative drugs fail, induce unacceptable side effects, or are clearly less effective, then the administration of a β-lactam antibiotic, using a desensitization protocol, may be justified. Infections in which this may be considered include subacute endocarditis due to enterococci, brain abscess, bacterial meningitis, or overwhelming infections (such as osteomyelitis or sepsis) with staphylococci or pseudomonad organisms, *Listeria* infections, neurosyphilis, or syphilis during pregnancy. Use of a desensitization protocol for penicillin skin-test-positive patients markedly reduces the risk of anaphylaxis.

β-lactam desensitization should only be performed in an intensive care setting. Any medical risk factor for anaphylaxis should be corrected. All β-adrenergic antagonists, including ophthalmologic drops, should be discontinued. Asthmatic patients should be under optimal control. An intravenous line should be established, and baseline electrocardiogram and spirometry should be performed. Continuous electrocardiogram monitoring should be instituted.

Protocols have been developed for β-lactam desensitization using both the oral and parenteral route (Tables 7.4 and 7.5) (30). If an oral preparation is available and the patient has a functional gastrointestinal tract, the oral route is preferred for desensitization. Results from oral desensitization have shown that approximately one-third of patients will develop a transient allergic reaction during desensitization (one-third) or during penicillin treatment after desensitization (two-thirds). These reactions are usually mild and self-limited in nature, but may be serious (21).

During desensitization, any dose that causes mild systemic reactions, such as pruritus, fleeting urticaria, rhinitis, or mild wheezing, should be repeated until the patient tolerates the dose without systemic symptoms or signs. More serious reactions, such as hypotension, laryngeal edema, or asthma, require appropriate treatment, and, if desensitization is continued, the dose should be decreased by at least ten-fold and withheld until the patient is stable (31).

Once desensitized, the patient's treatment with penicillin must not lapse, or the risk of an allergic reaction increases. If the patient requires a β-lactam antibiotic in the

Table 7.4   Protocol for oral desensitization of β-lactam antibiotic allergic patients*

Step	β-lactam drug (mg/mL)	Amount† (mL)	Dose given† (mg)	Cumulative dose (mg)
1	0.5	0.1	0.05	0.05
2	0.5	0.2	0.10	0.15
3	0.5	0.4	0.20	0.35
4	0.5	0.8	0.40	0.75
5	0.5	1.6	0.80	1.55
6	0.5	3.2	1.60	3.15
7	0.5	6.4	3.20	6.35
8	5.0	1.2	6.00	12.35
9	5.0	2.4	12.00	24.35
10	5.0	4.8	24.00	48.35
11	50.0	1.0	50.00	98.35
12	50.0	2.0	100.00	198.35
13	50.0	4.0	200.00	398.35
14	50.0	8.0	400.00	798.35

Observe patient for 30 minutes
Administer 1 g of same agent intravenously

*Interval between doses: 15 minutes.
†Drug suspension diluted in 30 mL of water for ingestion.
SOURCE: Reprinted from Sullivan (30) with permission.

Table 7.5 Protocol for parenteral desensitization of β-lactam antibiotic allergic patients*

Step	β-lactam drug (mg/mL)	Amount† (mL)	Dose given† (mg)	Cumulative dose (mg)
1	0.1	0.1	0.01	0.01
2	0.1	0.2	0.02	0.03
3	0.1	0.4	0.04	0.07
4	0.1	0.8	0.08	0.15
5	1.0	0.16	0.16	0.31
6	1.0	0.32	0.32	0.63
7	1.0	0.64	0.64	1.27
8	10	0.12	1.20	2.47
9	10	0.24	2.40	4.87
10	10	0.48	4.80	10
11	100	0.10	10	20
12	100	0.20	20	40
13	100	0.40	40	80
14	100	0.80	80	160
15	1,000	0.16	160	320
16	1,000	0.32	320	640
17	1,000	0.64	640	1,280

Observe patient for 30 minutes
Administer 1 g of same agent intravenously

*Interval between doses: 15 minutes.
†Doses administered subcutaneously (or intramuscularly or intravenously).
SOURCE Reprinted from Sullivan (30) with permission.

future and still remains skin-test-positive to penicillin reagents, desensitization would be required again. Patients have been maintained on long-term, low-dose penicillin therapy (usually b.i.d.-t.i.d.) to sustain a chronic state of desensitization.

CROSS-REACTIVITY AMONG DIFFERENT CLASSES OF β-LACTAM ANTIBIOTICS

Cephalosporins

Like penicillin, cephalosporins possess a β-lactam ring, but the five-membered thiazolidine ring is replaced by the six-membered dihydrothiazine ring (Figure 7.1). Shortly after cephalosporins came into clinical use, allergic reactions were reported, and the question of cross-reactivity between cephalosporins and penicillins was raised (32). To date, the degree of cross-reactivity between penicillins and cephalosporins remains a matter of considerable uncertainty. Complicating matters, the early cephalosporins were contaminated with trace amounts of penicillin (33), potentially leading to overestimates of the degree of cross-reactivity. Nevertheless, studies in both animals and humans clearly demonstrated cross-reactivity between penicillins and first-generation cephalosporins using immuno- and bioassays to evaluate IgE, IgM, and IgG antibodies (34–36). In general, the degree of clinical cross-reactivity is much lower than the in vitro cross-reactivity between penicillins and cephalosporins. Small numbers of penicillin skin-test-positive patients have been treated with cephalosporin antibiotics without allergic reactions (37,38). Very few cephalosporin skin-test-positive individuals have been challenged with cephalosporins to allow estimation of the predictive value of a positive skin test. Unfortunately, only native cephalosporins are currently available as skin test reagents; therefore, the utility of skin testing for cephalosporin allergy is limited.

The incidence of clinically relevant cross-reactivity between the penicillins and cephalosporins is probably small, but rare cases of life-threatening anaphylactic cross-reactivity have occurred. The risk of administering a first-generation cephalosporin to a penicillin-skin-test-positive patient is much lower than administering a penicillin antibiotic, but is not negligible. Antibodies to the second- and third-generation cephalosporins are often directed against the side chains rather than the ring structures, and therefore cross-reactivity with penicillins is less than with first-generation cephalosporins (30). Patients with positive skin tests to any penicillin reagent probably should not receive cephalosporin antibiotics unless alternative drugs are clearly less desirable. If cephalosporin drugs are to be used, they should be administered with caution and with adequate precautions.

Carbapenems

These are a new class of β-lactam antibiotics, of which imipenem is the prototype (Figure 7.1). Recent studies have shown that approximately 50% of penicillin-skin-test-positive patients have positive skin reactions to analogous imipenem determinants (39), which suggests appreciable cross-reactivity and indicates that these β-lactam antibiotics are relatively contraindicated in patients with positive penicillin skin tests.

Monobactams

The monobactams are a new group of β-lactam antibiotics that contain the monocyclic ring structure rather than the bicyclic structure of the penicillins, cephalosporins and carbapenems (Figure 7.1). The prototype monobactam licensed in the United States is aztreonam. In preclinical studies, negligible cross-reactivity in rabbits and in human subjects between aztreonam and penicillins or cephalosporins was found (40). When subjects with positive penicillin skin tests were skin tested with analogous aztreonam reagents, appreciable cross-reactivity was not found (41). In a subsequent trial, 20 patients with positive penicillin skin tests were treated with therapeutic doses of aztreonam; none had IgE-mediated reactions (42). Taken together, these data suggest weak cross-reactivity between aztreonam and other β-lactam antibiotics and indicate that aztreonam may be safely administered to most, if not all, penicillin-allergic subjects.

Unanswered Questions

Important clinical questions remain for future research in β-lactam allergy. These include (a) the further elucidation of when side-chain-specific allergies may be the cause of β-lactam reactions, (b) the possible identifications of genetic factors that predispose individuals to have β-lactam allergy, (c) the validation of testing procedures to evaluate clinical cross-reactivity between cephalosporin and penicillin antibiotics, and (d) the potential relationship of penicillin allergy to other medication reactions of structurally unrelated drugs.

REFERENCES

1 Gorevic PD. Drug-induced autoimmune disease. In: Kaplan A, ed. *Allergy.* New York: Churchill Livingston, 1985:480.

2 Schwartz HJ, Sher TH. Anaphylaxis to penicillin in a frozen dinner. *Ann Allergy* 1984; 52:342–343.

3 Parker CW. Drug therapy (first of three parts). *N Engl J Med* 1975;292:511–514.

4 Arndt KA, Jick H. Rates of cutaneous reactions to drugs. A report from the Boston Collaborative Drug Surveillance Program. *JAMA* 1976; 235:918–922.

5 Gell PGH, Coombs RRA. Classification of allergic reactions responsible for clinical hypersensitivity and disease. In: Gell PGH, Coombs RRA, Hachmann PJ, eds. *Clinical Aspects of Immunology.* Oxford: Blackwell Scientific Publications, 1975:761–781.

6 Levine BB. Immunologic mechanisms of penicillin allergy. A haptenic model system for the study of allergic diseases of man. *N Engl J Med* 1966;275:1115–1125.

7 Ishizaka T. Mechanisms of IgE-mediated hypersensitivity. In: Middleton E Jr, Reed CE, Ellis EF, Adkinson NF Jr, Yuninger JW, eds. *Allergy: Principles and Practice.* St. Louis: C. V. Mosby Co., 1988:71–93.

8 Idsoe O, Guthe T, Willcox RR, De Weck AL. Nature and extent of penicillin side-reactions, with particular reference to fatalities from anaphylactic shock. *Bull Wld Hlth Org* 1968; 38:159–188.

9 Jacobs RL, Geoffrey WR Jr, Fournier DC, Chilton RJ, Culver WG, Beckmann CH. Potentiated anaphylaxis in patients with drug-induced beta-adrenergic blockade. *J Allergy Clin Immunol* 1981;68:125–127.

10 Heckbert SR, Stryker WS, Coltin KL, Manson JE, Platt R. Serum sickness in children after antibiotic exposure: estimates of occurrence and morbidity in a health maintenance organi-zation population. *Am J Epidemiology* 1990; 132:336–342.

11 Levine B. Skin rashes with penicillin therapy: Current management. *N Engl J Med* 1972;286: 42–43.

12 Shapiro S, Siskin V, Slone D, Lewis GP, Jick H. Drug rash with ampicillin and other penicillins. *Lancet* 1969; Nov:7628.

13 Kerns DL, Shira JE, Go S, Summers RJ, Schwab JA, Plunket DC. Ampicillin rash in children. Relationship to penicillin allergy and infectious mononucleosis. *Am J Dis Child* 1973;125:187–190.

14 Eisen HN. Hypersensitivity to simple chemicals. In: Lawrence HS, ed. *Cellular and Humoral Aspects of the Hypersensitive States.* New York: P. B. Hoeber, 1959:111–126.

15 DiPiro JT, Hamilton RG, Adkinson NF Jr. Facilitation of penicilloation of proteins by serum cofactors. *J Aller Clin Immunol* 1990;85: 192 (abstract).

16 Sullivan TJ. Facilitated haptenation of human proteins by penicillin. *J Allergy Clin Immunol* 1989;83(abst.):255.

17 Levine BB, Redmond AP. Minor haptenic determinant-specific reagins of penicillin hypersensitivity in man. *Int Arch Allergy* 1969; 35:445–455.

18 Levine BB, Redmond AP, Fellner MJ, Voss HE, Levytska V. Penicillin allergy and the heterogeneous immune responses of man to benzylpenicillin. *J Clin Invest* 1966;45:1895–1906.

19 Levine BB. Effect of combinations of inbred strain, antigen, and antigen dose on immune responsiveness and reagin production in the mouse. A potential mouse model for immune aspects of human atopic allergy. *Int Arch Allergy Appl Immunol* 1970;39:156–171.

20 Adkinson NF Jr. Risk factors for drug allergy. *J Allergy Clin Immunol* 1984;74:567–572.

21 **Sullivan TJ, Yecies LD, Shatz GS, Parker CW, Wedner HJ.** Desensitization of patients allergic to penicillin using orally administered beta-lactam antibiotics. *J Allergy Clin Immunol* 1982;69:275–282.

22 **Adkinson NF Jr, Wheeler B.** Risk factors for IgE-dependent reactions to penicillin. In: Kerr JW, Ganderton MA, eds. *XI International Congress of Allergology and Clinical Immunology.* London: MacMillan Press Ltd., 1983:55–59.

23 **Sogn DD.** Prevention of allergic reactions to penicillin. *J Allergy Clin Immunol* 1987; 78:1051–1052.

24 **Adkinson NF Jr, Spence M, Wheeler B.** Randomized clinical trial of routine penicillin skin testing. *J Allergy Clin Immunol* 1984; 73:163.

25 **Sullivan TJ, Wedner HJ, Shatz GS, Yecies LD, Parker CW.** Skin testing to detect penicillin allergy. *J Allergy Clin Immunol* 1981; 68:171–180.

26 **Adkinson NF Jr.** Tests for immunological drug reactions. In: Rose NF, Friedman H, eds. *Manual of Clinical Immunology.* Washington, DC: American Society for Microbiology, 1986: 692–697.

27 **Weiss ME, Adkinson NF Jr.** Immediate hypersensitivity reactions to penicillin and related antibiotics. *Clin Allergy* 1988;18:515–540.

28 **Weiss ME, Adkinson NF Jr.** Beta-lactam allergy. In: Mandell LD, Douglas RG Jr, Bennett JE, eds. *Principles and Practice of Infectious Disease.* New York: Churchill Livingston Inc., 1989:264–269.

29 **Blanca M, Vega JM, Garcia J, Carmona MJ, Terados S, Avila MJ, Miranda A, Juarez C.** Allergy to penicillin with good tolerance to other penicillins: study of the incidence in subjects allergic to betalactams. *Clin Exper Allergy* 1990;20:475–481.

30 **Sullivan TJ.** Drug allergy. In: Middleton E, Reed C, Ellis E, Adkinson NF, Yunginger J, eds. *Allergy: Principles and Practice.* St. Louis: C.V. Mosby Co, 1989;1523–1534.

31 **Adkinson NF Jr.** Penicillin allergy. In: Lichtenstein LM, Fauci A, eds. *Current Therapy in Allergy, Immunology and Rheumatology.* Ontario, Canada: B.S. Decker, 1983:57–62.

32 **Grieco MH.** Cross-allergenicity of the penicillins and the cephalosporins. *Arch Intern Med* 1967;119:141–146.

33 **Pedersen-Bjergaard J.** Cephalothin in the treatment of penicillin sensitive patients. *Act Allergol* 1967;XXII:299–306.

34 **Petz L.** Immunologic cross-reactivity between penicillins and cephalosporins: A review. *J Infect Dis* 1978;137:S74–S79.

35 **Shibata K, Atsumi T, Itorivchi Y, Mashimo K.** Immunological cross-reactivities of cephalothin and its related compounds with benzylpenicillin (penicillin G). *Nature* 1966;212:419–420.

36 **Abraham GN, Petz LD, Fudenberg HH.** Immunohaematological cross-allergenicity between penicillin and cephalothin in humans. *Clin Exp Immunol* 1968;3:343–357.

37 **Solley GO, Gleich GJ, Van Dellen RG.** Penicillin allergy: clinical experience with a battery of skin-test reagents. *J Allergy Clin Immunol* 1982;69:238–244.

38 **Saxon A, Beall GN, Rohr AS, Adelman DC.** Immediate hypersensitivity reactions to beta-lactam antibiotics. *Ann Int Med* 1987;107: 204–215.

39 **Saxon A.** Immediate hypersensitivity reactions to beta-lactam antibiotics. *Rev Infect Dis* 1983; 5:S368.

40 **Adkinson NF Jr, Swabb EA, Sugerman AA.** Immunology of the monobactam aztreonam. *Antimicrobial Agents and Chemotherapy* 1984; 25:93–97.

41 **Saxon A, Hassner A, Swabb EA, Wheeler B, Adkinson NF Jr.** Lack of cross-reactivity between aztreonam, a monobactam antibiotic, and penicillin in penicillin-allergic subjects. *J Infect Dis* 1984;149:16–22.

42 **Adkinson NF Jr, Wheeler B, Swabb EA.** Clinical tolerance of the monobactam aztreonam in penicillin allergic subjects. Abstract (WS-26-4) presented at the 14th International Congress of Chemotherapy, June 23–28, 1984, Kyoto, Japan.

Periodontal diseases: gingivitis, juvenile periodontitis, adult periodontitis

RAY C. WILLIAMS

INTRODUCTION

Periodontal disease is a general term used to describe specific diseases that affect the gingiva, as well as the supporting connective tissue and alveolar bone that anchor the teeth in the jaws. The periodontal diseases are among the most common infectious diseases in humans. In the late 1800s, periodontal disease was called Rigg's disease and in the early 1900s became popularly known as "pyorrhea." This term denoted pus, periodontal pockets, loss of bone, and loss of teeth. Pyorrhea was thought to be an inevitable disease, and loss of teeth resulting from it part of the aging process (1). In the last 15 years, with the decline of dental caries in children aged six to 18 and better prevention programs for the general population, the role of periodontal disease in tooth loss has assumed even greater importance. As more teeth are retained due to reduced caries, more teeth are at risk to be affected by periodontal disease (2,3).

Research advances in recent years in the understanding of the etiology, pathogenesis, and treatment of periodontal disease are noteworthy. This review will describe periodontal diseases, including the bacterial etiology and the host responses to bacteria, and examine the treatment of periodontal disease. The final section will look at prospects for the future in the diagnosis and treatment of a ubiquitous group of diseases.

DEFINITIONS AND DISEASE CLASSIFICATION

The following terminology is used to describe the structures that comprise the periodontium. Figure 8.1 diagrams the periodontal structures. The tooth is suspended in the alveolar bone socket by collagen fibers. These suspensory collagen fibers, called the periodontal ligament, are embedded in both alveolar bone and in the cementum, which covers the outer surface of the tooth root. The periodontal ligament, the tooth root, and the alveolar bone socket are collectively referred to as the periodontium (4). These structures are also known as the attachment structures or the attachment apparatus.

146

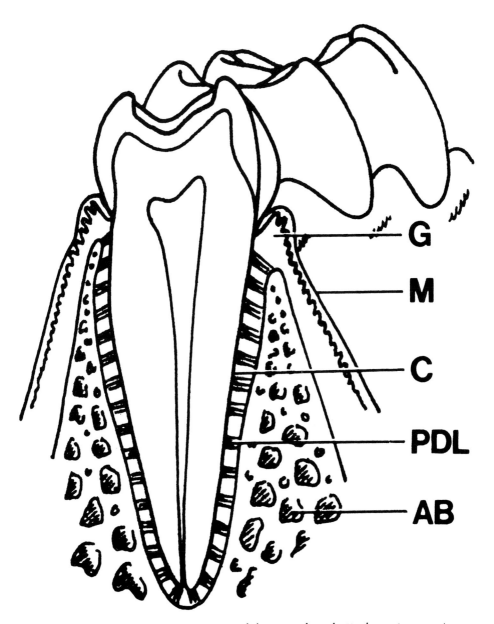

Figure 8.1   Schematic representation of the periodontal attachment apparatus structures, including the gingiva (G), the alveolar mucosa (M), the tooth root cementum (C), the periodontal ligament (PDL), and the alveolar bone (AB).

Overlying these supporting structures are the gingiva and the alveolar mucosa. Periodontal disease thus implies that the gingiva or the underlying attachment structures or both are affected.

Periodontal diseases have over the years been simplistically separated into those diseases that involve only the gingiva, i.e., "gingivitis," and those diseases that are also associated with the destruction of the underlying structures of the periodontium, i.e., "periodontitis" (5). Gingivitis is characterized clinically by increased redness, swelling, a change in the position of the gingival margin, and bleeding of the gingiva when patients brush their teeth or when the dentist gently probes the gingival sulcus (6). Acute necrotizing ulcerative gingivitis is a painful form of gingivitis. This disease was called trenchmouth or Vincent's infection in the 1920s and 1930s and is associated with sudden onset, pain, and tissue necrosis (7).

Other gingival diseases may be manifestations of systemic diseases or hormonal disturbances. Acute herpetic gingivostomatitis is a painful manifestation of primary herpes infection. Blood dyscrasias such as leukemia, autoimmune diseases such as pemphigus, and metabolic diseases such as diabetes can be associated with severe gingival inflammation. Pregnancy may also be associated with an increased incidence of gingivitis, and gingivitis is an almost universal occurrence at puberty (8–12). Various gingival diseases secondary to gingivitis may be observed in patients taking medications. For example, there may be hyperplasia and enlargement of the gingiva in patients taking phenytoin, cyclosporine, or nifedipine (13,14). Patients taking medicines that reduce salivary flow, such as anticholinergic, antidepressant, and antihistaminic drugs, frequently begin to experience painful gingivitis, as well as generalized inflammation of the oral mucosa (8).

In general, gingival diseases, especially gingivitis, are not considered as serious as the periodontal diseases that destroy the periodontal ligament and alveolar bone. When the inflammatory process of gingivitis extends into the periodontal ligament and alveolar bone, with destruction of both, then the periodontal disease is called periodontitis. As the periodontal ligament is destroyed and alveolar bone begins to resorb, the epithelium of the gingiva migrates along the root surface, following the destructive process, to form periodontal pockets. Thus, a patient with periodontitis has loss of connective tissue, resorption of alveolar bone, and periodontal pocket formation. As the disease progresses, there is increasing looseness and finally loss of the teeth.

In the 1970s and until around 1986, two main forms of periodontitis were recognized: juvenile periodontitis and chronic marginal periodontitis. In 1986 (15), there was a reclassification of periodontitis as follows:

I Juvenile periodontitis
  A. Prepubertal periodontitis
  B. Localized juvenile periodontitis
  C. Generalized juvenile periodontitis
II Adult periodontitis
III Necrotizing ulcerative gingivo-periodontitis
IV Refractory periodontitis

This reclassification helped establish the idea that different forms of periodontitis exist that go beyond the classical definitions. This reclassification has now been

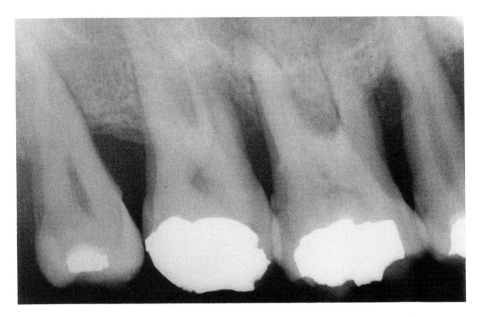

Figure 8.2   Radiographic example of moderate loss of alveolar bone about teeth (moderate periodontitis).

further expanded. At the recent World Workshop in Clinical Periodontics (16), it was recognized that extensive new data exist, and a new and expanded classification of different forms of periodontitis was recommended. This current classification is as follows:

   I Adult periodontitis
  II Early-onset periodontitis
     A. Prepubertal periodontitis
       1. Generalized
       2. Localized
     B. Juvenile periodontitis
       1. Generalized
       2. Localized
     C. Rapidly progressive periodontitis
 III Periodontitis associated with systemic disease
 IV Necrotizing ulcerative periodontitis
  V Refractory periodontitis

The most frequently encountered form of periodontitis, adult periodontitis (Figure 8.2), occurs in individuals at around age 35 and onward. Adult periodontitis is the disease most responsible for the loss of teeth, and its appropriate diagnosis and treatment is one of the greatest challenges facing dentistry today.

    Early-onset periodontitis is distinguished from adult periodontitis primarily by age:

age of onset prior to 35 years, rapid rate of progression, defects in host defense, and composition of the associated flora (17,18).

Prepubertal periodontitis is rare and appears soon after eruption of the primary dentition. This disease differs from the other early-onset types of periodontitis in the composition of the associated flora, onset between eruption of the primary teeth and puberty, and abnormalities in the host defense (19).

Juvenile periodontitis has as its most characteristic feature: (a) onset during the circumpubertal period, (b) familial distribution, (c) very little bacterial buildup, (d) a preponderance of *Actinobacillus actinomycetemcomitans* in the associated flora, and (e) the presence of abnormalities in leukocyte chemotaxis and bactericidal activity. The localized form is confined mostly to permanent first molars and/or incisors. In the generalized form, many other, if not all, teeth are involved (16–18). Figure 8.3 is a radiographic example of localized juvenile periodontitis in a 12-year-old girl.

Rapidly progressive periodontitis is similar to generalized juvenile periodontitis, but the age of onset is later (usually in the twenties or later). Also, familial distribution is not as prominent; pigmenting *Prevetalla* rather than *Actinobacillus actinomycetem-comitans* may be predominant in the flora; and the abnormalities in host defense may relate to random migration of the leukocytes rather than suppressed chemotaxis (16).

Several systemic diseases are reported to predispose persons to periodontitis. Among these are periodontitis associated with Down syndrome, type I diabetes, Papillon-LeFevre syndrome, and human immunodeficiency virus (HIV) infection (16,20).

Refractory periodontitis is a more and more commonly accepted term which implies a person with any form of periodontitis which is not responsive to any treatment provided, whatever the thoroughness or frequency (16,21).

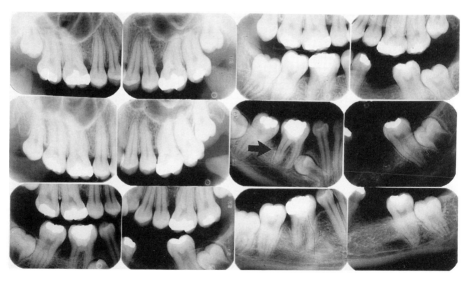

Figure 8.3. Radiographic example of localized juvenile periodontitis. The arrow points to an area of localized bone loss adjacent to the first molar.

EXAMINATION OF THE PATIENT

Examination of the patient for periodontal disease involves evaluating the gingiva for inflammation and the underlying attachment structures for pocket formation and bone loss. To diagnose gingivitis, visual assessment of color change of the gingiva is performed. In addition, the gingival sulcus is probed for the presence of bleeding. Bleeding in response to gentle probing, in addition to redness, is an indicator of gingivitis (6).

The periodontal probe, a small instrument calibrated in millimeters, is also used to detect and measure periodontal pocket formation. When the probe can be inserted beneath the gingiva 5 mm or more, the patient has periodontal pockets. Periodontal pocket formation indicates previous destruction of the periodontal structures, with resorption of alveolar bone. Dental radiographs are necessary to confirm and measure the extent of alveolar bone loss (Figure 8.2) Periodontal diseases are usually painless and asymptomatic; the first indication of gingivitis is often bleeding upon tooth brushing. The first indication of periodontitis may be loosening of teeth. Healthy-appearing, asymptomatic gingiva may be misleading because considerable loss of attachment structures underneath can occur without the patient's knowledge. Severe gingivitis, however, does not necessarily indicate that the underlying structures are being destroyed. The detection and diagnosis of periodontal disease rely on the dentist and hygienist.

EPIDEMIOLOGY OF PERIODONTAL DISEASES

For a number of years, there has been an ongoing effort to determine the incidence, prevalence, and natural history of periodontal disease in humans. Epidemiologic studies have documented that the severity of periodontal disease increases with age. In the absence of treatment, periodontitis, once initiated, will continue to progress, with the eventual loss of the teeth (22–24). Although gingivitis precedes periodontitis, it is not clear that in each case gingivitis will necessarily progress to periodontitis.

The National Institute of Dental Research (NIDR) 1985–1986 Survey of Employed and Senior Adults has continued to provide new insight into the prevalence of periodontal diseases in the United States (25). Recent findings from this study reveal that the prevalence of gingival bleeding was 44% in the employed population and the prevalence of attachment loss of 3 mm or more was 44%. Since most epidemiologic surveys underestimate periodontal disease, a significant effort has been made to further clarify these data. Beck and co-workers (26) and Hunt and co-workers (27) conducted epidemiologic surveys in an older population using the NIDR methodology in a full-mouth design, rather than examining half-mouths as was done in the NIDR study. Hunt reported that the half-mouth design consistently underestimated gingival bleeding and pocketing. Fox analyzed the effect of site selection on periodontal disease prevalence in a study of New England elders. Fox reported that the NIDR methodology had a sensitivity of 0.24 to detect pocketing of more than 6 mm (28). This means that, of all the subjects examined in the NIDR survey with pocketing of more than 6 mm, the NIDR methodology would have detected only 24% of them. Thus, Fox's work, as well as other studies such as those mentioned, show higher disease levels than reported initially from the NIDR survey. The studies also report that risks for a higher prevalence of periodontal disease include increased age, poor education, neglect of dental care, previous periodontal destruction, tobacco use, and diabetes (28).

The natural history of periodontal disease progression has been an ongoing component of study in the epidemiological research. One of the most noteworthy studies of disease progression was by Loe and co-workers (29). These epidemiologists documented the progression of periodontal disease in a population of Sri Lankan tea laborers who never had dental care. The subjects, aged 14 to 46 years, were studied over a 15-year period. Gingivitis was found to be widespread. Eight percent of the population demonstrated rapid progression of attachment loss, while 81% had moderate progression. In the majority of the population, seven teeth had been lost to periodontal disease by age 45. The finding that 11% of the population had virtually no disease suggests differences in susceptibility or level of infection. Others have examined the progression of periodontal disease in patients not treated for periodontal disease but who had access to routine dental treatment. For example, Becker and co-workers found that untreated patients presenting with moderate to advanced periodontal disease had progressive increases in pocket depth and alveolar bone loss over intervals of 18 to 115 months (30).

These studies demonstrate that, over time, untreated periodontal disease progresses, with eventual tooth loss. Since the early 1980s, the actual progression of periodontal disease has been postulated to be episodic, with periods of exacerbation and remission about individual teeth in an individual; this may not necessarily be the case. In a recent study (31), Jeffcoat and Reddy followed the course of periodontal disease in patients using an automated probe which could detect small amounts of disease progression. Thirty patients were examined regularly over a six-month period and the progression of attachment loss about the teeth noted. When small disease progression changes were measured, the prevalence of active disease was 29%, and 76% of those active sites lost attachment consistent with a continuous model for disease progression. This recent study employed more sensitive techniques for measuring disease progression and suggests that, as was popularly believed for decades, untreated periodontal disease likely progresses more or less continuously. Only a few tooth sites in the patients studied demonstrated bursts of disease activity (31).

ETIOLOGY

For about a hundred years, it has been recognized that periodontal diseases are caused by bacteria that are present on the tooth surface and under the gingiva. There has been a long and remarkable research effort to determine which bacteria are actually responsible for the disease (32).

During this hundred-year span of time, there have been three major cycles in dentistry's attitude toward the bacterial etiology of periodontal diseases. Figure 8.4 illustrates the time period. In the first part of the century, microbiologists, relying on culture methods available at the time, believed that certain microorganisms such as

100 YEARS OF PERIODONTAL MICROBIOLOGY

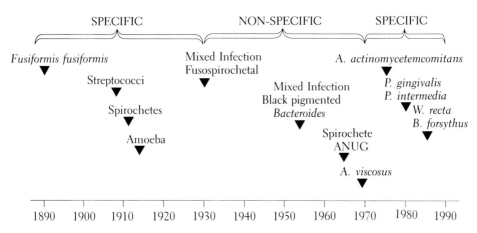

Figure 8.4 Schematic representation of 100 years of periodontal microbiology. (From Socransky SS, Haffajec AD. *J Periodontol* 1992;63:322–331, with permission.)

fusobacteria, amoebae, spirochetes, or streptococci were the primary etiologic agents. With each decade, however, the data linking these bacteria to the etiology of disease proved untrue (33). Thus, from 1930 to the early 1970s, the general belief prevailed that most bacteria on the teeth could cause periodontal disease or, alternatively, that there were minor or nonspecific contributors to disease etiology (33). In the early 1970s, there was a return to the belief that specific bacteria cause periodontal disease, following the pioneering studies of Socransky and Newman, who examined the bacteria in periodontal pockets of children with localized juvenile periodontitis (34). The bacteria present at a site of advanced bone loss and deep pocket formation, such as the first molar, were compared with the bacteria at an adjacent site with no periodontal disease, such as the premolar. Techniques were designed to study highly anaerobic and fastidious microorganisms. The findings were striking for the era and implicated *Actinobacillus actinomycetemcomitans* as a possible pathogen in this disease. Subsequently, many investigators have confirmed and extended these findings and have reported that, out of the more than 300 different types of bacteria that may reside in the oral cavity, only a few, either singly or in combinations, are responsible for the tissue destruction seen in periodontal disease (32–46).

In the late 1970s, the ability to designate specific bacteria as periodontal pathogens was greatly improved by the development of criteria for determining a species as an etiologic agent in periodontal disease. Five criteria were developed: association, elimination, host response, virulence factors, and animal studies (37). The criteria of association implies that the species should be found more frequently and in higher numbers in cases of the infection than in individuals without overt disease. Elimination

Table 8.1 Data that suggest *Porphyromonas gingivalis* as a possible etiologic agent of destructive periodontal diseases

Criterion	Findings
Association	Elevated numbers of organisms in lesions of periodontitis. Unusual in healthy or gingivitis subjects. Present on crevicular epithelial cells.
Elimination	Elimination or suppression resulted in successful therapy. Recurrent lesions harbored species.
Host response	Elevated serum antibody levels in periodontitis. Elevated local antibody response in periodontitis.
Virulence factors	Collagenase, trypsinlike activity, fibrinolysin, other proteases, phospholipase A, phosphatase, endotoxin, H_2S, NH_3, fatty acids and factors that adversely affect polymorphonuclear leukocytes.
Animal studies	Important role in experimental mixed infections. Studies in monkeys and dogs.

SOURCE From Reference 33, with permission.

is based on the concept that elimination of a species should be accompanied by a parallel remission of disease. The criterion of host response, especially the immunological response, implies that the host will produce antibodies or a cellular immune response directed specifically to the pathogenic bacterial species. Virulence factors may be potentially damaging metabolites produced by certain bacterial species which could provide clues to the pathogenicity of the bacterium. And animal studies may provide suggestive evidence that a microbial species plays a role in human disease (33,37,44).

At present, very clear differences in the types of bacteria residing under the gingiva in health and disease have been documented. At healthy sites, the bacteria are largely made up of gram-positive cocci, such as *Actinomyces* and *Streptococci* (35). Bacteria associated with gingivitis comprise increased numbers of *Actinomyces* species and reduced numbers of *Streptococci*. Also, *Fusobacterium nucleatum*, *Lactobacillus*, *Veillonella*, and *Treponema* species have been implicated in causing gingivitis (45).

Adult periodontitis is associated very strongly with *Porphyromonas gingivalis* (33,42). A summary of some of the data implicating this species is provided in Table 8.1. In addition, *Prevotella intermedia*, *Fusobacterium nucleatum*, *Campylobacter* species, *Bacteroides forsythus*, *Selenomonas sputigena*, *Eikenella corrodens*, *Peptostreptococcus* species, and spirochetes may also participate in active adult periodontitis (33). Table 8.2 presents data for these additional species.

As mentioned previously, in juvenile periodontitis, there is strong evidence that A. *actinomycetemcomitans* is one of the primary microorganisms responsible for this disease (33,34,42,44,46). Table 8.3 summarizes data implicating this microorganism in the etiology of juvenile periodontitis.

Table 8.2 Data that suggest additional species as possible etiologic agents of destructive periodontal diseases

	Association	Elimination	Host response	Virulence factors	Animal studies
P. intermedia	+++*	++	++	+++	+++
F. nucleatum	+++	+	+++	++	+
B. forsythus	+++	+	+		+
C. rectus	+++	++			
E. corrodens	+++	+		+	++
P. micros	+++	+	+		
Selenomonas sp	+++				
Eubacterium sp (E. brachy, E. nodatum, E. timidum)	++		++		
Spirochetes	+++	+++	+++	+++	+

*Indicates relative number of publications.
SOURCE From Reference 33, with permission.

Table 8.3 Data that suggest *Actinobacillus actinomycetemcomitans* as a possible etiologic agent of destructive periodontal diseases

Criterion	Findings
Association	Elevated numbers of organisms in lesions of juvenile periodontitis.
	Unusual in healthy or gingivitis subjects.
	Elevated numbers of organisms in some periodontitis lesions.
	Elevated numbers of organisms in active juvenile periodontitis lesions.
	Detected in prospective studies.
	Detected in apical area of pocket or in tissues of LJP* lesions.
Elimination	Elimination resulted in successful therapy.
	Recurrent lesions harbored species.
Host response	Elevated serum antibody levels in juvenile periodontitis.
	Elevated local antibody levels in juvenile periodontitis.
Virulence factors	Leukotoxin, collagenase, endotoxin, epitheliotoxin, fibroblast inhibitory factor, bone resorption inducing factor
Animal studies	Induce disease in gnotobiotic rat.

*LJP = localized juvenile periodontitis.
SOURCE From Reference 33, with permission.

PATHOGENESIS OF THE PERIODONTAL DISEASES

The pathogenesis of periodontal disease is a sequence of processes from health to the formation of characteristic lesions, including periodontal pocket formation, loss of the gingival and periodontal connective tissue attachments, and loss of the tooth-supporting alveolar bone (47–49). Several mechanisms may operate alone or cooperatively to produce the destruction of periodontal tissues.

Bacterial products that are present in the periodontal pocket may exert direct effects. These include histiolytic enzymes, endotoxins, exotoxins, and factors that are not toxic but interfere with cell function. Low-molecular-weight metabolites, such as sulfides and ammonia released by most bacteria in the periodontal pocket, may be cytotoxic in the periodontium. Collagenase and other neutral and acid proteases released by bacteria in the periodontal pocket may destroy collagens, proteoglycans, and connective tissue matrix. Also, bacteria may inhibit or interfere with the normal host defense mechanisms. Some bacteria can inactivate specific antibody, while others can prevent their own phagocytosis and killing by phagocytes (47–49). *Actinobacillus actinomycetemcomitans* produces a toxin that kills human neutrophils and, to a lesser extent, monocytes. Bacterial components such as endotoxin, lipoteichoic acid, and other molecules are potent stimulators of bone resorption (50–55).

Although bacterial substances per se may directly destroy the periodontal tissues, current knowledge reveals that periodontal bacteria cause destruction of the periodontal tissues by activation of host cells and systems to produce and release enzymes and other molecules that destroy the periodontal tissues; these host activities are guided and regulated by the mediators of inflammation. Equally important are components of the immune system, including the secretory immune system, the lymphocyte-macrophage-lymphokine axis, and the antibody-neutrophil-complement axis (48,52).

The role of the lymphocyte-macrophage-lymphokine axis in the susceptibility to and tissue destruction of periodontitis is still unclear. It has been proposed that the destruction of soft tissue and alveolar bone associated with periodontitis is a consequence of the activities of lymphoid cells activated by antigenic components of pocket bacteria. Lymphocytes activated by antigens or mitogens of the periodontal pathogens can stimulate the production of lymphokines. Stimulation of macrophages, either by bacterial products or by the lymphokine IL-2, results in the production of collagenase, leading to collagen dissolution. Stimulation of macrophages by lymphokines or bacterial products can lead to production of reactive-oxygen species that are toxic to local cells (48,52,56,57).

Much of the available evidence indicates that, if the immune system does participate in the destruction of the periodontium, it is likely through the production of interleukins such as osteoclast activating factor (IL-1B) and lymphotoxin (48,52,54–57). The loss of alveolar bone around the teeth is the major pathologic feature of periodontitis and leads directly to tooth loss. The bone destruction in periodontitis, mediated by osteoclasts, is induced and driven by bacterial substances that act directly on bone cells to induce and perpetuate bone resorption or activate other cells and systems to produce substances that induce and perpetuate bone destruction. The arachidonic acid metabolites, such as prostaglandins, as well as the cytokines, seem particularly important in the tissue destruction of periodontitis (52,58–61).

There is much interest in the role of the neutrophil-antibody-complement system in the pathogenesis of periodontal diseases. This axis is thought to be especially important in protecting the host against periodontal bacteria. In the mid-1970s, several landmark studies of patients with defects in neutrophil function indicated that those patients had

severe forms of periodontal disease. For example, patients with compromised neutrophil numbers or neutrophil function, such as those with agranulocytosis, Chédiak-
Higashi syndrome, or diabetes, have severe periodontal disease. Moreover, in severe
forms of periodontal disease in juveniles, such as localized juvenile periodontitis,
neutrophil chemotaxis is depressed (47,48,52,54,55,62,63).

TREATMENT

The primary goal in the treatment of periodontal disease is suppressing or altering the
etiologic bacteria, thus slowing progression of the disease process. In addition, treatment of periodontal disease seeks to regenerate the alveolar bone, periodontal ligament, and root cementum lost as a result of the disease and to prevent the recurrence of
active, progressive disease in patients previously treated (3). The single most important
factor in slowing or arresting disease progression is control of the etiologic bacteria by
mechanical removal. Several treatment regimens may be used, depending on the
severity of the disease. In general, the more advanced the destruction, the more
mechanical intervention will be necessary initially, and this may need to be augmented
with antibiotic treatment. It should also be noted that some patients do not respond to
current methods of mechanical or antibiotic treatment.

In patients with gingivitis but without loss of periodontal attachment, mechanical
removal of bacterial plaque with toothbrushing, supplemented with some type of
interproximal cleaning such as flossing, can remove bacteria and control gingivitis.
Such patients can be treated by their dentist or hygienist by scaling and polishing of the
teeth and instruction in personal oral hygiene, including effective use of the toothbrush
and other auxiliary devices (64).

Mild forms of periodontitis can also be treated with scaling, sometimes with the
addition of root planing, which involves scraping the tooth roots to smooth them and to
remove calculus and bacterial products. Root planing also removes bacterially infected
cementum. Regular scaling and root planing, combined with the patient's daily home
care procedures, can resolve gingivitis and can treat most mild forms of periodontitis
(64).

Once the loss of alveolar bone becomes more advanced, the gingival epithelium
migrates apically along the root to form periodontal pockets. Neither the patient nor
the dentist will be able to clean effectively down to the base of the periodontal pocket
where the disease process is occurring. Periodontal surgery may be necessary to allow
access to the roots for adequate calculus removal and root planing and to reduce the
depths of the periodontal pockets. Surgery is also necessary for access in bone grafting
and regenerative procedures that can stimulate new socket formation of alveolar bone
and periodontal ligament (65–67).

The most common surgical approach is the flap approach. An incision is made
around the necks of the teeth at or slightly apical to the gingival margin, and gingival
tissues are reflected. Once the flap is raised, efforts can be concentrated on removal of
granulation tissue, debridement of the root surface and correction of anatomic defects
created by the periodontal disease process. The gingival flaps are then replaced and

sutured. Healing results in a close adaptation of the gingiva via epithelial attachment to the root surface with much reduced pocket depths (65–71). It has become increasingly apparent in the last several years that mechanical therapy such as surgery is not enough to control certain types of periodontal disease. For example, certain forms of early-onset periodontitis and refractory forms of periodontal disease do not necessarily respond to mechanical treatment alone (21).

Antimicrobial adjuncts to mechanical therapy are becoming increasingly useful. Several antiseptic rinses, such as chlorhexidine, are effective in controlling bacterial plaque on the teeth, with a subsequent decrease in gingivitis (72). In periodontitis, specific periodontal organisms show a great variety of virulence properties and colonization patterns. Given the great variety of colonization mechanisms and virulence patterns and also the need for many different host protective mechanisms to eliminate these organisms, it is clear that mechanical therapy alone is likely not enough. Recently, several oral antibiotics have been particularly useful as adjuncts in the treatment of some types of periodontitis (73). For example, localized juvenile periodontitis has been treated with tetracycline hydrochloride and with a combination of amoxicillin and metronidazole (72–74). Other types of periodontal disease may also be treated with antibiotics. Table 8.4 summarizes antibiotic regimines used to treat several forms of this disease. Refractory periodontitis, for example, has been treated with antibiotics such as amoxicillin, metronidazole, clindamycin, amoxicillin-clavulanate, doxycycline, and ciprofloxacin (72–76).

Recently, there has been a rapid growth in research efforts to assess the efficacy of antibiotics and other antimicrobials placed subgingivally in slow-release vehicles to retard periodontal disease progression. A multicenter trial of tetracycline hydrochloride, locally delivered to periodontal pockets in an acrylic fiber, has been completed. In 113 patients with periodontitis, diseased sites were randomly assigned to one of four

Table 8.4   Systemic antibiotic regimens for periodontal diseases

Disease or condition	Regimen
Localized juvenile periodontitis	Tetracycline hydrochloride 1 g/d, 14–21 d
	Amoxicillin 1 g/d and metronidazole 750 mg/d, 7 d
Refractory periodontitis	Amoxicillin 1 g/d and metronidazole 750 mg/d, 7 d
	Augmentin (amoxicillin and clavulanic acid) and metronidazole 1 g of each for 8 d
	Clindamycin 650 mg/d, 7 d
	Augmentin
	Tetracycline 250–500 mg/d for long periods
	Doxycycline
	Metronidazole
	Culture and appropriate antibiotics; e.g., metronidazole 1 g/d; and ciprofloxacin 1 g/d for 8 d if culture shows enteric rods or pseudomonads

SOURCE From Reference 73, with permission.

treatment groups (tetracycline fiber, control fiber, scaling, or untreated). Disease progression was measured over a 60-day period. All treatment groups improved from baseline; the tetracycline fiber group exhibited significant improvement compared with the other groups with regard to pocket depth reduction, bleeding reduction, and attachment gain (77,78) Similar trials are underway to study the efficacy of local delivery of metronidazole, minocycline and the antiseptic sanguinarine (79). It seems very likely that, as the role of specific bacteria in disease causation is better understood, antibiotics, as well as other antimicrobials that eliminate these specific pathogens, will be used increasingly to treat periodontal disease and will be administered not only by mouth, but also locally (79).

PROSPECTS FOR THE FUTURE

There is much ongoing research in periodontology, and some areas show particular promise for the future management of periodontal disease. A decade of research has focused on new methods of diagnosing periodontal disease, with the hope that it will be possible to better identify persons at risk for periodontal disease, persons with actively progressing periodontal disease, and the response to treatment of periodontal disease (80). Douglas and Fox recently reviewed the goals of newer diagnostic tests in dentistry and expressed the hope that improved diagnosis will make the outcome of treatment more favorable (81).

The measurement of constituents of gingival crevicular fluid, an exudate similar to serum that flows out of the periodontal pocket, shows great promise for improved diagnosis of periodontitis. Crevicular fluid is easily collected, and components are now more readily measured at chairside using diagnostic test kits. Levels of enzymes such as elastase, collagenase, and aspartate aminotransferase, as well as hormones and other substances (prostaglandins and glycosaminoglycans), are reported to be very useful in monitoring the progression of periodontal disease and identifying patients at risk for disease progression (82).

Several microbiologic tests that employ enzyme reactions, DNA probes, or indirect immunofluorescent antibody techniques can detect specific bacteria within the periodontal pocket more readily than can conventional techniques such as culturing. Clinical trials are being conducted to determine the efficacy of these tests, which identify the presence of specific bacteria, in diagnosing active disease or patients at risk for subsequent active disease. Paquette and co-workers, for example, have reported a positive association between the BANA (N-α benzoyl-DL-arginine-2-naphthylamide) test, which detects *P. gingivalis* and *Treponema denticola*, and progression of adult periodontitis (83–85).

A decade of studies from animal models and human trials indicates that pharmacologic agents that block certain host responses involved in the pathogenesis of periodontal destruction can also block the progression of periodontal disease. The production of prostaglandins in the periodontal tissue is apparently an important mediator of periodontal alveolar bone loss. A number of studies indicate that cyclooxygenase inhibitors, such as flurbiprofen, can markedly reduce alveolar bone resorption in animal studies and human trials (86,87). Nonantibiotic, chemically altered tetracyclines are potent inhibitors of collagen destruction in experimental periodontitis in animals (88). This type of agent will likely prove efficacious in slowing human periodontal disease.

There is also exciting research focused on the regeneration of lost periodontal structures through various wound-healing techniques. Several polypeptide growth factors, such as platelet-derived growth factor and insulinlike growth factor-1, have been reported to induce a striking formation of new attachment structures around teeth in animals (89,90). Numerous studies have also been completed on the regeneration of the periodontal attachment structures, using techniques controlling the types of cells repopulating the root surface immediately following surgery. During periodontal surgery, a membrane such as a collagen or Teflon filter is placed around and over the tooth root and alveolar bone. The gingival tissue is returned to its presurgical position and sutured. During wound healing, the membrane prevents the gingival epithelium and connective tissue from contacting the tooth root, thus allowing the tooth root to be repopulated with cells originating from the periodontal ligament rather than the gingival tissue. This technique can lead to the reformation of new root cementum, periodontal ligament, and alveolar bone (91).

In addition, with the recognition that the periodontal diseases are bacterial infections, ongoing research efforts focus on finding the specific bacterial agents that actually cause the disease. In the future, these research findings should produce improved antiinfective strategies for preventing and treating periodontal disease.

ACKNOWLEDGMENTS

I thank Ms. Paula Sudduth, Ms. Anne Schmitt, and Dr. Vivek Doppalapudi for their help in the preparation of this manuscript. I also thank Mr. Steve Schmitt and Dr. Ellen Libert for help with figures. Part of this work was supported by NIDR Grants DE07010, DE08878, and K16 DE00275 and by grants from The Upjohn Company, Block Drug Company, The Institute of Molecular Biology, and the Oral-B Company.

REFERENCES

1   **Weinberger B.** *The History of Dentistry.* St. Louis: C.V. Mosby, 1948.

2   **Shaw JH.** Causes and control of dental caries. *N Engl J Med* 1987;317:996–1004.

3   **Williams RC.** Periodontal disease. *N Engl J Med* 1990;322:373–382.

4   **Williams RC, Zager NI.** The periodontium. In: Shaw JH, Sweeney EA, Cappuccino CC, Meller SM, eds. *Textbook of Oral Biology.* Philadelphia: W.B. Saunders, 1978:255–276.

5   **Klavan B.** *International Conference on Research in the Biology of Periodontal Disease.* Chicago, IL: 1977:134–135.

6   **Page RC.** Gingivitis. *J Clin Periodontol* 1986; 13:345–355.

7   **Goldhaber P, Giddon DB.** Present concepts concerning the etiology and treatment of acute necrotizing ulcerative gingivitis. *Int Dent J* 1964;14:468–496.

8   **Pindborg JJ.** Manifestations of systemic disorders in the periodontium. In: Lindhe J, ed. *Textbook of Clinical Periodontology.* 2nd edition. Copenhagen: Munksgaard, 1989: 282–296.

9   **Burket LW.** A histopathologic explanation for the oral lesions in the acute leukemias. *Am J Orthodontics* 1944;30:516–523.

10 **Chaundry AP, Sabes WR, Gorlin RJ.** Unusual oral manifestations of chronic lymphatic leukemias. *Oral Surg* 1962;15:446–449.

11 Shlossman M, Knowler WC, Pettit DJ, Genco RJ. Type 2 diabetes and periodontal disease. *J Am Dent Assoc* 1990;121:532–536.

12 Loe H, Silness J. Periodontal disease in pregnancy I. Prevalence and severity. *Acta Odont Scand* 1963;21:533–551.

13 Hassell TM. Epilepsy and the oral manifestations of phenytoin therapy. *Monograph in Oral Science*. New York: S. Karger, 1981.

14 Butler RT, Kalkwarf KL, Kaldahl WB. Drug-induced hyperplasia: phenytoin, cyclosporine, and nifedipine. *J Am Dent Assoc* 1987;114: 56–60.

15 Periodontal disease and treatment. *Current Procedural Terminology for Periodontics*. Chicago: American Academy of Periodontology, 1986;1–3.

16 Nevins M, Becker W, Kornman K, eds. *Proceedings of the World Workshop in Clinical Periodontics, Chicago*. American Academy of Periodontology, 1989:I-23–24

17 Genco RJ. Classification and clinical and radiographic features of periodontal disease. In: Genco RJ, Goldman HM, Cohen DW, eds. *Contemporary Periodontics*. Philadelphia: CV Mosby, 1990:63–81.

18 Page RC, Altman LC, Ebersole JL, Vandesteen G, Dahlberg W, Williams B, Osterberg S. Rapidly progressive periodontitis: a distinct clinical condition. *J Periodontol* 1983;54:197–209.

19 Page RC, Bowen T, Altman L, Vandesteen G, Ochs H, Mackenzie P, Osterberg S, Engel D, Williams B. Prepubertal periodontitis: Definition of a clinical disease entity. *J Periodontol* 1983;54:257–271.

20 Winkler JR, Grassi M, Murray PA. Clinical description and etiology of HIV-associated periodontal diseases. In: Robertson PB, Greenspan JS, eds. *Oral Manifestations of AIDS*. Littleton, MA: PSG Publishing, 1988:49–70.

21 Adams DF. Diagnosis and treatment of refractory periodontitis. *Current Opinion in Dentistry* 1992;2:33–38.

22 Johnson ES, Kelly JE, VanKirk LE. Selected dental findings in adults by age, race and sex, U.S. 1960–1962. *Vital Health Statistics* 1965; 11:1–13.

23 Douglas CW, Gillings M, Sollecito W, Gammon M. National trends in the prevalence and severity of the periodontal diseases. *J Am Dent Assoc* 1983;107:403–412.

24 Capilouto ML, Douglass CW. Trends in the prevalence and severity of periodontal diseases in the US: a public health problem? *J Pub Hlth Dent* 1988;48:245–251.

25 US Department of Health and Human Services, Public Health Service, National Institutes of Health. *Oral Health of United States Adults, the National Survey of Oral Health in US Employed Adults and Seniors: 1985–86, National Findings*. NIH pub no 87-2868. Washington, DC: GPO, Aug. 1987.

26 Beck JD, Koch GG, Rozier RG, Tudor GE. Prevalence and risk indicators for periodontal attachment loss in a population of older community-dwelling blacks and whites. *J Periodontol* 1990;61:521–528.

27 Hunt RJ, Levy SM, Beck JD. The prevalence of periodontal attachment loss in an Iowa population aged 70 and older. *J Pub Hlth Dent* 1990;50:251–256.

28 Fox CH. New considerations in the prevalence of periodontal disease. *Current Opinion in Dentistry* 1992;2:5–11.

29 Loe H, Anerud A, Boysen H, Smith M. The natural history of periodontal disease in man. The rate of periodontal destruction before 40 years of age. *J Periodontol* 1978;49:607–620.

30 Becker W, Berg L, Becker BE. Untreated periodontal disease: a longitudinal study. *J Periodontol* 1979;50:234–244.

31 Jeffcoat MK, Reddy MS. Progression of probing attachment loss in adult periodontitis. *J Periodontol* 1991;62:185–189.

32 Socransky SS. Relationship of bacteria to the etiology of periodontal disease. *J Dent Res* 1970;49:203–222.

33 Socransky SS, Haffajee AD. The bacterial etiology of destructive periodontal disease: current concepts. *J Periodontol* 1992;63:322–331.

34 Newman MG, Socransky SS, Savitt ED, Propas DA, Crawford A. Studies of the microbiology of periodontosis. *J Periodontol* 1976;47: 373–379.

35 Slots J. Microflora in the healthy gingival sulcus in man. *Scand J Dent Res* 1977;85:247–254.

36 Slots J. Predominant cultivable microflora of advanced periodontitis. *Scand J Dent Res* 1977;85:114–121.

37 Socransky SS. Criteria for the infectious agents in dental caries and periodontal disease. *J Clin Periodontol* 1979;6:16–21.

38 Slots J. Subgingival microflora and periodontal disease. *J Clin Periodontol* 1979;6:351–382.

39 Tanner ACR, Haffer C, Bratthall GT, Visconti RA, Socransky SS. A study of the bacteria associated with advancing periodontal disease in man. *J Clin Periodontol* 1979;6:278–307.

40 Slots J. Bacterial specificity in adult periodontitis—a summary of recent work. *J Clin Periodontol* 1986;13:912–917.

41 Moore WEC. Microbiology of periodontal disease. *J Periodontal Res* 1987;22:335–341.

42 Genco RJ, Zambon JJ, Christersson LA. The origin of periodontal infections. *Adv Dent Res* 1986;2:245–259.

43 Listgarten MA. Structure of microbial flora associated with periodontal health and disease in man. A light and electron microscopic study. *J Periodontol* 1976;47:1–18.

44 Socransky SS, Haffajee AD. Microbiological risk factors for destructive periodontal diseases. In: Bader JD, ed. *Risk Assessment in Dentistry*. Chapel Hill: U. North Carolina Dental Ecology; 1990:79–90.

45 Moore WEC, Holdeman LV, Smibert RM, Good J, Burmeister JA, Palcanis KG, Ranney RR. Bacteriology of experimental gingivitis in young adult humans. *Infect Immun* 1982;38:651–667.

46 Zambon JJ. *Actinobacillus actinomycetemcomitans* in human periodontal disease. *J Clin Periodontol* 1985;12:1–20.

47 Genco RJ, Slots J. Host responses in periodontal diseases. *J Den Res* 1984;63:441–451.

48 Genco RJ. Pathogenesis and host responses in periodontal disease. In: Genco RJ, Goldman HM, Cohen DW, eds. *Contemporary Periodontics*. St. Louis: CV Mosby, 1990;184–193.

49 Genco RJ. Host responses in periodontal diseases: current concepts. *J Periodontol* 1992;63:338–355.

50 Shenker BJ, Kushner ME, Tsai CC. Inhibition of fibroblast proliferation by *Actinobacillus actinomycetemcomitans*. *Infect Immun* 1982;38:986–992.

51 Shenker BJ, Tsai CC, Taichman NS. Suppression of lymphocyte responses by *Actinobacillus actinomycetemcomitans*. *J Periodontal Res* 1982;17:462–465.

52 Page RC. Pathogenic mechanisms. In: Schluger S, Yuodelis R, Page RC, Johnson RH, eds. *Periodontal Diseases*. Philadelphia: Lea and Febiger, 1989:221–262.

53 Raisz LG, Nuki K, Alander CB, Craig RG. Interactions between bacterial endotoxin and other stimulators of bone resorption in organ culture. *J Periodontal Res* 1981;16:1–7.

54 Listgarten MA. Pathogenesis of periodontitis. *J Clin Periodontol* 1986;13:418–425.

55 Listgarten MA. Nature of periodontal diseases: pathogenic mechanisms. *J Periodontal Res* 1987;22:172–178.

56 Horton JE, Raisz LG, Simmons HA, Oppenheim JJ, Mergenhagen SE. Bone resorbing activity in supernatant fluid from cultured human peripheral blood leukocytes. *Science* 1972;177:793–795.

57 Dewhirst FE, Stashenko PP, Mole JE, Tamotsu T. Purification and partial sequence of human osteoclast-activating factor: identity with interleukin-1-beta. *J Immunol* 1985;135:2562–2568.

58 Goldhaber P, Rabadjija L, Beyer W, Kornhauser A. Bone resorption in tissue culture and its relevance to periodontal disease. *J Am Dent Assoc* 1973;87:1027–1033.

59 Goodson JM. A potential role of prostaglandins in the etiology of periodontal disease. In: Kahn RH, Lands WEM, eds. *Prostaglandins and Cyclic AMP*. New York: Academic Press, 1973:215–216.

60 Ranney RR. Immunologic mechanisms of pathogenesis in periodontal diseases: an assessment. *J Periodontal Res* 1991;26:243–254.

61 Page RC. The role of inflammatory mediators in the pathogenesis of periodontal disease. *J Periodontal Res* 1991;26:230–242.

62 Cianciola LR, Genco RJ, Patters MR, McKenna J, Van Oss CJ. Defective polymorphonuclear leukocyte function in a human periodontal disease. *Nature* 1977;265:445–447.

63 Clark RA, Page RC, Wilde G. Defective neutrophil chemotaxis in juvenile periodontitis. *Infect Immun* 1977;18:694–700.

64 Ciancio SG. Non-surgical periodontal treatment. In: Nevins R, Becker W, Kornman K, eds. *Proceedings of the World Workshop of Clinical Periodontics*. Chicago: Amer Acad Perio, 1989;II-1–12.

65 McHugh WD. *Surgical Therapy for Periodontitis*. National Institute of Dental Research, Bethesda: GPO, 1981.

66 Rabbani GM, Ash MM, Caffesse RG. The effectiveness of subgingival scaling and root planing in calculus removal. *J Periodontol* 1981;52:119–123.

67 Kalkwarf KL. Tissue attachment. In: Nevins R, Becker W, Kornman K, eds. *Proceedings of the World Workshop in Clinical Periodontics*. Chicago: Amer Acad Perio, 1989;V-1–19.

68 Schluger S. Osseous resection: a basic principle in periodontal surgery. *Oral Surg* 1949;2:316–325.

69 Caffesse RG. Resective procedures. In: Nevins R, Becker W, Kornman K, eds. *Proceedings of the World Workshop of Clinical Periodontics*. Chicago: Amer Acad Perio, 1989;IV-1–21.

70 Barrington EP. An overview of periodontal surgical procedures. *J Periodontol* 1981;52:518–528.

71 **Barrington EP.** Moderate chronic adult periodontitis: current concepts. In: Wilson T, Kornman K, Newman M, eds. *Advances in Periodontics.* Chicago: Quintessence, 1992: 144–147.

72 **Rees TD.** Adjunctive therapy. In: Nevins R, Becker W, Kornman K, eds. *Proceedings of the World Workshop in Clinical Periodontics.* Chicago: Amer Acad Perio 1989;X-1–31.

73 **Genco RJ.** Using antimicrobial agents to manage periodontal diseases. *J Am Dent Assoc* 1991;122:31–38.

74 **Slots J, Rams TE.** Antibiotics in periodontal therapy: advantages and disadvantages. *J Clin Periodontol* 17:479–493.

75 **Ciancio S.** Antibiotics in periodontal care. In: Newman MG, Kornman KS, eds. *Antibiotic/ Antimicrobial Use in Dental Practice.* Chicago: Quintessence, 1990;136–147.

76 **Loesche WJ, Schmidt E, Smith BA, Morrison EC, Caffesse RG, Hujoel P.** Effect of metronidazole on periodontal treatment needs. *J Periodontol* 1991;62:247–257.

77 **Goodson JM, et al.** Multi-center evaluation of tetracycline fiber therapy I. Experimental design. *J Periodontal Res* 1991;26:361–370.

78 **Goodson JM, et al.** Multi-center evaluation of tetracycline fiber therapy II. Clinical response. *J Periodontal Res* 1991;26:371–379.

79 **Fiorellini JP, Paquette DW.** The potential role of controlled-release delivery systems for chemotherapeutic agents in periodontics. *Current Opinion in Dentistry* 1992;2:63–79.

80 **Fine DH.** Incorporating new technologies in periodontal diagnosis into training programs and patient care: a critical assessment and a plan for the future. *J Periodontol* 1992;63:383–393.

81 **Douglas CH, Fox CH.** Determining the value of a periodontal test kit. *J Periodontol* 1991;62: 721–730.

82 **Curtis MA, Gillett IR, Griffeths GS, Maiden MFJ, Sterne JAC, Wilson DT, Wilton JMA, Johnson NW.** Detection of high-risk groups and individuals for periodontal diseases. Laboratory markers from analysis of crevicular fluid. *J Clin Periodontol* 1989;16:1–11.

83 **Savitt ED, Strzempko MN, Vaccaro KK, Peros WJ, French CK.** Comparison of cultural methods and DNA probe analysis for the detection of *Actinobacillus actinomycetemcomitans, Bacteroides gingivalis* and *Bacteroides intermedius* in subgingival plaque samples. *J Periodontol* 1988; 59:431–438.

84 **Zambon JJ, Reynolds HS, Chen P, Genco RJ.** Rapid identification of periodontal pathogens in subgingival dental plaque. Comparison of indirect immunofluorescence microscopy with bacterial cultures for detection of *Bacteroides gingivalis. J Periodontol* 1985;56:32–40.

85 **Paquette DN, Fiorellini JP, Howell TH, Weber HP, Williams RC.** Periodontal disease and health as monitored with sequential probing and the BANA test. *J Dent Res* 1992 (in press, abstract).

86 **Williams RC.** The use of non-steroidal antiinflammatory drugs in periodontal disease. In: Lewis AJ, Furst DE, eds. *New Antiinflammatory Drugs: Mechanisms and Clinical Use.* New York: Marcel Dekker, 1987:143–155.

87 **Howell TH, Williams RC.** Altering periodontal disease progression with non-steroidal antiinflammatory drugs. *Crit Rev Oral Biol Med* 1992:72:856 (abstract).

88 **Golub LM, Ramamurthy N, McNamara TF, Gomes B, Wolff M, Cesino A, Kapoor A, Zambon J, Ciancio S, Schneir M, Perry H.** Tetracyclines inhibit tissue collagenase activity. A new mechanism in the treatment of periodontal disease. *J Periodontal Res* 1984;19: 651–655.

89 **Lynch SE, Williams RC, Polson AM, Howell TH, Reddy MS, Zappa VE, Antoniades HN.** A combination of platelet-derived and insulinlike growth factors enhances periodontal regeneration. *J Clin Periodontol* 1989;16:545–548.

90 **Schallhorn RG.** Present status of osseous grafting procedures. *J Periodontol* 1977;48: 570–576.

91 **Nyman S, Gottlow J, Lindhe J, Karring T, Wennstrom J.** New attachment formation by guided tissue regeneration. *J Periodontal Res* 1987;22:252–254.

Diagnosis and management of perianal and perirectal infection in the granulocytopenic patient

KENNETH V. I. ROLSTON
GERALD P. BODEY

INTRODUCTION

Infection poses the greatest risk to the neutropenic cancer patient. It is the proximate cause of death in 50% of patients with solid tumors and lymphomas and in 75% of patients with acute leukemia (1). During the last two decades, improvements in the supportive care of neutropenic cancer patients has resulted in a decrease in infection-related morbidity and mortality. Nonetheless, tissue infections such as pneumonitis, neutropenic colitis, and perianal/perirectal infections are still associated with substantial morbidity and mortality, particularly when caused by aerobic, gram-negative bacilli.

The gastrointestinal tract serves as an important focus for bacterial and fungal infections, especially in patients with cancer. These patients frequently receive antineoplastic therapy that is often associated with gastrointestinal side effects such as mucosal erosion and diarrhea. Disruption of normal anatomical barriers, combined with the myelosuppressive effects of chemotherapy, renders patients at considerable risk of developing infections that originate from the gastrointestinal tract. Perirectal infections, however, are still relatively uncommon even in cancer patients, and the proper management of these infections is controversial. It is well accepted that perirectal infection is an urgent problem requiring prompt therapy; most of the controversy regarding the management of this infection centers around the necessity of surgical intervention.

PATIENT POPULATION AND PREDISPOSING FACTORS

The majority of patients with cancer who develop perirectal infections have underlying hematological malignancies, although these infections are being observed with increasing frequency in patients with solid tumors (Table 9.1) (2–7). They have been estimated to occur in 10% of patients with leukemia at autopsy examination and up to 23% of patients with acute leukemia undergoing chemotherapy. Tissue infiltration with leukemic cells is more common in monocytic leukemias than in other varieties of leukemia.

Table 9.1   Underlying diagnosis in cancer patients with perirectal infections

Diagnosis	NCI series*		M. D. Anderson series[†]	
	No.	%	No.	%
Leukemia	27	61	50	82
Acute lymphocytic	10		10	
Acute myelogenous	10		30	
Chronic lymphocytic	2		3	
Chronic myelogenous	2		4	
Other leukemia	3		3	
Solid tumors	17	39	11	18
Lymphomas	7		2	
Sarcomas	4		2	
Lung carcinoma	4		1	
Other solid tumors	2		6	
Total no. of patients	44		61	

*Reference 4.
[†]Reference 17.

Perirectal infections have been observed to be particularly common in patients with acute monocytic and acute myelomonocytic leukemia, suggesting that leukemic infiltration of tissues might play a role in the pathogenesis of these infections (2).

The vast majority of perirectal infections occurred during relapse of leukemia (4). They may occur in newly diagnosed patients with leukemia or during initial remission induction chemotherapy. Occasionally, they may serve as the presenting sign of acute leukemia (8). A few of these infections occur in patients with lymphoma or disseminated solid tumors, and they are almost never seen during periods of remission.

The most common predisposing factor is neutropenia, which is found in over 90% of patients who develop perirectal infections (4). The depth of neutropenia also appears to be important. VanHeuverzwyn et al. found that, among patients with hematologic diseases, perirectal infections developed in 11% who had severe neutropenia (<500 neutrophils/mm^3) but in only 0.4% of patients who did not (9). Since many solid tumors are now being treated with very intensive and myelosuppressive chemotherapeutic regimens and occasionally with bone marrow transplantation, which produce prolonged periods of severe neutropenia, the incidence of perirectal infections has increased in such patients.

CLINICAL FEATURES

The predominant presenting symptom is rectal pain that is aggravated by the act of defecation. Most patients (>95%) are febrile, often with a hectic or septic temperature pattern. Hypotension or frank septic shock may occur in up to 10% of patients,

Table 9.2 Common clinical findings in neutropenic patients with perirectal infections

Findings	Percentage
Local	
Pain/tenderness	74
Fluctuance	50–55
Drainage	35–50
Fissure	43
Hemorrhoids	31
Erythema/cellulitis	30
Induration	28
Necrosis	26
True abscess	<10
General	
Fever	97
Associated bacteremia	61–87
Diarrhea	26
Constipation	11
Shock	5–10

SOURCE From References 4, 17.

particularly in those with gram-negative bacteremia (Table 9.2). The perirectal lesion is usually discrete, erythematous, and indurated, and fluctuance may be elicited as the infection progresses. True abscess formation is rare, probably as a consequence of severe neutropenia (10). The lesion may extend into the rectum, resulting in extensive local necrosis and sloughing of tissue. Up to 50% of patients may develop a serosanguinous or bloody discharge. In some instances, only local erythema and cellulitis are observed, and development of a discrete perirectal lesion does not occur.

The infection often arises at the site of a preexisting fissure or hemorrhoid, and, due to the blunting of inflammatory responses in neutropenic patients, the severity of the local process may not be fully appreciated. Prior intestinal dysfunction, such as diarrhea or constipation, is not uncommon and may facilitate the development of infection. Persistence of hemorrhoids or rectal fissures may serve as a focus for relapses or recurrent infections after the acute episode has been treated successfully.

MICROBIOLOGY

The majority of these infections are polymicrobial. The organisms isolated most often are aerobic, gram-negative bacilli of enteric origin, especially *Pseudomonas aeruginosa* and *Escherichia coli* (Table 9.3). *P. aeruginosa* in particular has the propensity for invading the walls of blood vessels and causing vasculitis and tissue necrosis (11,12). Gram-positive organisms, particularly coagulase-negative *Staphylococci* and the *Enterococci*, are also frequently present. Superinfections with *Candida* species are not

Table 9.3   Microorganisms frequently isolated
from perirectal infections in cancer patients

Gram negatives
Escherichia coli
Pseudomonas aeruginosa
Klebsiella species
Proteus species
Citrobacter species
Enterobacter species
Serratia species

Gram positives
Coagulase-negative *Staphylococcus* species
Staphylococcus aureus
Enterococcus species

Anaerobes
Bacteroides fragilis
Clostridium species

Yeast
Candida species

uncommon. The role of anaerobic organisms in this infection has not been fully
defined because anaerobic cultures have not often been obtained. When anaerobes are
isolated, the predominant organisms are *Bacteroides* species and *Clostridium* species
(4,13). Most of these are isolated from the local perianal lesions. When the infection
has been associated with septicemia, anaerobes have been cultured from blood infrequently. Septicemia is almost always caused by single or multiple gram-negative bacilli. In our experience, approximately 85% of these infections are polymicrobial,
while a single organism is isolated from about 15%. More than two organisms are
isolated from approximately 50% of lesions.

TREATMENT

The proper management of perirectal infection consists of antimicrobial therapy, general measures, and surgical intervention (see Table 9.4). The administration of broad-
spectrum antibiotics and symptomatic therapy is accepted practice. The use and timing
of surgical intervention continues to be debated. Newer modalities such as monoclonal
antibodies and the cytokines may be beneficial and need to be evaluated.

Antimicrobial therapy

Various antimicrobial combinations have been used to provide coverage against enteric gram-negative bacilli, gram-positive cocci, and anaerobes. Combinations of an

Table 9.4 Therapy of perirectal infections in neutropenic cancer patients

Symptomatic therapy
Sitz baths
Warm compresses
Stool softeners
Analgesics, antipyretics

Antimicrobial therapy
Broad-spectrum antimicrobial combinations
    Aminoglycoside + antipseudomonal penicillin or ticarcillin/clavulanate
    Aminoglycoside + extended-spectrum cephalosporin or monobactam
    Specific gram-positive and/or anaerobic drugs (vancomycin, clindamycin, metronidazole)
    Antifungal or antiviral drugs
    Oral, nonabsorbable, gut-sterilizing regimens

Surgery
Needle aspiration
Incision and drainage
Wide debridement

Other measures
Radiation (?)
Granulocyte transfusions
Gut-sterilizing regimens
Monoclonal antibodies against endotoxins
Cytokines (G-CSF; GM-CSF)

aminoglycoside (tobramycin, amikacin) with an antipseudomonal penicillin (mezlocillin, piperacillin) or an extended-spectrum cephalosporin with activity against *P. aeruginosa* (ceftazidime, cefoperazone) are commonly used. Newer β-lactam agents with broad antimicrobial activity (imipenem, ticarcillin/clavulanate) are also useful. Vancomycin, clindamycin, and metronidazole are used frequently to provide specific gram-positive and anaerobic coverage. Antifungal therapy (amphotericin B, fluconazole, 5-flucytosine) or antiviral therapy (acyclovir) might occasionally become necessary. Gut-sterilizing oral antibiotic regimens may have some value in reducing contamination of ulcerated lesions by fecal flora. In some patients, a diverting colostomy may become necessary. Symptomatic treatment consists of sitz baths or warm compresses, the use of stool softeners, and analgesics.

Surgery

Anorectal infection in patients without neutropenia has classically been treated with prompt surgical intervention (14). However, in neutropenic patients, a more conservative approach has usually been recommended with respect to surgical procedures due to the frequent presence of thrombocytopenia in these patients, which substantially increases the risk associated with surgery. Needle aspiration may be performed to relieve pain and to collect specimens for culture. If an abscess is present, it should be incised and drained, but most patients do not develop abscesses. In these situations, surgery may not be beneficial and could actually be detrimental. Serious surgical complications such as severe hemorrhage, sloughing, extension of soft tissue infection, and poor wound healing have been reported following incision and drainage in such patients. In a review of 57 episodes of perirectal infections in 44 patients with malignant diseases at the National Cancer Institute, it was concluded that surgery should be performed only in the presence of obvious fluctuance or a significant amount of necrotic tissue, or in the face of progression of the local infection and/or continued sepsis after an adequate trial of antibiotic therapy (4). However, in a recent report of 16 leukemic patients with perirectal infections, relief of symptoms and recovery followed a more aggressive approach (15). Five patients had spontaneous drainage, whereas 10 patients underwent surgical incision and drainage because spontaneous drainage had not occurred. The lesions consisted of necrotic cavities with tissue debris. Scant watery or serosanguinous fluid was drained, resulting in relief of pain, resolution of fever, minimal complications of surgery, and good wound healing. These investigators and others have recommended early surgical intervention even in the absence of fluctuant lesions (15,16). Our own experience at the University of Texas M. D. Anderson Cancer Center favors aggressive surgical intervention; we recommend obtaining a surgical opinion early in the course of infection (17).

In addition to antibiotics, symptomatic therapy, and surgery, treatment of the affected area with local radiation has been attempted in the past. However, a randomized, double-blind study failed to confirm the utility of this approach in 35 leukemic patients with anorectal infections (18). With the current availability of effective chemotherapy, the likelihood of local radiation being of added benefit is minimal. Patients who recover from perianal or perirectal infections that originated from hemorrhoids or anal fissures should undergo hemorrhoidectomy or fissurectomy when they achieve a remission of their underlying disease. If this is not done, they are likely to have recurrent infections when their disease recurs or with subsequent courses of chemotherapy.

Other therapeutic modalities

The overall mortality associated with perirectal infections is in the range of 15–35%, with many deaths occurring in patients with bacteremia and septic shock. In this situation, patients may benefit from the administration of monoclonal antibodies directed against endotoxins (although this form of therapy has not been specifically evaluated in this setting). In the neutropenic patient, resolution of infection often depends on the neutrophil count. As the patient's neutrophil count increases, an abscess may develop at the site of infection, requiring incision and drainage. Persistence of severe neutropenia is associated with substantial mortality. In the series from the National Cancer Institute, 88% of episodes of perirectal infection associated with more than 28 days of neutropenia ended fatally, and 65% of episodes in patients with neutropenia lasting more than seven days had a similar outcome (4). In contrast, only 13% of patients with perirectal infection and neutropenia lasting less than seven days died ($p = 0.0004$). In our own experience, greater than 90% of deaths occur in patients who are severely neutropenic for more than 15 days. Selected patients with severe and persistent neutropenia might benefit from granulocyte transfusions (19). Some investigators have administered granulocytes locally into the perirectal lesions in order to maximize the concentrations of these cells at the site of infection. This form of treatment, however, has not been definitively studied. Newer therapeutic modalities such as granulocyte macrophage colony stimulating factor (GM-CSF) and granulocyte colony stimulating factor (G-CSF) have been shown to reduce the duration of chemotherapy-induced neutropenia (20). Whether these agents will be useful in reducing the incidence of infection or in improving the outcome of an established infection remains to be seen.

SUMMARY AND RECOMMENDATIONS

Perirectal infection is an uncommon but serious complication in neutropenic cancer patients. Conservative medical management of this infection with antibiotics and supportive measures is successful in a substantial number of patients. Broad-spectrum antimicrobial regimens directed against aerobic gram-negative bacilli, anaerobes, and the enterococci, form the cornerstone of therapy. We recommend the combination of an antipseudomonal β-lactam and an aminoglycoside for optimal efficacy and potential for reducing the emergence of resistant organisms (21). Symptomatic management includes the administration of stool softeners, analgesics, and sitz baths. Gut-sterilizing, oral antimicrobial regimens may be useful in reducing fecal contamination at local ulcerated lesions. Prompt and aggressive surgical incision and drainage is of benefit in patients not responding to conservative management. Granulocyte transfusions or the cytokines (G-CSF, GM-CSF) should probably be used routinely in patients with severe and persistent neutropenia, since the neutrophil plays a critical role in combating these infections. Monoclonal antibodies directed against endotoxins may be of benefit in patients with gram-negative bacteremia and/or septic shock.

REFERENCES

1   **Bodey GP.** Infections in cancer patients. *Cancer Treat Rev* 1975;2:89–128.

2   **Schimpff SC, Wiernik PH, Block JB.** Rectal abscesses in cancer patients. *Lancet* 1972; 2:844–847.

3   **Sehdev MK, Dowling MD Jr, Seal SH, Sterans MW Jr.** Perianal and anorectal complications in leukemia. *Cancer* 1973;31:149–152.

4   **Glenn J, Cotton D, Wesley R, Pizzo P.** Anorectal infections in patients with malignant diseases. *Rev Infect Dis* 1988;10:42–52.

5   **Birnbaum W, Ahlquist R.** Rectal infections and ulcerations associated with blood dyscrasias. *Am J Surg* 1955;90:367–372.

6   **Earle MF, Fossieck BE Jr, Cohen MH, Ihde DC, Bunn PA Jr, Minna JD.** Perirectal infections in patients with small cell lung cancer. *JAMA* 1981;246:2464–2466.

7   **Merrill JM, Brereton HD, Kent CH, Johnson RE.** Anorectal disease in patients with non-haematological malignancy. *Lancet* 1976;1: 1105–1107.

8   **Kott I, Urca I.** Perianal abscess as a presenting sign of leukemia. *Dis Colon Rectum* 1969; 12:338–339.

9   **Vanheuverzwyn R, Delannoy A, Michaux JL, Dive C.** Anal lesions in hematologic diseases. *Dis Colon Rectum* 1980;23:310–312.

10 **Bodey GP, McKenna RJ Jr.** Surgical considerations in the immunocompromised cancer patient. In: McKenna R, Murphy GP, eds. *Fundamentals of Surgical Oncology.* New

York: Macmillan Publishing Company, 1986: 114–140.

11 Givler RL. Necrotizing anorectal lesions associated with *Pseudomonas* infection in leukemia. *Dis Colon Rectum* 1969;12:438–440.

12 Rolston K, Bodey GP. *Pseudomonas aeruginosa* infection in cancer patients. *Cancer Investigation* 1992;10:43–59.

13 Brook I, Martin WJ. Aerobic and anaerobic bacteriology of perirectal abscesses in children. *Pediatrics* 1980;66:282–284.

14 Hagihara P, Howard R. Anal and perianal infections. In: Simmons R, Howard R, eds. *Surgical Infectious Diseases.* New York: Appleton-Century-Crofts, 1982:987–995.

15 Barnes SG, Sattler FR, Ballard JO. Perirectal infections in acute leukemia: improved survival after incision and debridement. *Ann Intern Med* 1984;100:515–518.

16 Silen W. Rectal abscesses in cancer patients (letter). *Lancet* 1973;1:553.

17 Rolston K, Paulino A, Elting L, Joshi J, Bodey GP. Perirectal infections in cancer patients (Abstract no. 966). In: *Programs and Proceedings of the 27th Interscience Conference on Antimicrobial Agents and Chemotherapy.* New York: October 5–7, 1987.

18 Levi JA, Schimpff SC, Slawson RG, Wiernik PH. Evaluation of radiotherapy for localized inflammatory skin and perianal lesions in adult leukemia: a prospectively randomized double-blind study. *Cancer Treat Rep* 1977;61: 1301–1305.

19 Clift RA, Buckner CD. *Granulocyte Transfusions in Infectious Complications of Neoplastic Disease, Controversies in Management.* Brown Arthur E, Armstrong Donald, eds. York Medical Books, 1985:269–279.

20 Crawford J, Ozer H, Stoller I, et al. Reduction by granulocyte colony-stimulating factor of fever and neutropenia induced by chemotherapy in patients with small-cell lung cancer. *New Engl J Med* 1991;325:164–170.

21 Rolston K, Berkey P, Bodey GP, et al. A comparison of imipenem to ceftazidime with or without amikacin as empiric therapy in febrile neutropenic patients. *Arch Intern Med* 1992; 152:283–291.

Hemolytic uremic syndrome: clinical picture and bacterial connection

JULIE PARSONNET
PATRICIA M. GRIFFIN

INTRODUCTION

Definition and spectrum of HUS and TTP

Hemolytic uremic syndrome (HUS) and thrombotic thrombocytopenic purpura (TTP) constitute two acute syndromes of thrombotic microangiopathy. HUS, a leading cause of renal failure in children, is characterized clinically by microangiopathic hemolytic anemia, thrombocytopenia, renal failure, and variable central nervous system (CNS) symptoms (1). TTP, a disease of adults, is defined by the same tetrad of findings as HUS, with the addition of fever and more prominent neurologic findings. Although differences in the clinical and epidemiologic features of these two illnesses distinguish them from one another, they appear to represent the same pathogenic process: deposition of hyaline thrombi in small blood vessels with consumption coagulopathy.

HUS, has long been thought to be caused by an infectious agent. Its seasonal distribution, its occurrence in epidemics and familial clusters, and its association with diarrhea all suggest an infectious disease (2). Numerous gastrointestinal pathogens, in particular Shiga-like, toxin-producing strains of *Escherichia coli* (enterohemorrhagic *E. coli*) (3–7) and *Shigella dysenteriae* type 1 (8–13) have been implicated in disease causation. HUS has also been attributed to nongastrointestinal infections, as well as to defects in serum complement (1), chemotherapy (14), and immunosuppressants in organ transplantation (Table 10.1) (15–17).

Unlike HUS, TTP has not been consistently associated with specific underlying disease processes, infectious or noninfectious (18–20). A small minority of TTP cases are preceded by diarrheal disease and may be identical in pathogenesis to classical HUS. Because HUS is so typically linked to infectious agents, while TTP has only rarely been correlated with a preceding infectious disease, this chapter will focus on the former syndrome. It should be understood, however, that some TTP cases are undoubtedly synonymous with HUS.

Table 10.1 Categories of HUS

Categories	Percentage of occurrence
I. Diarrhea-related (classical) HUS	85–95
II. Non-diarrhea-related HUS	5–15
A. Postinfectious	5–10
B. Immunosuppression-related	<5
1. Chemotherapy	
2. Complement deficiency	
3. Transplant immunosuppression	
C. Pregnancy or oral-contraceptive related	Rare
D. Hereditary	Rare

Epidemiology of HUS

HUS was first reported in 1955 in Switzerland (21). Since then, foci of endemic disease have been identified in temperate climates throughout the developed world (19). Regions that report significant disease risk include the northwestern United States, western Canada, northern Europe, and South Africa. In Argentina, the risk of HUS in children less than four years old may be as high as 21.7 per 100,000 per year (22). Regions of high risk within countries exist as well. In Canada, in 1986–1988, the annual incidence of HUS in the western province of Alberta was 2.78 per 100,000, three times the incidence in the province of Ontario (0.97 per 100,000) (23).

Although HUS can occur at any age, most cases worldwide occur in children younger than five years old. In developed countries, HUS has a summer peak incidence and occurs most frequently in children from higher socioeconomic groups (19,23–25). Some investigations suggest a slight female predilection for HUS (23,25,26).

Since its description, the reported incidence of HUS has increased (19). While improved recognition of the syndrome may account for some of this increase, the severity of clinical presentation makes it unlikely that the rise can be attributed to improved recognition alone (27). In King County, Washington, the incidence of HUS in children less than 15 years old increased from 0.69 per 100,000 between 1971 and 1975 to 1.77 in 1976–1980 (27). In Minnesota, the incidence of HUS in children less than 18 years old increased from 0.5 per 100,000 in 1979 to 2.0 in 1988 (28). The increase was most marked for children less than five years old (from 1.6 cases per 100,000 in 1979 to 5.8 cases per 100,000 in 1988). Similar increases have been seen in the Netherlands (29) and the United Kingdom (30).

INFECTIONS ASSOCIATED WITH HUS

While many infections have been linked to HUS (Table 10.2), only three, *Shigella dysenteriae* type 1, *Escherichia coli* O157:H7, and *Streptococcus pneumoniae*, have been extensively studied. Other enterohemorrhagic *E. coli* besides *Escherichia coli*

Table 10.2   Infections associated with the hemolytic uremic syndrome

---

Infections strongly associated with HUS
Escherichia coli O157:H7
Shigella dysenteriae type 1
Streptococcus pneumoniae
Infections possibly associated with HUS
Other Shigalike, toxin-producing *E. coli*
Salmonella typhi
Infections anecdotally associated with HUS (partial list)
Aeromonas hydrophila
Campylobacter jejuni
Shigella flexneri
Yersinia entercolitica
Yersinia pseudotuberculosis
Enteroviruses
Adenovirus
Multiple viruses

O157:H7 have been implicated, but evidence for their association with HUS is less compelling. The remaining infectious pathogens can best be termed anecdotally related to a microangiopathic process.

Shigella dysenteriae type 1

In 1973, Ullis et al. reported hemolytic anemia and thrombocytopenia associated with S. *dysenteriae* type 1 infection (the Shiga bacillus) in a Guatemalan child (12). Although the investigators called the hematologic picture disseminated intravascular coagulation, in retrospect, this may be the first reported case of HUS caused by an infectious agent. Over the subsequent two decades, HUS from S. *dysenteriae* type 1 has been identified as the primary cause of acute renal failure in children of the Indian subcontinent (11).

Because resources are often quite limited in countries with endemic S. *dysenteriae* type 1 infection, the risk of HUS in infected patients is difficult to estimate. In Vellore, India, 40 (13%) of 320 patients admitted to the hospital with "bacillary dysentery" developed HUS (11). Unfortunately, stool cultures were performed only on 29 of the 40 patients, and only 10 had positive cultures; of these, nine patients' stools grew S. *dysenteriae* type 1, and one grew *Shigella flexneri*. While it is likely that the remaining dysentery patients also were infected with *Shigella* sp, other infectious and noninfectious etiologies cannot be excluded.

In Bangladesh, 9 (4%) of 241 patients hospitalized for S. *dysenteriae* type 1 infection developed hemolytic uremic syndrome (defined as blood urea nitrogen > 100 mg/dL). An additional 19 patients (8%) had hemolysis with mild renal insufficiency (13). None of the 34 adults in the study developed hematologic or renal complications.

A similar pattern for HUS due to S. *dysenteriae* type 1 was recently observed in the United States. In a 1988 outbreak of S. *dysenteriae* type 1 infections among U.S.

tourists to Mexico, two (5%) of 42 patients, including one child (age seven years) and one adult (age 57 years), developed HUS. An additional child (age two years) developed severe hemolysis, thrombocytopenia, and hematuria without renal failure (10). Because sicker patients would be more likely to seek medical care, both of these studies may overestimate the risk of HUS secondary to *S. dysenteriae* type 1.

Several studies demonstrate that a profound leukemoid reaction with *S. dysenteriae* type 1 infection marks persons at risk for HUS (11,13). Similarly, intestinal obstruction, previous use of antibiotics to which *S. dysenteriae* type 1 is resistant, and severe bloody diarrhea may indicate persons at high risk for complication by HUS (9,11,13,31).

Shiga-like toxin-producing *E coli*

While *S. dysenteriae* type 1 is responsible for the majority of cases of HUS in developing regions, in the industrialized world, the organisms most closely associated with HUS belong to the species *Escherichia coli*. *E. coli* can be classified into four pathogenic groups: enterotoxigenic, enteropathogenic, enteroinvasive, and Shiga-like toxin producers (32). This section will focus on the last of these, the Shiga-like, toxin-producing *E. coli* (SLTEC). The term enterohemorrhagic *E. coli* (EHEC) refers to a defined subset of SLTEC that cause hemorrhagic colitis, produce one or more phage-encoded, Shigalike toxins, possess a 60-megadalton virulence plasmid, and produce attaching-effacing lesions in an animal model (19).

***E coli* O157:H7**   In 1982, two outbreaks of a distinctive bloody diarrheal syndrome led to the identification of *E. coli* O157:H7 as a cause of human disease (33). But while *E. coli* O157:H7 can be called a "new" pathogen, it is not considered rare. In surveillance studies in the United States, Canada, and the United Kingdom, it has been cultured from between 0.5% and 1.7% of diarrheal stool samples, making it more common than *Shigella* and *Yersinia* sp (34–38). If only bloody stools are evaluated, *E. coli* O157:H7 may account for 15% of diarrheal pathogens (39,40). Paradoxically, however, this relatively common diarrheal pathogen is rare in the developing world (19,41).

Infection with *E. coli* O157:H7 may produce a spectrum of diseases, from asymptomatic carriage to hemorrhagic colitis. Typical illness begins with nonbloody diarrhea and severe abdominal cramps. Abdominal symptoms may be sufficiently severe to lead to surgical intervention (23,28,42). In the majority of cases, the stools become bloody on the second or third day of illness, with the amount of blood ranging from streaks to stools that are essentially all blood; unlike bacillary dysentery, mucus is not a feature of *E. coli* O157:H7 diarrhea (5,34,43). Approximately half the patients experience nausea and vomiting. Fever occurs in fewer than one-third of patients and is typically low grade; high fever is a sign of more severe illness (5). Diarrhea usually resolves spontaneously six to eight days after onset (5,43).

In 1980, Karmali first noted the association of EHEC with HUS when he isolated a Shiga-like, toxin-producing *E. coli* from the bowel of a patient with fatal HUS (44). Numerous subsequent studies have shown a consistent association between infection and microangiopathy (45–49). Thirty to 75% of HUS patients had serologic, microbiologic, or toxicologic evidence of SLTEC infection, and between 8% and 63% were found to have specifically *E. coli* O157:H7 in their stools (23,28,44,46–49). The lower isolation rate of *E. coli* O157:H7 in the earlier studies may be partially attributed to the facts that cultures were often taken late in the course of illness and that culture methods had not yet been optimized. In one study, a remarkable 96% of cultures taken from HUS patients during the first six days of diarrheal illness yielded *E. coli* O157:H7 (49). Thus, it appears that *E. coli* O157:H7 is a more common cause of HUS in developed areas than are all the other causes combined (19).

Outbreaks of *E. coli* O157:H7 infections have facilitated understanding of its relationship to HUS. Between 1982 and 1990, 12 outbreaks were investigated in the United States, affecting 654 people (19). The majority of cases resulted from eating bacterially contaminated foods of bovine origin, although some cases, in particular those in day care and chronic care facilities, were attributable to person-to-person transmission (19). In the combined studies, 21% of patients were hospitalized (range: 2% to 73%), and 4% developed HUS or TTP (range: 0% to 19%); 2% of outbreak patients died. Since only a small minority of *E. coli* O157:H7-infected patients progress to HUS, factors in addition to infection must play a part in disease pathogenesis. Reported risk factors for developing microangiopathy among patients with *E. coli* O157:H7 infection include very young or old age, female sex, mental retardation, P antigen expression by red blood cells, bloody diarrhea, fever, elevated leukocyte count early in the diarrheal illness, use of antimotility agents, and use of antimicrobial therapy for the diarrhea (19). Many of these risk factors remain controversial. Only extremes of age have been consistently linked to development of HUS (4,5,39,50).

Other enterohemorrhagic *E. coli*   Little is known about non-O157 SLTEC serotypes and human disease. Over 25 non-O157 SLTEC serotypes have been isolated from humans with diarrhea. No single non-O157 serotype predominates, but *E. coli* O26:H11 is the most frequently reported (19).

A two-year survey of diarrheal stools in Canada found that 36 (0.7%) of 5,415 specimens grew non-O157 SLTEC, a higher isolation rate than that of *Shigella* (0.5%); seven (19%) of the 36 specimens with non-O157 SLTEC, however, also grew *E. coli* O157:H7 (37). Significant differences in the clinical manifestations of illness due to non-O157 SLTEC and *E. coli* O157:H7 were observed; 42% of patients with diarrhea due to non-O157 SLTEC had bloody diarrhea, compared with 97% for patients with *E. coli* O157:H7. Diarrhea also lasted longer in patients with non-O157 SLTEC (nine versus six days).

Rates of non-O157 SLTEC infection similar to those in the Canadian study have been found in Korean children (0.9%) (51), Chilean children (52), and Thai adults (53). In Argentina, a non-O157 SLTEC was detected in one (2.3%) of 44 children with diarrhea, but 11 (25%) had free fecal toxin or seroconversion to Shiga-like toxin. The authors believed that non-O157 SLTEC may be an important cause of diarrhea in that area (22).

Pneumococcus

The only gram-positive bacterium associated with HUS is *Streptococcus pneumoniae*. Including the first two cases described in 1977 (54), 16 cases of pneumococcal infection with HUS have been reported (55–58). In 13 cases, the age of the child was specified;

all were previously healthy children less than five years old; 85% were less than two years old. Over 90% were bacteremic, usually with a primary pulmonary source.

Infants with pneumococcus-related HUS are sicker than children with classical diarrheal HUS. All reported patients required dialysis, and the total mortality rate was quite high (40%). Whether the poor prognosis of this HUS form relates to the very young age of the patients or to the pathogen itself is not known. Because pneumococcal HUS is rare, there have been no systematic studies, and true incidence of this complication remains unknown.

Infections sporadically associated with HUS

Numerous other organisms have been linked to development of HUS, although none has been more than anecdotally reported (Table 10.1), including diarrheal (59–64) and nondiarrheal pathogens (57,65–69). For some, such as *Salmonella typhi*, the data is the most convincing. In one study, six (12.5%) of 48 patients with typhoid developed HUS (70). For other organisms, such as *Aeromonas hydrophila* and *Campylobacter jejuni*, the prodromal illness is compatible with the classical prodrome, and there is a potential pathogenic mechanism (both organisms may produce low levels of Shigalike toxins), but a causal association remains uncertain (62,71). Reports of patients with *E. coli* O157:H7-associated HUS who had evidence of concomitant infection with *Blastocystis hominis*, adenovirus, and *Salmonella* dictate caution in ascribing causality to other organisms when SLTEC were not sought (19). Further epidemiologic and laboratory studies are needed to define the possible role of these other organisms in HUS.

PATHOGENESIS OF INFECTION-ASSOCIATED HUS

The underlying process in HUS is thrombotic microangiopathy. Arterioles and capillaries become occluded with hyaline thrombi composed of platelet aggregates and fibrin. This causes consumption of platelets and coagulation factors, destruction of red blood cells, and finally anoxic damage to the organs supplied by the obstructed vessels. There is no evidence of a vasculitis or inflammation specific to the vascular endothelium (20).

Although pathogenesis of the thrombotic process is not well understood, recent research on virulence properties of *S. dysenteriae* type 1 and EHEC grants insight into disease mechanism. Three pathogenetic factors appear be intertwined in the disease process: cytotoxin, endotoxin, and leukocytes. Separately, these factors may be insufficient to cause illness, but their combined effects provide a credible scenario for disease pathogenesis.

Toxins and endothelial damage

Two types of toxins have been considered pathogenic in HUS: the Shiga-like toxins and endotoxin.

Shiga toxin and Shiga-like toxins   SLTEC produce two cytotoxins, Shiga-like toxin I (SLT I) and Shiga-like toxin II (SLT II). These SLT (also known as verotoxins) are so named because of their close resemblance to the Shiga toxin produced by *S.*

dysenteriae type 1 (30,71). While the gene for Shiga toxin in *S. dysenteriae* type 1 is chromosomal, genes for SLTs are phage-encoded, which suggests that *E. coli* may have acquired these toxins through phage-mediated transfer (72).

SLT I is is genetically and antigenically indistinguishable from Shiga toxin. SLT II, on the other hand, is antigenically distinct and shows 58% overall DNA homology with SLT I (71). Despite this difference, Shiga, SLT I, and SLT II share the same receptor and have similar structures and modes of action. Five smaller B subunits bind to the glycolipid cell surface receptor, globotriosylceramide (Gb3). Following binding and internalization, the active subunit catalyzes cleavage of ribosomal RNA, disrupting protein synthesis and causing cell death (71).

In vitro, Shiga toxin is directly toxic to rapidly dividing human umbilical endothelial cells (73). The toxin binds to Gb3 endothelial cell receptors and decreases protein synthesis, an effect that can be neutralized by anti-Shiga toxin antibody. Endothelial cell damage caused by the cytotoxins may contribute to pathogenesis of HUS by causing necrosis of the microvasculature in the intestine and facilitating entry of the cytotoxins and endotoxin into the bloodstream (74). Subsequent cytotoxin damage to systemic endothelial cells can precipitate thrombosis by systemically decreasing endothelial prostacyclin generation and fibrinolysis, increasing endothelial factor VIII release, and causing appearance on the cell surface of von Willebrand factor (2,20,75). While this hypothesis is plausible, Shiga toxin has not been demonstrated to be toxic to the slowly dividing endothelial cells of human glomeruli, only to rapidly dividing tissue culture cells (73). Identification of free toxin in the circulation would lend further credence to a role for Shiga in HUS, but, to date, free toxins have not been identified in the blood of patients with EHEC or *S. dysenteriae* type 1 infection.

Several retrospective studies show that strains of *E. coli* O157:H7 that produce SLT II or both SLTs are much more likely to induce HUS than strains producing SLT I only (47,76). This is surprising in light of the association of *S. dysenteriae* type 1, which only produces Shiga toxin (a toxin identical to SLT I), with HUS. Further studies focusing on the differences between the SLTs are needed to advance understanding of their independent roles in human disease.

Endotoxin   Endotoxin, with or without Shiga toxin or SLT, may play a part in microangiopathy and its renal, hematologic, and neurologic consequences. While it is not known whether endotoxin circulates in the blood of patients with enterohemorrhagic *E. coli* infection, in one study, nine of 18 patients hospitalized in Bangladesh with *Shigella* infection and hemolysis had circulating endotoxin by the limulus assay (13).

In tissue culture, LPS directly damages glomerular endothelial cells (77). Louise and Obrig hypothesized that some of endotoxin's deleterious effects are mediated through the production of tumor necrosis factor (TNF) (78). TNF, like SLT, is directly cytotoxic. Together, TNF and Shiga toxin are synergistically cytotoxic to cultured cells, an effect neutralized by antibodies directed against either toxin. The investigators speculate that Shiga toxin primes the endothelial cell for damage by TNF.

In addition to its cytotoxic effects, TNF induced by endotoxin may alter endothelial cell surface proteins, such as thrombomodulin and membrane-associated tissue factor, and cause release of tissue plasminogen activator. These changes transform the normally inactive endothelial cell to a thrombogenic cell (20).

Leukocytes and tissue damage

In children with S. *dysenteriae* type 1, *E. coli* O157:H7 infection, and perhaps *Salmonella typhi* infection, a leukemoid reaction appears to increase risk for development of HUS (13,26,50,70). Leukocytes are now thought to play a part in mediating the thrombotic process. In a rabbit model, animals injected with endotoxin developed glomerular fibrin deposition, renal cortical necrosis, and renal insufficiency. Leukopenia protected rabbits from these effects (79). Neutrophils from patients with HUS are more adherent to endothelial cells than are neutrophils from unmatched controls (80). Antibodies directed against the neutrophil surface proteins minimize this attachment and limit endothelial damage in tissue culture.

Some investigators postulate that endotoxin is responsible for leukocyte-related damage. Activation of leukocytes by endotoxin releases cytokines and free radicals that could potentially augment cell damage (74). In vivo, leukocytes may only serve as mediators of endotoxin-related endothelial injury.

Neuraminidase

Cytotoxins and endotoxin may explain HUS related to *E. coli* O157:H7 and *Shigella*, but they cannot account for HUS seen with S. *pneumoniae*. For the pneumococcus, the enzyme neuraminidase has been suggested as the critical causative factor (54). All pathogenic pneumococci produce neuraminidase, a low-molecular-weight protein that facilitates tissue invasion by cleaving cell membrane glycoproteins and glycolipids (81). Some investigators maintain that neuraminidase cleaves terminal sialic acid residues, exposing the T (Thomsen-Friedenreich) antigen on capillary walls, platelets, and red cells to circulating anti-T IgM (54). This results in agglutination of cells and platelets and thrombosis of small vessels. In support of this hypothesis, peanut lectin, which binds to exposed T antigen, also binds to renal tissue and red blood cells of patients with HUS (55). Furthermore, IgM deposits are found in affected glomeruli (56). Neuraminidase production by pneumococcus is the norm, however, and HUS associated with infection is rare. Other pathogenic factors in pneumococcal HUS still need to be investigated.

P_1 blood group antigen

Pentaosyceramide, the P_1 blood group antigen, is a globoseries glycolipid, capable of binding Shiga toxin and the Shiga-like toxins (82). In one study, patients with weaker expression of P_1 on red blood cells had higher rates of HUS, possibly because P_1 was not available to bind circulating toxin and prevent endothelial exposure (83).

CLINICAL PRESENTATION

Prodrome

HUS has long been noted to succeed prodromal illnesses, usually diarrheal in nature. In four recent series, the proportion of HUS cases with a diarrheal prodrome varied from

86% to 95% (22–24,28); 75% of these patients described bloody diarrhea (23,24). In some patients, gastrointestinal complaints may mimic an acute abdomen and provoke unnecessary laporatomy. Intussusception and rectal prolapse may occur (24,26,28).

In less than 10% of cases, HUS may succeed or coincide with a respiratory illness (24,28,82). Two of 21 children with HUS in a U.S. hospital presented with primary pulmonary symptoms and pneumonia (82). In bone marrow transplant patients with HUS, respiratory findings are common. In one study, six of ten bone marrow transplant patients with HUS presented with respiratory complaints ranging from mild cough and dyspnea to frank hemoptysis and respiratory failure (16). All six patients had at least one underlying infection, including herpes simplex (2), *Aspergillus* (2), *Candida* (1), *Pseudomonas* (1), and hepatitis B (1).

HUS usually occurs six to 10 days after the diarrheal prodrome begins and, in scattered reports, three to five after onset of respiratory symptoms (19,55,56,84). A small number of cases of HUS will occur without prodromal illness. Some of these may be the rare instances of familial or recurrent HUS (85).

Hematologic abnormalities

While renal and neurologic diseases may vary in their intensity, as the syndrome name implies, marked disruption of blood elements is a sine qua non of HUS. All patients with HUS have evidence of microangiopathic hemolytic anemia. In one series, the mean serum hemoglobin in 67 children was 5.9 g/dL (57). Schistocytes will be found on the blood smear, and blood chemistries will show evidence of intravascular hemolysis (elevated lactate dehydrogenase (LDH) and unconjugated bilirubin, decreased haptoglobin). Thrombocytopenia is seen in 83% to 96% of patients with thrombotic microangiopathy and often is sufficiently grave to cause purpura, petechiae, and life-threatening gastrointestinal hemorrhage (20,86).

Coagulation factors are not prominently affected in HUS. In one-quarter of patients, fibrin-split products may be mildly elevated, but other clotting factors generally remain unaltered (20). The mild fibrinogen consumption compared with the degree of thrombocytopenia distinguishes HUS from disseminated intravascular coagulation (84). Levels of complement components C3 and C4 may be depressed (13).

Some patients with the typical diarrheal prodrome will develop abnormal hematologic values in the absence of uremia or neurologic complications (87). This "incomplete" HUS has been reported with both *E. coli* O157:H7 and *S. dysenteriae* type 1 infection (10,13,26).

Renal and metabolic abnormalities

To meet the definition of HUS, all patients with HUS must have some degree of uremia, although an absolute value for elevated blood urea has not been defined. Seventy-five to 95% of children with HUS will have some degree of oligoanuria within one week of disease onset (23,24,57). Proteinuria and hematuria are almost invariable, and proteinuria may reach the nephrotic range. Hyponatremia is seen in the majority of children, and a quarter have hyperkalemia. Fifty percent to 75% will require dialysis during the acute stages of disease (23,24,57).

Acute renal failure appears to be attributable to two distinct histopathologic patterns of vascular pathology. In persons with a diarrheal prodrome, the predominant lesion is glomerular capillary thrombosis with arteriolar necrosis (57,84). A variable degree of renal cortical necrosis results. In older patients and those without the typical prodrome, intimal proliferation with luminal stenosis involves larger vessels of the preglomerular vasculature. This latter type of disease has a poorer prognosis and is not thought to be reversible (57).

One-third of children develop hypertension, and a cardiomyopathy has also been described in rare instances (24,57,84). There are anecdotal reports of diabetes mellitus occurring after HUS, but no causal relationship has been established (24).

Neurologic abnormalities

Central nervous system signs and symptoms in HUS include irritability, seizures, drowsiness, ataxia, reduced consciousness, paralysis, and coma (28,84). These alterations may result directly from CNS microangiopathy but more commonly are consequent to hypertension, CNS hemorrhage, or metabolic abnormalities (e.g., uremia, hyponatremia). Seizures are the most common neurologic manifestation in HUS and occur in 20% to 50% of children (23,24,28). In one study, over half of the patients with seizures had concomitant hypertension and/or hyponatremia (24).

Prognosis

HUS is a life-threatening disease, with a mortality rate ranging from 3% to 7% (23,24, 28,57,84). Deaths most commonly occur in the very young and the very old and are usually ascribed to CNS complications and/or discontinuation of renal dialysis (24,88). Persons with a diarrheal prodrome have a better prognosis than those without diarrhea (83,89). In cases with a diarrhea prodrome, prolonged anuria indicates greater risk of a poor outcome (57,83,90). HUS associated with pneumococcal sepsis has a particularly poor outcome.

In children who survive acute illness, the long-term outcome from HUS is usually favorable. Less than 2% progress to end-stage renal failure, and between 2% and 10% have hypertension without renal failure (24,90,91). One-third of patients, however, will have increased albumin excretion years after the acute illness, and one-fifth will have a reduced glomerular filtration rate (90,91). Children who suffered a neurologic insult may be left with residual damage, including developmental, cognitive, motor, or behavioral problems (84).

DIAGNOSIS OF HUS-RELATED INFECTION

Culture

Stools from patients with diarrhea-related HUS should be cultured for routine enteric pathogens (*Salmonella*, *Shigella*, *Campylobacter*) and for *E. coli* O157:H7. Because *E. coli* O157:H7 does not ferment sorbitol rapidly, sorbitol MacConkey agar can be used to screen clinical stool specimens quickly (40). Coliform colonies that are colorless at 24 hours on sorbitol MacConkey agar can then be identified using direct agglutination with commercially available latex-conjugated O157 antisera (92). Stools from children with recent travel to a less developed area should be cultured specifically for S. *dysenteriae* type 1. Unlike the other *Shigella* sp, S. *dysenteriae* type 1 may be fragile on routinely used media (salmonella-shigella and xylose-lactose-deoxycholate agars), and nonselective media such as tergitol-7 and MacConkey agar enhance isolation (10). Although an association between HUS infection and *Aeromonas hydrophila* has not been established, in regions where E. *coli* O157:H7 is rare, stools might also be cultured on media selective for *Aeromonas hydrophila* (32). Cultures should be done as early in the illness as possible. E. *coli* O157:H7 is easily isolated from feces in the first week after symptoms begin, but becomes difficult to isolate thereafter (93).

Detection of other SLTEC is more problematic since serotyping of E. *coli* is only possible at large reference laboratories. Identification of free SLT in stools, however, allows nonspecific detection of SLTEC. Sensitive enzyme-linked immunosorbent assays for detection of SLTs in culture or stool extracts and DNA probes for SLTEC genes have been created (94–97). The polymerase chain reaction is also being developed for detection of Shiga and Shigalike toxins (98,99). Unfortunately, none of these assays is yet commercially available. Marketing of these tests may eventually facilitate diagnosis of SLTEC in hospital and public health laboratories.

Patients without a diarrheal prodrome are unlikely to have E. *coli* O157:H7 or *Shigella* infection (19). In these patients, blood cultures should be performed, particularly if respiratory symptoms are present.

Serology

Antibodies to lipopolysaccharide of O157 have been detected in sera of patients with recent E. *coli* O157:H7 infection and may be useful in determining the cause of hemolytic uremic syndrome (100,101). In an outbreak setting, an IgG ELISA for anti-O157 antibody was over 90% sensitive and specific for patients with recent culture-confirmed infection (102).

TREATMENT

The mainstays of treatment of HUS are supportive. Patients frequently require packed red blood cells and attention to metabolic abnormalities such as hyponatremia. Platelet transfusions may worsen the microangiopathy and are only recommended when platelet counts are extremely low or when active bleeding occurs. Children with diarrhea-related HUS may be significantly hypovolemic and may require volume replacement with crystalloid. Some authors suggest that vigorous volume replacement and diuresis may prevent additive renal insult by urate and hemoglobin (84). Children who remain anuric despite volume replacement will require dialysis.

Although patients with S. *typhi* or S. *pneumoniae* will clearly require antimicrobial therapy, the question of antibiotic use in patients with diarrheal HUS remains unresolved. Poor outcome associated with antibiotic use was first reported with *Shigella*-related HUS. Treatment with an antimicrobial agent to which the infecting organism was resistant accelerated progression to HUS (9,10). In two studies of *E. coli* O157:H7 infections, treatment with trimethoprim-sulfamethoxazole was also associated with an increased risk of HUS or TTP (50,76). Two other studies, however, showed a protective effect of antibiotics (4,28). Some investigators have reported that subinhibitory concentrations of antimicrobial agents can increase production of Shiga-like toxin (103,104). Prospective studies are needed to determine the risk and benefits of antimicrobial drug therapy for diarrhea due to *Shigella* and *E. coli* O157:H7.

Antimotility agents in diarrhea-related HUS, like antibiotics, are also controversial. Receiving an antimotility agent for more than 24 hours was a risk factor in one study (4). Until further studies of these agents are done, their use is unwarranted.

Increasingly, plasma exchange is being recommended for treatment of TTP. Several studies show dramatically improved prognoses in adult patients who have undergone this therapy (105,106). It is speculated that the provision of new plasma provides thombolytic components of the coagulation system that interrupt the production of new hyaline thrombi. One study has shown excellent outcome in HUS-infected children treated with plasma infusion (107). Because most children with HUS resolve their disease spontaneously, however, plasma exchange is not generally used, and its role in treatment should be addressed in randomized trials.

CONCLUSION

HUS, a major cause of acute renal failure in young children, can be divided into HUS with and without diarrhea. HUS with diarrhea accounts for approximately 90% of cases and appears to be occurring with increasing frequency in the United States. The majority of cases is attributable to bacterial infection, principally to infection with a newly identified pathogen, *E. coli* O157:H7. Infections with this organism, which is largely transmitted by consumption of contaminated foods of bovine origin, appear to be increasing parallel to the apparent increase in HUS infections (19).

While treatment of HUS remains largely supportive, infectious disease practitioners must remain alert to cases of bloody diarrhea and diarrhea-related HUS in the community. The characteristic syndrome of hemorrhagic colitis should warn health care providers of a possible outbreak of *E. coli* O157:H7 infections. Stool cultures early in the course of illness can prompt recognition of infection, allow identification of exposed groups, and limit transmission of a potentially fatal infection.

REFERENCES

1 Kaplan BS, Proesmans W. The hemolytic uremic syndrome of childhood and its variants. *Semin Hematol* 1987;24:148–160.

2 Kavi J, Wise R. Causes of haemolytic uraemic syndrome. *BMJ* 1989;298:65–66.

3 Neill MA, Tarr PL, Clausen CR, et al. *Escherichia coli* O157:H7 as the predominant pathogen associated with the hemolytic uremic syndrome: a prospective study in the Pacific Northwest. *Pediatrics* 1987;80:37–40.

4 Cimolai N, Carter JE, Morrison BJ, et al. Risk factors for the progression of *Escherichia coli* O157:H7 enteritis to hemolytic-uremic syndrome. *J Pediatr* 1990;116:589–592.

5 Griffin PM, Ostroff SM, Tauxe RV, et al. Illnesses associated with *Escherichia coli* O157:H7 infections. *Ann Intern Med* 1988;705:705–712.

6 Gransden WR, Damm MAS, Anderson JD, et al. Haemorrhagic cystitis and balanitis associated with verotoxin-producing *Escherichia coli* O157:H7 (Letter). *Lancet* 1985;2:150.

7 Karmali MA, Steele BT, Petric M, et al. Sporadic cases of haemolytic-uraemic syndrome associated with faecal cytotoxin and cytotoxin-producing *Escherichia coli* in stools. *Lancet* 1983;1:619–620.

8 Raghupathy P, Date A, Shastry JCM, et al. Haemolytic-uraemic syndrome complicating *Shigella* dysentery in south Indian children. *Br Med J* 1978;1:1518–1521.

9 Butler T, Islam MR, Azad MAK, et al. Risk factors for development of hemolytic uremic syndrome during shigellosis. *Pediatrics* 1987; 110:894–897.

10 Parsonnet J, et al. *Shigella dysenteriae* type 1 in U.S. tourists to Mexico. *Lancet* 1988;2: 543–545.

11 Rahaman MM, Jamiul Alam AKM, Islam MR, et al. Shiga bacillus dysentery associated with marked leukocytosis and erythrocyte fragmentation. *Johns Hopkins Med J* 1975;136:65–70.

12 Ullis KC, Rosenblatt RM. Shiga bacillus dysentery complicated by bacteremia and disseminated intravascular coagulation. *J Pediatr* 1973;83:90–93.

13 Koster F, Levin J, Walker L, et al. Hemolytic-uremic syndrome after shigellosis: Relation to endotoxemia and circulating immune complexes. *N Engl J Med* 1978;927–933.

14 Gradishar WJ, Vokes EE, Ni K, et al. Chemotherapy-related hemolytic-uremic syndrome after the treatment of head and neck cancer. A case report. *Cancer* 1990;66:1914–1918.

15 Giroux L, Smeesters C, Corman J, et al. Hemolytic uremic syndrome in renal allografted patients treated with cyclosporin. *Can J Physiol Pharm* 1987;65:1125–1131.

16 Juckett M, Perry EH, Daniels BS, Weisdorf DJ. Hemolytic uremic syndrome following bone marrow transplantation. *Bone Marrow Transplant* 1991;7:405–409.

17 Rabinowe SN, Soiffer RJ, Tarbell NJ, et al. Hemolytic-uremic syndrome following bone marrow transplantation in adults with hematologic malignancies. *Blood* 1991;77: 1837–1844.

18 Ridolfi RL, Bell WR. Thrombotic thrombocytopenic purpura: report of 25 cases and review of the literature. *Medicine* 1981;60:413–428.

19 Griffin PM, Tauxe RV. The epidemiology of infections caused by *Escherichia coli* O157:H7, other enterohemorrhagic *E. coli*, and the associated hemolytic uremic syndrome. *Epidemiol Rev* 1991;13:80–92.

20 Case Records of the Massachusetts General Hospital (Case 30-1991). *N Engl J Med* 1991; 325:265–273.

21 Gasser C, Gautier E, Steck A, et al. Hamolytisch-uramische syndrome: Bilaterale nierenrindennekrosen bei akuten erworbenen hamolytischen anamien. *Schweiz med Wschr* 1955; 85:205–209.

22 Lopez EL, Diaz M, Grinstein S, et al. Hemolytic uremic syndrome and diarrhea in Argentine children: the role of Shiga-like toxins. *J Infect Dis* 1989;160:469–475.

23 Rowe PC, Orrbine E, Wells GA, et al. The epidemiology of hemolytic uremic syndrome in Canadian children, 1986–1988. *J Pediatr* 1991; 119:218–224.

24 Milford DV, Taylor CM, Guttridge B, et al. Haemolytic uraemic syndromes in the British Isles 1985–8: association with verocytotoxin producing *Escherichia coli*. Part 1: Clinical and epidemiological aspects. *Arch Dis Child* 1990; 65:716–721.

25 Waters HR. Enterohemorrhagic *Escherichia coli* and hemolytic uremic syndrome—the Alberta experience. *Can Dis Weekly Report* 1989;15:9–12.

26 Rowe PC, Walop W, Lior H, Mackenzie AM. Haemolytic anaemia after childhood *Escherichia coli* O157:H7 infection: are females at increased risk? *Epidemiol Infect* 1991; 106:523–530.

27 Tarr PI, Neill MA, Allen J, et al. The increasing incidence of the hemolytic-uremic syndrome in King County, Washington: lack of evidence for ascertainment bias. *Am J Epidemiol* 1989;129: 582–586.

28 Martin DL, MacDonald KL, White KE, et al. The epidemiology and clinical aspects of the hemolytic uremic syndrome in Minnesota. *N Engl J Med* 1990;323:1161–1167.

29 Van Wieringen PM, Monnens LAH, Schretlen EDAM. Haemolytic-uraemic syndrome. Epidemiologic and clinical study. *Arch Dis Child* 1974;49:432–437.

30 PHLS Communicable Disease Surveillance Center. Haemolytic uraemic syndrome surveillance. British paediatric surveillance unit/ CDSC surveillance scheme. *Communicable Disease Report* 1990;90/21:1

31 Bennish ML, Azad AK, Yousefzadeh D. Intestinal obstruction during shigellosis: incidence, clinical features, risk factors and outcome. *Gastroenterol* 1991;101:626–634.

32 Farmer JJ, Kelly MT. Enterobacteriaceae. In: Balows A, Hausler WJ, Herrman KL, Isenberg HD, Shadomy HJ, eds. *Manual of Clinical Microbiology*. Washington DC: American Society of Microbiology, 1991.

33 Riley LW, Remis RS, Helgerson SD, et al. Hemorrhagic colitis associated with a rare *Escherichia coli* serotype. *N Engl J Med* 1983;308:681–685.

34 MacDonald KL, O'Leary MJ, Cohen ML, et al. *Escherichia coli* O157:H7, an emerging gastrointestinal pathogen: Results of a one-year prospective population-based study. *JAMA* 1988;259: 3567–3570.

35 Marshall WF, McLimans CA, Yu PK, et al. Results of a 6-month survey of stool cultures for *Escherichia coli* O157:H7. *Mayo Clinic Proc* 1990;65:787–792.

36 Cahoon FE, Thompson JS. Frequency of *Escherichia coli* O157:H7 isolation from stool specimens. *Can J Microbiol* 1987;33:914–915.

37 Pai CH, Ahmed N, Lior H, et al. Epidemiology of sporadic diarrhea due to verocytotoxin-producing *Escherichia coli*: a two-year prospective study. *J Infect Dis* 1988;157:1054–1057.

38 Walker CW, Upson R, Warren RE. Haemorrhagic colitis: detection of verotoxin producing *Escherichia coli* O157 in a clinical microbiology laboratory. *J Clin Pathol* 1988;41:80–84.

39 Pai CH, Gordon R, Sims HV, et al. Sporadic cases of hemorrhagic colitis associated with *Escherichia coli* O157:H7: clinical, epidemiologic, and bacteriologic features. *Ann Intern Med* 1984;101:738–742.

40 March SB, Ratnam S. Sorbitol-MacConkey medium for detection of *Escherichia coli* O157: H7 associated with hemorrhagic colitis. *J Clin Microbiol* 1987;23:869–872.

41 Seriwatana J, Brown JE, Echeverria P, et al. DNA probes to identify shiga-like toxin I- and II-producing enteric bacterial pathogens isolated from patients with diarrhea in Thailand. *J Clin Microbiol* 1988;26:1614–1615.

42 Neill MA, Agosti J, Rosen H. Hemorrhagic colitis with *Escherichia coli* O157:H7 preceding adult hemolytic uremic syndrome. *Arch Intern Med* 1985;45:2215–2217.

43 Riley LW. The epidemiologic, clinical and microbiologic features of hemorrhagic colitis. *Ann Rev Microbiol* 1987;41:383–407.

44 Karmali MA, Steele BT, Petric M, et al. Sporadic cases of haemolytic-uraemic syndrome associated with faecal cytotoxin and cytotoxin-producing *Escherichia coli* in stools. *Lancet* 1983;1:619–620.

45 Remis RS, MacDonald KL, Riley LW, et al. Sporadic cases of hemorrhagic colitis associated with *Escherichia coli* O157:H7. *Ann Intern Med* 1984;101:624–626.

46 Karmali MA, Petric M, Lim C, et al. The association between idiopathic hemolytic uremic syndrome and infection by verotoxin-producing *Escherichia coli*. *J Infect Dis* 1985;151:775–782.

47 Scotland SM, Rowe B, Smith HR, et al. Vero cytotoxin-producing strains of *Escherichia coli* from children with haemolytic uraemic syndrome and their detection by specific DNA probes. *J Med Microbiol* 1988;25:237–243.

48 Klenthous H, Smith HR, Scotland SM, et al. Haemolytic uraemic syndrome in the British Isles, 1985–5: association with verocytotoxin producing *Escherichia coli*. Part 2: microbiological aspects. *Arch Dis Child* 1990;65:722–727.

49 Tarr PI, Neill MA, Clausen CR, et al. *Escherichia coli* O157:H7 and the hemolytic uremic syndrome: importance of early cultures in establishing the etiology. *J Infect Dis* 1990; 162:553–556.

50 Pavia AT, Nichols CR, Green DP, et al. Hemolytic-uremic syndrome during an outbreak of *Escherichia coli* O157:H7 infections in institutions for mentally retarded persons: clinical and epidemiologic observations. *J Pediatr* 1990;116:544–551.

51 Kim KH, Suh IS, Kim JM, et al. Etiology of childhood diarrhea in Korea. *J Clin Microbiol* 1989;27:1192–1196.

52 Levine MM, Xu J, Kaper JB, et al. A DNA probe to identify enterohemorrhagic *E. coli* of 157:H7 and other serotypes that cause hemorrhagic colitis and hemolytic uremic syndrome. *J Infect Dis* 1987;156:175–182.

53 Bettelheim KA, Brown JE, Lolekha S, et al. Serotyes of *Escherichia coli* that hybridized with DNA probes for genes encoding Shiga-like toxin I, Shiga-like toxin II, and serogroup O157 enterohemorrhagic *E. coli* fimbriae isolated from adults with diarrhea in Thailand. *J Clin Microbiol* 1990;28:293–295.

54 Klein PJ, Bulla M, Newman RA, et al. Thomsen-Friedenreich antigen in haemolytic uraemic syndrome. *Lancet* 1977;1:24–25.

55 Feld LG, Fildes RD. Pneumococcal pneumonia and hemolytic uremic syndrome. *Pediatr Infect Dis J* 1987;6:693–694.

56 Alon U, Adler SP, Chan JCM. Hemolytic uremic syndrome associated with Streptococcus pneumoniae. *Am J Dis Child* 1984; 138:496–499.

57 Loirat C, Sonsino F, Moreno AV, et al. Hemolytic-uremic syndrome: An analysis of the natural history and prognostic features. *Acta Paediatr Scand* 1984;73:505.

58 Begue R, Dennehy PH, Peter G. Hemolytic uremic syndrome associated with Streptococcus pneumoniae. *N Engl J Med* 1991;325:133–134.

59 Prober CG, June B, Hoder L. Yersinia pseudotuberculosis septicemica. *Am J Dis Child* 1979;33:623–624.

60 Tsukahara H, Hayashi S, Nakamura K, et al. Haemolytic uremic syndrome associated with Yersinia entercolitica infection. *Pediatr Nephrol* 1988;2:309–314.

61 Chamovitz BN, Hartsein AI, Alexander SR, et al. Campylobacter jejuni-associated hemolytic-uremic syndrome in a mother and daughter. *Pediatrics* 1983;71:253–256.

62 Delans RJ, Biuso JD, Saba SR, et al. Hemolytic uremic syndrome after Campylobacter-induced diarrhea in an adult. *Arch Intern Med* 1984;144:1074–1076.

63 San Joaquin EH, Pickett DA. Aeromonas-associated gastroenteritis in children. *Pediatr Infect Dis J* 1988;7:53–57.

64 Bogdanovic R, Cobeljic M, Markovic M et al. Hemolytic uremic syndrome associated with Aeromonas hydrophila enterocolitis. *Pediatr Nephrol* 1991;5:293–295.

65 Blachar Y, Leibovitz E, Levin S. The interferon system in two patients with hemolytic uremic syndrome associated with adenovirus infection. *Acta Paediatr Scand* 1990;79:108–109.

66 Austin TW, Ray CG. Coxsackie virus group B infections and the hemolytic-uremic syndrome. *J Infect Dis* 1971;127:698–701.

67 Ray GC, Tucker VL, Harris HJ, et al. Enteroviruses associated with the hemolytic-uremic syndrome. *Pediatrics* 1970;46:378–384.

68 O'Regan S, Robitaille P, Mongean JG, et al. The hemolytic uremic syndrome associated with ECHO 22 infection. *J Pediatr* 1980;19:25–27.

69 Bryce RP, Preiksaitis JK, Devine RD, et al. Haemolytic uraemic syndrome: evidence for multiple viral infections in a cluster of ten cases. *J Med Virol* 1983;12:51–59.

70 Baker NM, Mills AE, Rachman I, Thomas JEP. Haemolytic uraemic syndrome in typhoid fever. *BMJ* 1974;2:84–87.

71 O'Brien AD, Holmes. Shiga and Shiga-like toxins. *Microbiological Rev* 1987;51:206–220.

72 Strockbine NA, Marques LRM, Newland JW, et al. Two toxin-converting phages from Escherichia coli O157:H7 strain 933 encode anti-

73 Obrig TG, Del Vecchio PJ, Brown JE, et al. Direct cytotoxic action of Shiga toxin on human vascular endothelial cells. *Infect and Immun* 1988;55:2373–2378.

74 Tesh VL, O'Brien AD. The pathogenic mechanisms of Shiga toxin and the Shiga-like toxins. *Molecular Microbiol* 1991;5:1817–1822.

75 Karch H, Bitzan M, Pietsch R, et al. Purified verotoxins of Escherichia coli O157:H7 decrease prostacyclin synthesis by endothelial cells. *Microbiol Pathogenesis* 1988;5:215–221.

76 Ostroff SM, Neill MA, Lewis JH, et al. Toxin genotypes and plasmid profiles as determinants of systemic sequelae in Escherichia coli O157:H7 infections. *J Infect Dis* 1989;160:884–888.

77 Raghu G, Striker L, Striker G. Lipopolysaccharide-mediated injury to cultured human glomerular endothelial cells. *Clin Immunol Immunopathol* 1986;38:275–281.

78 Louise CB, Obrig TG. Shiga toxin-associated hemolytic uremic syndrome: combined cytotoxic effects of Shiga toxin, interleukin-1β, and tumor necrosis factor alpha on human vascular endothelial cells in vitro. *Infect Immun* 1991;59:4173–4179.

79 Butler T, Rahman H, Al-Muhmud KA, et al. An animal model of hemolytic uremic syndrome in shigellosis: lipopolysaccharides of Sh. dysenteriae 1 and Sh. flexneri produce leucocyte-mediated renal cortical necrosis in rabbits. *Br J Exp Path* 1985;66:7–15.

80 Forsyth KD, Simpson AC, Fitzpatrick MM, et al. Neutrophil-mediated endothelial injury in haemolytic uraemic syndrome. *Lancet* 1989:411–414.

81 Kelly RT, Farmer S, Greiff D. Neuraminidase activities of clinical isolates of Diplococcus pneumoniae. *J Bacteriol* 1967;94:272–273.

82 Boyd B, Lingwood C. Verotoxin receptor glycolipid in human renal tissue. *Nephron* 1989;51:1207–1210.

83 Taylor CM, Milford DV, Rose PE, et al. The expression of blood group P1 in post-enteropathic haemolytic uraemic syndrome. *Pediatr Nephrol* 1990;4:59–61.

84 Neild GH. Haemolytic uraemic syndrome. *Nephron* 1991;59:194–205.

85 Milford DV, Taylor CM. New insights into the haemolytic uraemic syndromes. *Arch Dis Child* 1990;65:713–715.

86 Loirat C, Sonsino F, Moreno AV, et al. Hemolytic-uremic syndrome: An analysis of the natural history and prognostic features. *Acta Paediatr Scand* 1984;73:505–501.

87 **Dolislager D, Tune B.** The hemolytic-uremic syndrome. *Am J Dis Child* 1978;132:55–58.

88 **Krishnan C, Fitzgerald VA, Dakin SJ, Gehme RJ.** Laboratory investigation of outbreak of hemorrhagic colitis caused by *Escherichia coli* O157:H7. *J Clin Microbiol* 1987;1043–1047.

89 **Trompeter RS, Schwartz R, Chantler C, et al.** Haemolytic-uraemic syndrome: an analysis of prognostic features. *Arch Dis Child* 1983; 58:101–105.

90 **Siegler RL, Milligan MK, Burningham TH, et al.** Long-term outcome and prognostic indicators in the hemolytic uremic syndrome. *J Pediatrics* 1991;118:195–200.

91 **Fitzpatrick MM, Shah V, Tompeter RS, et al.** Long term renal outcome of childhood haemolytic uraemic syndrome. *BMJ* 1991;303:489–492.

92 **Chapman PA.** Evaluation of commercial latex slide test for identifying *Escherichia coli* O157. *J Clin Pathol* 1989;42:1109–1110.

93 **Wells JG, Davis BR, Wachsmuth JK, et al.** Laboratory investigation of hemorrhagic colitis outbreaks associated with a rare *Escherichia coli* serotype. *J Clin Microbiol* 1983;18:512–520.

94 **Downes FP, Green JH, Greene K, et al.** Development and evaluation of enzyme-linked immunosorbent assays for detection of Shiga-like toxin I and Shiga-like toxin II. *J Clin Microbiol* 1989;27:1292–1297.

95 **Karmali MA.** Laboratory diagnosis of verotoxin-producing *Escherichia coli* infections. *Clin Microbiol Newsletter* 1987;9:65–70.

96 **Perera LP, Marques RM, O'Brien D.** Isolation and characterization of monoclonal antibodies to Shiga-like toxin II of enterohemorrhagic *E. coli* and use of the monoclonal antibodies in a colony enzyme-linked immunosorbent assay. *J Clin Microbiol* 1988;26:2127–2131.

97 **Newland JW, Neill RJ.** DNA probes for Shiga-like toxins I and II and for toxin-converting bacteriophages. *J Clin Microbiol* 1988;26:1292–1297.

98 **Jackson MP.** Detection of Shiga toxin-producing *Sh. dysenteriae* type 1 and *Escherichia coli* by using polymerase chain reaction with incorporation of digoxigenin-11-dUTP. *J Clin Microbiol* 1991;29:1910–1914.

99 **Pollard DR, John WM, Lior H, et al.** Rapid and specific detection of verotoxin genes in *Escherichia coli* by the polymerase chain reaction. *J Clin Microbiol* 1990;28:540–545.

100 **Chart H, Scotland SM, Rowe B.** Serum antibodies to *Escherichia coli* serotype O157:H7 in patients with hemolytic uremic syndrome. *J Clin Microbiol* 1989;27:285–290.

101 **Chart H, Smith HR, Scotland SM, et al.** Serological identification of *Escherichia coli* O157:H7 infection in haemolytic uraemic syndrome. *Lancet* 1991;337:138–140.

102 **Barrett TJ, Green JH, Griffin PM, et al.** Enzyme-linked immunosorbent assays for detecting antibodies to Shiga-like toxin I, Shiga-like toxin II, and *Escherichia coli* O157:H7 lipopolysaccharide in human serum. *Curr Microbiol* 1991;23;195–198.

103 **Karch H, Strockbine NA, O'Brien AD.** Growth of *Escherichia coli* in the presence of trimethoprim-sulfamethoxazole facilitates detection of Shiga-like toxin producing strains by colony blot assay. *FEMS Microbiol Lett* 1986;35:141–145.

104 **Walterspiel JN, Ashkenazi S, Morrow AL, Cleary TG.** Effect of subinhibitory concentrations of antibiotics on extracellular Shiga-toxin I. *Infection* 1992;20:25–29.

105 **Bell WR, Braine HG, Ness PM, Kickler TS.** Improved survival in thrombotic thrombocytopenic purpura-hemolytic uremic syndrome: clinical experience in 108 patients. *N Engl J Med* 1991;325:398 -403.

106 **Rock GA, Shumak KH, Buskard NA, et al.** Comparison of plasma exchange with plasma infusion in the treatment of thrombotic thrombocytopenic purpura. *N Engl J Med* 1991; 325:393–397.

107 **Isiani R, Appiani AC, Edifonti AM, et al.** Hemolytic uremic syndrome: therapeutic effects of plasma infusion. *BMJ* 1982;285: 1304–1306.

Clinical features and treatment of infection due to mycobacterium fortuitum/chelonae complex

ELIZABETH J. McFARLAND
DANIEL R. KURITZKES

Mycobacterium fortuitum and *Mycobacterium chelonae* are rapidly growing mycobacteria (Runyon's Group IV) that are important causes of cutaneous, pulmonary, and nosocomial infection. Together, they account for the vast majority of human disease due to this group of mycobacteria. Though often referred to as opportunistic pathogens, given the appropriate portal of entry, these common soil microbes can cause serious disease even in immunologically competent hosts. Whereas fatal cases are uncommon, rapidly growing mycobacteria can produce chronic infections with significant morbidity that require prolonged therapy. Their importance as potential nosocomial pathogens in particular has been underscored by the growing number of case reports. This chapter reviews the clinical manifestations of *M. fortuitum/chelonae* complex infection and discusses potential improvements in treatment brought about by the introduction of the quinolones and newer macrolide antibiotics.

MICROBIOLOGY

Organisms of the *M. fortuitum/chelonae* complex were first isolated from amphibians: *M. fortuitum* from frogs (hence its original designation as *Mycobacterium ranae*) (1) and *M. chelonae* from turtles (2). (*M. chelonae* has been known variously as *Mycobacterium abscessus*, *Mycobacterium bostelense*, *Mycobacterium friedmanii*, and *Mycobacterium chelonei* in the past (3).) *M. fortuitum* is ubiquitous in nature, having been isolated from water, soil, and dust (4–6); the precise ecological niche of *M. chelonae* is not known. The rapidly growing mycobacteria are distinguished from other mycobacteria by the appearance of nonpigmented colonies within three to five days when cultures are inoculated onto blood or chocolate agar plates. Colonies may take up to several weeks to appear during primary isolation, however (7). When mycobacterial infection is suspected on clinical grounds, recovery from specimens may be aided by the use of Lowenstein-Jensen agar. Because some strains of *M. chelonae* fail to grow at 35°C, culture sensitivity may be improved by incubation at 28°C to 30°C. Although less fastidious in their growth requirements than other mycobacteria, the rapidly growing species are more susceptible to decontaminants such as sodium hydroxide. Overuse of this agent in processing sputum samples may limit recovery from clinical specimens (8,9). These organisms are also more easily decolorized by acid alcohol, a property that makes them more difficult to stain than the slowly growing mycobacteria.

Three biovariants of *M. fortuitum* have been described: *fortuitum, peregrinum,* and an unnamed variant known as the "third biovariant complex" (10). *M. chelonae* also comprises three subspecies: *abscessus, chelonae,* and an unnamed third group, the "*M. chelonae*-like organisms." Differentiation as to species, subspecies, and biovariant is accomplished by biochemical tests, as described by Silcox et al. (10). These tests are generally available only through reference laboratories such as the Mycobacteriology Branch of the Centers for Disease Control and Prevention (Atlanta, GA). No specific organ tropism or clinical manifestations are associated with any one member of the *M. fortuitum/chelonae* complex, with the exception of disseminated disease, which is most frequently due to *M. chelonae* subsp *abscessus*. Specific identification of isolates is important, however, because susceptibility to antibiotics differs among the subgroups.

Antimicrobial susceptibility

Members of the *M. fortuitum/chelonae* complex are resistant to most agents used in the treatment of tuberculosis (except aminoglycosides), but are inhibited by certain standard antimicrobial agents at drug concentrations that are readily achievable in serum. Because of their rapid growth, susceptibility testing of these organisms can be performed using routine clinical microbiological techniques. Wallace and co-workers have shown that agar and broth microdilution methods work well when applied to *M. fortuitum* and *M. chelonae* (11,12). Susceptibility testing by disk diffusion on Mueller-Hinton agar can be used accurately for determining minimum inhibitory concentrations (MICs) for *M. fortuitum*. However, *M. chelonae* grows poorly on this medium. Because species identification of an isolate is generally incomplete by the time susceptibility tests are set up, the broth microdilution method is still used by most laboratories engaged in antimycobacterial drug testing.

The susceptibility of *M. fortuitum/chelonae* complex subgroups to antimicrobial agents known to be effective against these organisms is shown in Table 11.1. No single agent was active against all isolates. Although each species subgroup has a typical pattern of susceptibility, variability within each subgroup necessitates testing of all clinically significant isolates to confirm drug susceptibility.

Amikacin has the greatest activity of the aminoglycosides against all five subgroups, but is most active against the *M. fortuitum* variants ($MIC_{50} \leq 1$ $\mu g/mL$). Tobramycin has good activity only against *M. fortuitum* biovariant *peregrinum* and *M. chelonae* subsp *chelonae* (MIC_{50} 4 $\mu g/mL$).

Among the β-lactams and related antibiotics, imipenem is the most active. At 8 $\mu g/mL$, all isolates of *M. fortuitum* biovar *fortuitum* were inhibited (14). Ninety percent of isolates from the third biovariant complex were inhibited at a concentration of 4 $\mu g/mL$ (14). Cefoxitin is active against nearly all isolates of *M. fortuitum* biovariants *fortuitum* and *peregrinum* (MIC_{50} 8 $\mu g/mL$ and 32 $\mu g/mL$, respectively) if the intermediate

Table 11.1 Antimicrobial susceptibility of rapidly growing mycobacteria

Susceptible ‖ Intermediate	≤16 (32)	≤8 (16–32)	≤16 (32)	≤8	≤0.5 (1–4)	<1 (1–4)	≤1 (2–8)	≤32 (64)	≤2
Species	Amikacin	Cefoxitin	Cefmetazole	Imipenem	Erythro*	Clarithro†	Doxycycline	Sulfa‡	Cipro§
M. fortuitum									
biovar *fortuitum*	99%	2% (99%)	82% (100%)	100%	0% (1%)	100%	33% (46%)	95%	9%
peregrinum	100%	88% (100%)	—	—	0% (25%)	100%	38% (63%)	100%	—
Third biovariant complex	100%	26% (79%)	—	95%	0%	35% (81%)	5% (26%)	100%	100%
M. chelonae									
subsp *abscessus*	95% (98%)	29% (82%)	27% (76%)	57%	1% (19%)	100%	0% (4%)	0% (4%)	0%
chelonae	88% (97%)	0% (0%)	0%	39%	9% (82%)	100%	0% (26%)	3%	0%

NOTE: Percent of strains susceptible to commonly used antibiotics (data compiled from References 9,13–17). Numbers in parentheses denote the percent of strains susceptible using the cut-off for intermediate susceptibility.

*Erythro = erythromycin.

†Clarithro = clarithromycin.

‡Sulfa = sulfamethoxazole.

§Cipro = ciprofloxacin.

‖Susceptible and intermediate breakpoints (μg/mL) are as given in References 9,13–15,17.

susceptibility breakpoint of ≤32 μg/mL is used; only 80% of strains belonging to the third biovariant complex (MIC$_{50}$ 16 μg/mL) are susceptible to cefoxitin (13). Cefmetazole, a second-generation cephalosporin, is two to four times more potent in vitro than cefoxitin. By contrast, cefotetan has poor activity against this group of organisms (14). The *M. chelonae* subgroups are more resistant to β-lactam antibiotics. Imipenem inhibited only 57% of *M. chelonae* subsp *abscessus* and 39% of *M. chelonae* subsp *chelonae* isolates (breakpoint 8 μg/mL). Although approximately 80% of *M. chelonae* subsp *abscessus* isolates are susceptible (MIC$_{50}$ 16 μg/mL), cefoxitin is ineffective against *M. chelonae* subsp *chelonae*. None of the newer semisynthetic penicillins (e.g., piperacillin, azlocillin, mezlocillin) or monobactams (aztreonam) are effective against the *M. fortuitum/chelonae* complex.

Erythromycin is effective against 88% of *M. chelonae* subsp *chelonae* isolates (MIC$_{50}$ 2 μg/mL), but has no activity against most strains of the *M. fortuitum* complex (MIC$_{50}$ ≥ 16 μg/mL). The newer macrolides, azithromycin, clarithromycin, and roxithromycin, all show superior activity against rapidly growing mycobacteria when compared with erythromycin. Clarithromycin is the most potent agent of this class, inhibiting all strains of *M. chelonae* subsp *abscessus*, *M. chelonae* subsp *chelonae*, *M. chelonae*-like organisms, and *M. fortuitum* biovar *peregrinum* at ≤1 μg/mL (15). Nearly all strains of *M. fortuitum* behavior *fortuitum* are inhibited at 4 μg/mL, but isolates of the third biovariant complex of *M. fortuitum* are heterogenous in their susceptibility, with MICs exceeding 8 μg/mL.

Most strains of the *M. fortuitum* complex are susceptible to sulfamethoxazole (MIC$_{50}$ ≤ 2 μg/mL), whereas *M. chelonae* strains are nearly all resistant. The tetracyclines have variable activity against *M. fortuitum/chelonae* complex organisms. Doxycycline and minocycline are more active than tetracycline against *M. fortuitum* biovariants, but all are ineffective against *M. chelonae* subsp *abscessus*.

Ciprofloxacin and ofloxacin have good in vitro efficacy against isolates of the *M. fortuitum* complex (MIC$_{90}$ 1 μg/mL). Norfloxacin and enoxicin are less active, however, with MIC$_{90}$s of 4 μg/mL (16,17). Isolates in the *M. chelonae* subgroups are generally resistant to the quinolones (MICs 8 to ≥18 μg/mL).

CLINICAL MANIFESTATIONS

Pulmonary disease

For many years, doubt persisted as to whether rapidly growing mycobacteria recovered from sputum samples were colonizers or etiologic agents of disease (18). It is now well established that *M. fortuitum* and *M. chelonae* do indeed cause pulmonary infection. Wallace and colleagues have the largest published experience with pulmonary disease due to these organisms (9,19,20). In their series, the majority of cases were patients over 50 years of age, but pediatric cases have been reported (21). Although individual cases have been reported in the setting of ankylosing spondylitis (22), chronic obstructive lung disease (23), malignancy (24), previous tuberculosis (7), and rheumatic diseases (19), underlying lung disease is not a usual finding. An association with achalasia and lipoid pneumonia has been suggested by several investigators (25–29), who postulate that fats and oils aspirated into the lung enhance the growth of these organisms. Of note is the absence of any inceased risk of M. *fortuitum/chelonae* complex pneumonia in patients with human immunodeficiency virus (HIV) infection.

Chronic cough is the most frequent symptom of pulmonary infection with rapidly growing mycobacteria. Weight loss has been noted in several reports, but is uncommon in the experience of Wallace and colleagues (20). Low-grade fever occurs commonly, but night sweats are usually absent. Hemoptysis is unusual, most likely because cavitary disease is seldom encountered. A few patients complain of shortness of breath, but respiratory compromise is seldom a presenting symptom.

There is no specific pattern on chest radiograph associated with M. *chelonae* or M. *fortuitum* infection (Figure 11.1). Most often, patchy bilateral infiltrates are seen, which may be mistaken for fibrotic lung disease or bronchiectasis (9,19). Hilar adenopathy and pleural effusion are generally absent (9). Radiographs from patients in whom infection is associated with achalasia show dense infiltrates in areas of aspiration (27). Cavitary disease has been described but is present in fewer than 20% of cases (20,30–32).

Although M. *fortuitum* and M. *chelonae* account for 10% of nontuberculous myco-

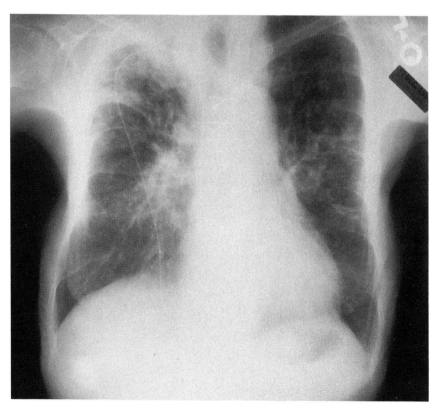

Figure 11.1 Pulmonary infection due to M. *chelonae* in a woman treated with prednisone for rheumatoid arthritis. (Courtesy of Dr. Patricia Simone, National Jewish Center for Immunology and Respiratory Medicine, Denver, Colorado.)

bacteria isolated from sputum, fewer than half of these isolates are thought to be clinically significant (19,24,33). Diagnosis of pulmonary infection due to rapidly growing mycobacteria should therefore be made according to standards established by the American Thoracic Society (34). Repeated isolation of the same species of mycobacterium in association with an infiltrate on a chest radiograph is sufficient evidence to establish a diagnosis. Because of the difficulty in staining organisms of the *M. fortuitum/chelonae* complex, acid-fast smears of sputum may be negative. In patients with underlying lung disease, transbronchial biopsy may be needed to confirm the diagnosis. Histological examination of biopsy specimens reveals acute inflammation with polymorphonuclear leukocytes, as well as granulomatous inflammation with giant cell formation. Areas of necrosis and microabscess formation are seen often, but caseous necrosis of granulomas is less frequently observed (19).

The clinical course of pulmonary infection with *M. fortuitum* or *M. chelonae* is quite variable. In the majority of patients, disease progresses at an indolent pace. Periods of disease activity with productive cough and pulmonary infiltrates alternate with asymptomatic intervals during which pulmonary infiltrates may resolve even without specific antimicrobial therapy (20,23). Deaths from progressive infection have been reported in patients with severe underlying disease or with inadequate antimicrobial therapy (19,25,28,32). For additional details on *M. chelonae* pulmonary infections, the reader may consult several excellent reviews (9,20,35).

Primary cutaneous disease

Skin and soft tissue infections account for the majority of disease due to *M. fortuitum/chelonae* complex. A history of antecedent trauma can be elicited in most cases. In particular, penetrating trauma that results in contamination of the wound with soil predisposes to infection with these organisms. Injuries from automobile accidents, farm equipment, nails, and bullets have all been reported in association with *M. chelonae* and *M. fortuitum* infection (19,36,37). Infection can also result from less serious injury, such as superficial abrasion (38) or from hypodermic injection (39,40,41). Localized soft tissue infections complicating surgical procedures are well described and are discussed in the section on nosocomial infections.

Unlike pulmonary disease, cutaneous infections with rapidly growing mycobacteria occur with equal frequency in all age groups. In the typical patient, nodular lesions with scant serous drainage appear four to six weeks after the initial injury (Figure 11.2). The lesions are only mildly tender, with minimal surrounding cellulitis. Fever and other systemic manifestations are usually absent. Infections tend to remain localized in patients with normal immunity. Occasionally, lesions may progress to frank abscess formation with fluctuance (42–45). Gram and acid-fast stains of draining fluid are usually negative, but organisms are readily demonstrated by culture. On occasion, skin biopsy or incision and drainage of a nodule may be required to establish the diagnosis.

Disseminated disease

Disseminated infection is a rare manifestation of disease due to rapidly growing mycobacteria. Of 125 cases of *M. fortuitum/chelonae* complex infection reported by Wallace.

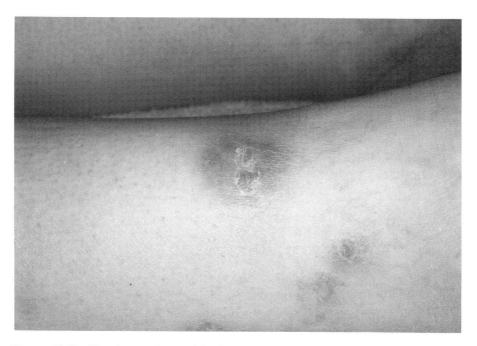

Figure 11.2 Skin lesion due to *M. chelonae* in a woman with mixed connective tissue disorder. (Courtesy of Dr. Patricia Simone, National Jewish Center for Immunology and Respiratory Medicine, Denver, Colorado.)

et al. (19), only nine involved dissemination. Additional case reports of disseminated infection have appeared, but no other large series have been published (46–52).

Most cases of disseminated disease occur in immunocompromised patients or in patients with serious underlying disease (9). A primary focus of infection usually cannot be identified, but spread from pulmonary disease and from a primary cutaneous lesion have been reported (48,50,53). A large proportion of the cases of disseminated *M. fortuitum/chelonae* complex infection occurs in patients who have undergone renal transplantation or who are on chronic hemodialysis (19). Disseminated disease has also been described in patients with malignancy and in those receiving high-dose steroid therapy (19,54). By contrast, disseminated infection with rapidly growing mycobacteria among patients with acquired immune deficiency syndrome (AIDS) is distinctly unusual (55). Only ten cases of *M. fortuitum/chelonae* complex infection were noted in a survey of 1,984 cases of disseminated nontuberculous mycobacterial disease in patients with AIDS (56). It is interesting to speculate whether the relative paucity of cases relates to the low virulence of these organisms or is due to differences in host immune responses to rapidly growing mycobacteria, as compared with *M. tuberculosis* and *M. avium* complex, which are common pathogens in HIV-infected individuals. All species of *M. fortuitum/chelonae* complex have been reported to cause disseminated disease, but isolates of *M. chelonae* predominate.

The clinical manifestations of disseminated disease are distinctive. Most patients present with multiple erythematous subcutaneous nodules that typically involve the extensor surfaces of the arms and legs. Lesions frequently suppurate and drain serous fluid from which organisms can be isolated (9). Occasionally, skin lesions can become invasive, developing into large subcutaneous abscesses (51,57) or progressing to osteomyelitis (48,49). Dissemination to visceral organs, however, is rare (9).

Mortality of disseminated *M. fortuitum/chelonae* complex infection is high, even with antibiotic therapy. In many cases, death results from underlying disease (19,49,55). Although cures have been noted in some cases, infection frequently relapses when antibiotics are discontinued (47,48,50,52,53,55).

Nosocomial infections

Nosocomial infections are an important clinical manifestation of infection with *M. fortuitum/chelonae* complex. Indeed, the first recognition of *M. fortuitum* as a human pathogen was in association with abscesses at injection sites (58). These infections can be considered in two groups: postoperative wound infections and infections of prosthetic devices. Included in this last category are infections of indwelling intravenous and intraperitoneal catheters.

The majority of nosocomial infections due to rapidly growing mycobacteria occur sporadically, but epidemics following cardiac bypass surgery (59–61) and augmentation mammaplasty (62,63) have been reported. Cases in the United States appear to be clustered in Texas and the southern coastal states (64,65). The isolation from individual patients of strains genetically related to *M. fortuitum/chelonae* complex isolates cultured from environmental sources suggests that these infections are due to environmental contaminants (60,64). Contaminated aqueous solutions are implicated most frequently as the cause of common source outbreaks (66). Strains of *M. fortuitum/chelonae* complex can be isolated from tapwater and are resistant to many disinfectants, including 2% aqueous formaldehyde and 2% alkaline glutaraldehyde (67,68). Nosocomial outbreaks with identified sources of organisms are summarized in Table 11.2.

A large number of the reported cases of postsurgical wound infection have occurred following cardiac surgery. A survey of cardiac surgeons identified 87 cases of infection due to rapidly growing mycobacteria (74). Most patients presented with sternal wound

Table 11.2 Nosocomial outbreaks of *M. fortuitum/chelonae* complex infection

Source (cleaning solution)	Clinical disease	Reference
Ultrasonic bath (Cari Clean in tapwater)	Otitis media	69
Peritoneal dialysis machines	Peritonitis	70
Ice tapwater	Median sternotomy wound infection	61
Hemodialysis machines (Formaldehyde 2%)	Systemic infection	71
Gentian violet	Postsurgical wound infection	63
High-flux dialysis (Renalin 2.5%)	Systemic infection	72
Electromyography needles (tapwater)	Muscle abscess	73
Povidone-iodine 10%	Nasal cellulitis	66

SOURCE Adapted from Soto et al. (66).

infection following coronary artery bypass graft surgery. In one fatal case, sternotomy wound infection with *M. fortuitum* progressed to mediastinitis and aortitis (75). Infection of prosthetic heart valves with these organisms is less common but is associated with a high mortality. Most cases of *M. fortuitum/chelonae* complex prosthetic valve endocarditis have occurred with porcine heterografts (76); infection of mechanical prosthetic valves has also been reported (74,77). Reports of other implanted devices infected by *M. fortuitum/chelonae* include prosthetic joints, pacemakers, Marlex mesh, and penile prostheses (78–80).

A variety of minor surgical procedures may be complicated by *M. fortuitum/chelonae* complex infection, particularly when chemical methods are used to sterilize surgical instruments. Scleral abscess, keratitis, granulomatous eye disease, and nasolacrimal gland infection have been reported following ophthalmologic procedures (68,81–85). Inadequate sterilization of otologic instruments led to an outbreak of otitis media due to *M. chelonae* in an office practice (69). Failure of 10% povidone-iodine to kill *M. chelonae* was considered the likely culprit in an outbreak of postsurgical nasal cellulitis (66). An outbreak of soft tissues abscesses due to *M. fortuitum* related to electromyographic testing has also been reported (73).

Infection of indwelling venous catheters with *M. fortuitum/chelonae* complex is well documented (9,19,86–88). Catheter infections may be accompanied by exit site infections or manifest as mycobacteremia alone. Rapidly growing mycobacteria have been described as a cause of peritonitis and tunnel site infections of peritoneal catheters in patients treated by intermittent or continuous ambulatory peritoneal dialysis (70,89–92). Outbreaks of *M. chelonae* infection associated with hemodialysis have also been noted, particularly in patients treated with high-flux dialysis machines (91,92).

Clinical features of postsurgical wound infections due to rapidly growing mycobacteria are similar to those of cutaneous infections. Patients present with erythema, swelling, mild tenderness, and serous drainage at the surgical site several weeks to months after the procedure (78). Failure of the wound to heal or dehiscence of a previously closed wound are important clinical clues. Acid-fast organisms can often be demonstrated in smears of wound drainage and will grow on routine medium in five to seven days. The microbiology laboratory should be alerted, however, so that cultures will not be discarded as negative after only two days.

Patients with *M. fortuitum/chelonae* complex prosthetic valve endocarditis (PVE) are indistinguishable clinically from other forms of this disease. They present with fevers, peripheral embolic phenomena, and heart murmurs. Blood cultures are routinely positive. The mortality of PVE due to rapidly growing mycobacteria is high even with prompt institution of appropriate antimicrobial therapy.

TREATMENT

Treatment of infections due to *M. fortuitum/chelonae* complex organisms must be individualized, depending on the clinical setting and the antimicrobial susceptibility of the isolate. Because of the variability in antimicrobial susceptibility, all clinically significant isolates of rapidly growing mycobacteria should be sent to a reference laboratory for testing. The broad susceptibility of M. *fortuitum* biovariants makes therapy relatively straightforward. Whereas suitable oral agents were previously unavailable for multiply-resistant strains of M. *chelonae*, the newer macrolides such as clarithromycin may play an important role in treatment of resistant isolates.

For serious infections, empiric therapy based on susceptibility patterns listed in Table 11.1 may be used initially while awaiting definitive culture results. A combination of cefoxitin and amikacin administered intravenously provides coverage of the majority of isolates of M. *fortuitum* and provides at least one active drug (amikacin) against isolates of M. *chelonae*. Cefmetazole has greater activity in vitro than does cefoxitin, but comparative clinical trials are needed to determine whether this greater potency translates into better clinical outcomes. Most experts recommend a minimum of four to eight weeks of combination therapy for susceptible isolates, with cefoxitin continued for a minimum of 12 weeks (78). The choice of antibiotics can be refined when the results of susceptibility tests become available. After 12 weeks of intravenous therapy, oral therapy can be substituted if possible and continued for another 12 weeks, for a minimum six-month course of antibiotics.

Treatment of pulmonary disease due to M. *fortuitum* follows the guidelines cited above. Amikacin and cefoxitin are given intravenously for at least four to eight weeks, followed by oral therapy with a combination of sulfamethoxazole with doxycycline, ciprofloxicin, or ofloxacin (20). The majority of pulmonary infections, however, are due to M. *chelonae* subsp *abscessus* (9), which is resistant to most oral agents, including the quinolones. For these patients, treatment should be based on the extent of disease, susceptibility of the isolate, and the patient's age and overall health status. Patients whose isolates are susceptible to erythromycin should be treated initially with oral erythromycin, together with amikacin plus cefoxitin given intravenously for a minimum of four to six weeks (20). If disease is circumscribed and the patient is a surgical candidate, excision of the lesion might be considered after this period of initial antibiotic therapy. Erythromycin should then be continued for six to 12 months postoperatively. Patients who are not surgical candidates should be treated for at least 12 months with erythromycin after the initial period of intravenous therapy (20).

In the past, a more conservative approach was taken towards patients with pulmonary disease whose isolates were erythromycin resistant. Because most patients are in their sixties and pulmonary disease progresses slowly, hospitalization during periods of exacerbation and treatment with intravenous antibiotics, along with chest percussion, postural drainage, and bronchodilators, were recommended (9,20). The availability of clarithromycin should prompt a reexamination of this approach. Isolates of M. *chelonae* subsp *abscessus* appear to be uniformly susceptible at MICs $\leq$ 1 μg/mL, including those that are erythromycin resistant (15). Although clinical experience with this agent in the treatment of M. *chelonae* pulmonary infections is limited, the in vitro data are grounds for cautious optimism that clarithromycin will provide substantial benefit to these patients.

Skin and soft tissue infections can be managed less aggressively if the infection is localized. Approximately 10% to 20% of skin infections may resolve spontaneously over six to 12 months (9). Treatment with a single oral agent, depending on the susceptibility of the isolate, is usually sufficient without subjecting the patient to hospitalization or long-term intravenous therapy with its attendant toxicities. Treatment is usually continued for three to six months. Emergence of resistance to therapy is not a frequent problem with erythromycin, sulfamethoxazole, or doxycycline, but emergence of resistance to ciprofloxacin has been reported (9,93). Surgical debridement is a critical adjunct to antimicrobial therapy. Abscesses should be incised and completely drained; wounds should be packed so as to prevent premature closure of the skin, which can result in renewed abscess formation with draining sinus tracts (78). For highly resistant species of M. chelonae, complete excision of the lesion may be curative (9,78).

Recommendations for the treatment of disseminated disease are based largely on case reports of successful therapy. As with other serious infections due to M. fortuitum/chelonae complex, initial intravenous treatment with amikacin and cefoxitin is recommended (9). Patients with large abscesses or bone infection generally require debridement in addition to antibiotic therapy (48,57). Subsequent treatment with a variety of regimens employing combinations of oral antibiotics, with and without continued intravenous antibiotics, has been reported. The oral agents most frequently used have been erythromycin, trimethoprim-sulfamethoxazole, and doxycycline (9,53,52). Successful treatment with ciprofloxacin, in combination with other antibiotics, has been reported in several cases (47–49). The duration of therapy in these reports ranged from three to 13 months, but prolonged therapy is the rule. Although symptoms in most cases can be controlled with appropriate antibiotics, patients often relapse when treatment is stopped, and death due to the underlying disease frequently ensues.

The treatment of postsurgical infection varies with the location and extent of tissue involvement. Antibiotic selection follows the same guidelines discussed above. In general, successful treatment has been accomplished only with combined surgical debridement, removal of prosthetic devices and other foreign bodies, and antibiotic therapy. In some cases, such as median sternotomy infection, debridement must be extensive. Successful treatment of intravenous catheter sepsis and tunnel infections requires removal of the catheter in addition to antibiotic therapy (86–88). Infection of prosthetic heart valves has been uniformly fatal without valve replacement (74). In the case of prosthetic joint infection, sterilization usually requires removal of the prosthesis. Subsequent joint replacement should be delayed until aspirate cultures of the involved joint are documented as negative for several weeks after discontinuing antibiotics (79).

CONCLUSIONS

As is clear from the preceding discussion, treatment of M. fortuitum/chelonae complex infections does not follow a set approach. Since most cases are sporadic, controlled trials of specific therapeutic regimens are difficult to organize. The quinolones and the newer macrolides may offer additional options to the standard antibiotics currently available. Additional clinical experience with these agents is needed, however, to determine their place in the treatment of the stubborn infections due to these organisms.

REFERENCES

1 **Kuster E.** Uber Kaltblütertuberkulose. *Muenchener Medizinische Wochenschrift* 1905;52: 57–59.

2 **Moore M, Frerichs B.** An unusual acid fast infection of the knee with subcutaneous abscesslike lesions of the gluteal region. *J Invest Dermatol* 1953;20:33–169.

3 **Sneath PHA, Nair NS, Sharpe ME, Holt HG, eds.** *Bergey's Manual of Systemic Bacteriology.* Baltimore: Williams and Wilkins, 1986; 1452–1457.

4 **Wolinsky E, Rynearson TK.** Mycobacteria in soil and their relation to disease-associated strains. *Am Rev Respir Dis* 1968;97: 1032–1037.

5 **Goslee S, Wolinsky E.** Water as a source of potentially pathogeneic mycobacteria. *Am Rev Respir Dis* 1976;113:287–292.

6 **Dawson DK.** Potential pathogens among strains of mycobacteria isolated from house dusts. *Med J Aust* 1971;1:679–681.

7 **Tsukamura M, Nakamura E, Kurita I, Nakamura T.** Isolation of *Mycobacterium chelonei* subspecies chelonei (*Mycobacterium bostelense*) from pulmonary lesions of 9 patients. *Am Rev Respir Dis* 1973;108:683–685.

8 **Gruft H, Henning HG.** Pulmonary mycobacteriosis due to rapidly growing acid fast bacillus, *Mycobacterium chelonae. Am Rev Respir Dis* 1972;105:618–620.

9 **Wallace RJ Jr.** The clinical presentation, diagnosis, and therapy of cutaneous and pulmonary infections due to the rapidly growing mycobacteria, *M. fortuitum* and *M. chelonae. Clin Chest Med* 1989;10:419–429.

10 **Silcox VA, Good RC, Floyd MM.** Identification of clinically significant *Mycobacterium fortuitum* complex isolates. *J Clin Microbiol* 1981;14:686–691.

11 **Wallace RJ Jr, Dalovisio JR, Pankey GA.** Disk diffusion testing of susceptibility of *Mycobacterium fortuitum* and *Mycobacterium chelonae* to antibacterial agents. *Antimicrob Agents Chemother* 1979;16:611–614.

12 **Swenson JM, Thornsberry C, Silcox VA.** Rapidly growing mycobacteria: testing of susceptibility to 34 antimicrobial agents by broth microdilution. *Antimicrob Agents Chemother* 1982;22:186–192.

13 **Swenson JM, Wallace RJ Jr, Silcox VA, Thornsberry C.** Antimicrobial susceptibility of five subgroups of *Mycobacterium fortuitum* and *Mycobacterium chelonae. Antimicrob Agents Chemother* 1985;28:807–811.

14 **Wallace RJ Jr, Brown BA, Onyi GO.** Susceptibilities of *Mycobacterium fortuitum* biovar.

fortuitum and the two subgroups of *Mycobacterium chelonae* to imipenem, cefmetazole, cefoxitin, and amoxicillin-clavulinic acid. *Antimicrob Agents Chemother* 1991;35:773–775.

15 **Brown BA, Wallace RJ Jr, Onyi GO, De Rosas V, Wallace RJ III.** Activities of four macrolides, including clarithromycin, against *Mycobacterium fortuitum, Mycobacterium chelonae,* and *M. chelonae*-like organisms. *Antimicrob Agents Chemother* 1992;36:180–184.

16 **Gay JD, DeYoung DR, Roberts GD.** In vitro activities of norfloxacin and ciprofloxacin against *Mycobacterium tuberculosis,* M. *avium* complex, *M. chelonei,* M. *fortuitum,* and *M. kansasii. Antimicrob Agents Chemother* 1984; 26:94–96.

17 **Leysen DC, Haemers A, Pattyn SR.** Mycobacteria and the new quinolones. *Antimicrob Agents Chemother* 1989;33:1–5.

18 **Awe RJ, Gangadharam PR, Jenkins DE.** Clinical significance of *Mycobacterium fortuitum* infections in pulmonary disease. *Am Rev Respir Dis* 198;108:1230–1234.

19 **Wallace RJ Jr, Swenson JM, Silcox VA, Good RC, Tschen JA, Stone MS.** Spectrum of disease due to rapidly growing mycobacteria. *Rev Infect Dis* 1983;5:657–679.

20 **Griffith DE, Wallace RJ Jr.** Pulmonary disease due to rapidly growing mycobacteria. *Semin Respir Med* 1988;9:505–513.

21 **Paone RF, Mercer LC, Glass BA.** Pneumonectomy secondary to *Mycobacterium fortuitum* in infancy. *Ann Thorac Surg* 1991;51: 1010–1011.

22 **Gacad G, Massaro D.** Pulmonary fibrosis and Group IV mycobacteria infection of the lungs in ankylosing spondylitis. *Am Rev Respir Dis* 1974;109:274–278.

23 **Sopko JA, Fieselmann J, Kasik JE.** Pulmonary disease due to *Mycobacterium chelonei* subspecies *abscessus*: A report of four cases. *Tubercle* 1980;61:165–169.

24 **Rolston KVI, Jones PG, Fainstein V, Bodey GP.** Pulmonary disease caused by rapidly growing mycobacteria in patients with cancer. *Chest* 1985;87:503–506.

25 **Banerjee R, Hal R, Hughes GRV.** Pulmonary *Mycobacterium fortuitum* infection associated with achalasia of the oesophagus: case report and review of the literature. *Br J Dis Chest* 1970;64:112–118.

26 **Burke DS, Ullian RB.** Megaesophagus and pneumonia associated with *Mycobacterium chelonei*: a case report and a literature review. *Am Rev Respir Dis* 1977;116:1101–1107.

27 **Aronchick JM, Miller WT, Epstein DM, Gefter WB.** Association of achalasia and pulmonary *Mycobacterium fortuitum* infection. *Radiology* 1986;10:85–86.

28 **Verghese G, Shepherd R, Watt P, Bruce JH.** Fatal infection with *Mycobacterium fortuitum* associated with oesophageal achalasia. *Thorax* 1988;43:151–152.

29 **Irwin RS, Pratter MR, Corwin RW, Farrugia R, Teplitz C.** Pulmonary infection with *Mycobacterium chelonei:* Successful treatment with one drug based on disk diffusion susceptibility data. *J Infect Dis* 1982;145:722.

30 **Ichiyama S, Tsukamura M.** Ofloxacin and the treatment of pulmonary disease due to *Mycobacterium fortuitum*. *Chest* 1987;92:1110–1112.

31 **Pacht ER.** *Mycobacterium fortuitum* lung abscess: Resolution with prolonged trimethoprim/sulfamethoxazole therapy. *Am Rev Respir Dis* 1990;141:1599–1601.

32 **Nussbaum JM, Heseltine PNR.** Fatal pulmonary infection with *Mycobacterium fortuitum*. *West J Med* 1900;152:423–425.

33 **O'Brien RJ, Geiter LJ, Snider DE.** The epidemiology of nontuberculous mycobacterial diseases in the United States. Results from a national survey. *Am Rev Respir Dis* 1987;135:1007–1014.

34 **American Thoracic Society.** Diagnostic standards and classification of tuberculosis and other mycobacterial diseases (14th edition). *Am Rev Respir Dis* 1981;123:343–351.

35 **Singh N, Yu VL.** Successful treatment of pulmonary infection due to *Mycobacterium chelonae:* Case report and review. *Clinical Infectious Diseases* 1992;14:156–61.

36 **Subbarao EK, Tarpay MM, Marks MI.** Soft-tissue infections caused by *Mycobacterium fortuitum* complex following penetrating injury. *Am J Dis Child* 1987;141:1018–1020.

37 **Miller AC, Commens CA, Jaworski R, Packham D.** The turtle's revenge: a case of soft tissue *Mycobacterium chelonae* infection. *Med J Aust* 1990;153:681–697.

38 **Levine N, Rothschild JG.** Treatment of *Mycobacterium chelonae* infection with controlled localized heating. *J Am Acad Dermatol* 1991;24:867–870.

39 **Hand WL, Sanford JP.** *Mycobacterium fortuitum*—A human pathogen. *Ann Intern Med* 1970;73:971–977.

40 **Clapper WE, Whitcomb J.** *Mycobacterium fortuitum* abscess at an injection site. *JAMA* 1967;202:550.

41 **Borghans JG, Stanford JL.** *Mycobacterium chelonei* in abscesses after injection of diphtheria-pertussis-tetanus-polio vaccine. *Am Rev Respir Dis* 1973;107:1–8.

42 **Woods GL, Washington JA.** Mycobacteria other than *Mycobacterium tuberculosis:* Review of microbiologic and clinical aspects. *Rev Infect Dis* 1987;9:275–294.

43 **Hendrick SJ, Jorizzo L, Neton RC.** Giant *Mycobacterium fortuitum* abscess associated with systemic lupus erythematosus. *Arch Dermatol* 1986;122:695–697.

44 **Westmoreland D, Woodwards RT, Holden PE, James PA.** Soft tissue abscess caused by *Mycobacterium fortuitum*. *J Infection* 1990;20:223–225.

45 **Crick JC, Vandevelde AG.** *Mycobacterium fortuitum* midpalmar space abscess: A case report. *J Hand Surg* 1986;11A:438–440.

46 **Lazo-de-la-Vega SA, Ponce-de-Leon S, Sifuentes J,Ruiz-Palacios GM.** Cutaneous manifestation of disseminated infection by *Mycobacterium fortuitum* biovariant "third group". *J Am Acad Derm* 1987;16:1058–1060.

47 **Gutknecht DR.** Treatment of disseminated *Mycobacterium chelonae* infection with ciprofloxacin. *J Am Acad Derm* 1990;23:1179–1180.

48 **Burns DN, Rohatgi PK, Rosenthal R, Seiler M, Gordin FM.** Disseminated *Mycobacterium fortuitum* successfully treated with combination therapy including ciprofloxacin. *Am Rev Respir Dis* 1990;142:468–470.

49 **Drabick JJ, Duffy PE, Samlaska CP, Scherbenske JM.** Disseminated *Mycobacterium chelonae* subspecies *chelonae* infection with cutaneous and osseous manifestations. *Arch Dermatol* 1990;126:1064–1067.

50 **Nelson BR, Rapini RP, Wallace RJ, Tschen JA.** Disseminated *Mycobacterium chelonae* ssp. *abscessus* in an immunocompetent host and with a known portal of entry. *J Am Acad Derm* 1989;20:909–912.

51 **LaBorde H, Rodrique S, Catoggio PM.** *Mycobacterium fortuitum* in systemic lupus erythematosus. *Clin Exper Rheum* 1989;7:292–293.

52 **Cooper JF, Lichtenstein MJ, Graham BS, Schaffner W.** *Mycobacterium chelonae:* a cause of nodular skin lesions with a proclivity for renal transplant recipients. *Am J Med* 1988;86:173–177.

53 **Fonseca E, Alzate C, Canedo T, Contreras F.** Nodular lesions in disseminated *Mycobacterium fortuitum* infection. *Arch Dermatol* 1987;123:1603–1604.

54 **Wolinsky E.** Nontuberculous mycobacteria and associated disease. *Am Rev Respir Dis* 1979;119:107–159.

55 Sack JB. Disseminated infection due to *Mycobacterium fortuitum* in a patient with AIDS. *Rev Infect Dis* 1990;12:961–963.

56 Horsburgh CR Jr., Selik RM. The epidemiology of disseminated nontuberculous mycobacterial infection in the acquired immunodeficiency syndrome (AIDS). *Am Rev Respir Dis* 1989;139:4–7.

57 Katayama I, Nishioka K, Nishiyama S. *Mycobacterium fortuitum* infection presenting as a widespread cutaneous abscess in a pregnant women. *Internatl J Derm* 1990;29:383–384.

58 Da Costa Cruz J. "Mycobacterium fortuitum" un novo bacilo acido resistente pathogenico par o homem. *Acta Medica Rio de Janeiro* 1938; 1:297–301.

59 Robicsek F, Daugherty HK, Cook JW, et al. *Mycobacterium fortuitum* epidemics after open heart surgery. *J Thorac Cardiovasc Surg* 1978; 75:91–96.

60 Hoffman PC, Fraser DW, Robicsek F, O'Bar PR, Mauney CU. Two outbreaks of sternal wound infection due to organisms of the *Mycobacterium fortuitum* complex. *J Infect Dis* 1981;143:533–542.

61 Kuritsky JN, Bullen MG, Broome CV, Silcox BA, Good RC, Wallace RJ. Sternal wound infections and endocarditis due to organisms of the *Mycobacterium fortuitum* complex. *Ann Intern Med* 1983;98:938–939.

62 Clegg HW, Foster MT, Sanders EW, Baine WB. Infection due to organisms of the *Mycobacterium fortuitum* complex after augmentation mammaplasty: clinical and epidemiologic features. *J Infect Dis* 1983;147:427–433.

63 Safranek TJ, Jarvis WR, Carson LA, Cusick LB, Bland LA, Swenson JM, Silcox VA. *Mycobacterium chelonae* wound infections after plastic surgery employing contaminated gentian violet skin-marking solution. *N Engl J Med* 1987;317:197–201.

64 Wallace RJ Jr, Musser JM, Hull SI, Silcox VA, Steele LC, Forrester GD, Labidi A, Selander RK. Diversity and sources of rapidly growing Mycobacteria associated with infection following cardiac surgery. *J Infect Dis* 1989;159:708–715.

65 Wallace RJ, Steele L, Labidi A, et al. Heterogeneity among isolates of rapidly growing mycobacteria responsible for infections following augmentation mammaplasty despite case clustering in Texas and Florida. *J Infect Dis* 1989;160:281–288.

66 Soto LE, Bobadilla M, Villalobos Y, Sifuentes J, Avelar J, Arrieta M, Ponce de Leon S. Postsurgical nasal cellulitis outbreak due to *Mycobacterium chelonae*. *J Hosp Infect* 1991;19:99–106.

67 Carson LA, Peterson NJ, Favero MS, Aguero SM. Growth characteristics of atypical mycobacteria in water and their comparative resistance to disinfectants. *Appl Environ Microbiol* 1978;36:839.

68 Pope J Jr, Sternberg P, McLane NJ, Potts DW, Stulting RD. *Mycobacterium chelonae* scleral abscess after removal of a scleral buckle. *Am J Ophthalmol* 1989;107:557–558.

69 Lowry PW, Jarvis WR, Oberle AD, Bland LA, Silberman R, Bocchini JA, Dean HD, Swenson JM, Wallace RJ. *Mycobacterium chelonae* causing otitis media in an ear-nose-and-throat practice. *NEJM* 1988;319:978–982.

70 Band JD, Ward JI, Fraser DW, et al. Peritonitis due to a *Mycobacterium chelonei* like organism associated with intermittent chronic peritoneal dialysis. *J Infect Dis* 1982;145:9–17.

71 Bolan G, Reingold AL, Carson LA, et al. Infection with *Mycobacterium chelonei* in patients receiving dialysis and using processed hemodializers. *J Infect Dis* 1985;152:1013–1019.

72 Lowry PW, Beck-Sague CM, Bland LA, Aguero SM, Arduino MJ, Minuth AN, Murray RA, Swenson JM, Jarvis WR. *Mycobacterium chelonae* infection among patients receiving high-flux dialysis in a hemodialysis clinic in California. *J Infect Dis* 1990;161:85–90.

73 Nolan CM, Hashisaki PA, Dundas DF. An outbreak of soft-tissue infection due to *Mycobacterium fortuitum* associated with electromyography. *J Infect Dis* 1991;163:1150–1153.

74 Robicsek F, Hoffman PC, Masters TN, Daugherty HK, Cook JW, Selle JG, Mauney CU, Hinson P. Rapidly growing nontuberculous mycobacteria: a new enemy of the cardiac surgeon. *Ann Thor Surg* 1988;46:703–710.

75 Schlossberg D, Aaron T. Aortitis caused by *Mycobacterium fortuitum*. *Arch Intern Med* 1991;151:1010–1011.

76 Centers for Disease Control. Follow-up on mycobacterial contamination of porcine heart valve prostheses—United States. *MMWR* 1978;27:92–98.

77 Chow WH, Leung WH, Tai TLY, Lee WT, Cheung KL. Echocardiographic diagnosis of an aortic root abscess after *Mycobacterium fortuitum* prosthetic valve endocarditis. *Clin Cardiol* 1991;14:273–275.

78 Wallace RJ, Swenson JM, Silcox VA, Bullen MG. Treatment of nonpulmonary infections due to *Mycobacterium fortuitum* and *Mycobacterium chelonei* on the basis of in vitro susceptibilities. *J Infect Dis* 1985;152:500–514.

79 Herold RC, Lotke PA, MacGregor RR. Prosthetic joint infections secondary to rapidly

growing *Mycobacterium fortuitum*. *Clin Ortho Related Res* 1987;216:184–186.

80 Edelstein H, McCabe RE. *Mycobacterium fortuitum* infection in a patient with a penile prosthesis. *Scan J Urol Nephrol* 1990;24: 315–316.

81 Newman PE, Goodman RA, Waring GO III, Finton RJ, Wilson LA, Wright J, Cavanagh HD. A cluster of cases of *Mycobacterium chelonei* keratitis associated with outpatient office procedures. *Am J Ophthalmol* 1984; 97:344–348.

82 Dugel PU, Holland GN, Brown HH, Pettit TH, Hofbauer JD, Simons KB, Ullman H, Bath PE, Foos RY. *Mycobacterium fortuitum* keratitis. *Am J Ophthalmol* 1988; 105:661–669.

83 Fong-Rong H. Infectious crystalline keratopathy caused by *Mycobacterium fortuitum* and *Pseudomonas aeruginosa*. *Am J Ophthalmol* 1990;109:738–739.

84 Rootman DS, Insler MS, Wolfley DE. Canaliculitis caused by *Mycobacterium chelonae* after lacrimal intubation with silicone tubes. *Can J Ophthalmol* 1989;24:221–222.

85 Katowitz JA, Kropp TM. *Mycobacterium fortuitum* as a cause for nasolacrimal obstruction and granulomatous eyelid disease. *Ophthalmol Surg* 1987;18:97–99.

86 Svirbely JR, Buesching WJ, Ayers LW, Baker PB, Britton AJ. *Mycobacterium fortuitum* infection of a Hickman catheter site. *Am Soc Clin Pathol* 1983;80:733–735.

87 Hoy JF, Rolston KVI, Hopfer RL, Bodey GP. *Mycobacterium fortuitum* bacteremia in patients with cancer and long-term venous catheters. *Am J Med* 1987;83:213–217.

88 Brady MT, Marcon JF, Maddux H. Broviac catheter-related infection due to *Mycobacterium fortuitum* in a patient with acquired immunodeficiency syndrome. *Ped Infect Dis J* 1987;6:492–494.

89 Woods GL, Hall GS, Schreiber MJ. *Mycobacterium fortuitum* peritonitis associated with continuous ambulatory peritoneal dialysis. *J Clin Microbiol* 1986;23:786–788.

90 Merlin TL, Tzamaloukas AH. *Mycobacterium chelonae* peritonitis associated with continuous ambulatory peritoneal dialysis. *Am J Clin Pathol* 1989;91:717–720.

91 Soriano F, Rodriguez-Tudela JL, Gomez-Garces JL, Velo M. Two possibly related cases of *Mycobacterium fortuitum* peritonitis associated with continuous ambulatory peritoneal dialysis. *Eur J Clin Microbiol Infect Dis* 1989;8:895–897.

92 LaRocco MT, Mortensen JE, Robinson A. *Mycobacterium fortuitum* peritonitis in a patient undergoing chronic peritoneal dialysis. *Diagn Microbiol Infect Dis* 1986;4:161–164.

93 Wallace RJ Jr, Hull SI, Bobey DG, et al. Mutational resistance as the mechanism of acquired drug resistance to aminoglycosides and antibacterial agents in *Mycobacterium fortuitum* and *Mycobacterium chelonei*. *Am Rev Respir Dis* 1985;132:409–416.

Fish and shellfish poisoning

ARVID E. UNDERMAN
JOHN M. LEEDOM

INTRODUCTION

A cholesterol-conscious public, spurred on by the 1988 Surgeon General's report on reducing dietary fat, has increasingly eschewed red meat in favor of fish. However, this increased consumption is not without its own hazards.

A recent article asks, "Is Our Fish Fit to Eat?"(1). Its focus was on exogenous contamination by bacteria, heavy metals such as mercury, and a variety of organic pesticides. The special problem of fish contaminated by polychlorinated dibenzodioxins and dibenzofurans (PCBs) has also been studied (2). Suffice it to say, the conclusions reached are enough to send even the die-hard, diet-conscious consumer back to a repast of red meat!

Less commonly, there also exists a potential for poisoning from endogenous seafood-associated biotoxins. This subject has recently been reviewed in both journals and texts (3–7).

Various names and classifications for this type of poisoning have been used, but none are entirely satisfactory. "Pelagic paralysis," while physiologically and alliteratively pleasing, is etymologically and ecologically incorrect (8). "Pelagic" refers to the open seas; however, marine biotoxins nearly always occur in association with organisms found in coastal or coral reef waters. Perhaps "neritic neurotoxins" would be acceptable?

Another classification is based on the location of the toxin (6). Thus, ichthyosarcotoxin is found in muscle, ichthyocrinotoxins in glands, ichthyootoxins in gonads and roe, and ichthyohemotoxins in hemolymph. Though no doubt understandable to "ichthyologists," there is something "fishy" about these cumbersome terms, which, by definition, exclude shellfish.

In this discussion, these poisonings will be separated into two groups, based on the producer of the biotoxins. In the first group, the biotoxins originate primarily in dinoflagellates; in the second, they are produced by bacteria or bacterial decomposition. This grouping takes into consideration the close structural and phylogenetic relationship of many of the toxins.

As knowledge increases, multiple toxins will be implicated in these poisonings. Thus, it might be best to consider them as syndromes rather than specific entities.

DINOFLAGELLATE-RELATED SYNDROMES

Dinoflagellates are single-celled microalgae whose taxonomy is considered debatable. Some authorities might classify them as protozoa. They usually have cellulose-containing walls, most are photosynthetic, and they abound in all oceans. Some are free floating, while others are fixed. Only a small proportion produce biotoxins, and these species are predominantly shore and reef associated. These biotoxins may be concentrated in the fish food chain; in mollusks, which filter feed, they are present during periods of high seawater dinoflagellate density. Usually, this occurs in warmer months. Thus, mussels originating in coastal waters of California are banned from May through October.

Dinoflagellate-associated syndromes to be considered include: ciguatera fish poisoning, paralytic, neurotoxic, and diarrhetic shellfish poisoning, followed by amnesic shellfish poisoning.

Ciguatera fish poisoning

Background   Ciguatera poisoning is a syndrome characterized by gastrointestinal, neurologic, musculoskeletal, and (less commonly) cardiovascular symptoms following ingestion of fish. These fish originate in tropical waters and usually exceed six pounds.

The name is attributed to the naturalist Don Antonio Parra, who in 1787 described typical symptoms in himself and his family following a meal of cooked fish. This illness resembled one that was common to colonists of the Spanish Antilles, who ascribed it to ingestion of "cigua" or turban-shelled snails (*Turbo pica*) (9,10). Similar illnesses had previously been described in sailors of the explorer de Quiros, as well as Captain Cook himself, during their Pacific voyages (8).

Epidemiology   Ciguatoxic fish are restricted to oceans between latitudes 35° on either side of the equator (10,11). Nevertheless, with air transport, poisoning may occur anywhere. An increased incidence may be associated with disruption of coral reef ecology by dredging or military activity (12). Relatively few of the 400 species of bony fish that have been described as ciguatoxic account for the majority of cases; they include snappers, jacks, barracuda, grouper, and parrot fish species (11).

In North America, ciguatera is the most commonly reported toxin-caused food poisoning. In Florida and the Virgin Islands, its estimated annual incidence has been 0.5 and 36.5 per thousand (13,14). In Puerto Rico, 7% of inhabitants have reported ciguatoxic symptoms (15). Cases have been reported in California, North Carolina, Vermont, Washington, Hawaii, Texas, Georgia, and Canada (16–23). However, with the exception of Hawaii, North Carolina, Georgia, and Texas, either the fish were imported or the patients had travelled. In the Caribbean and Indo-Pacific, the incidence is often high enough to require importation of fish rather than eating those from native waters. In Florida, barracuda has been banned (13).

Pathogenesis and toxinology   Ciguatoxin was first isolated and its chemical nature defined by Scheuer in 1967 (24). It is a fat-soluble, polycyclic, quaternary ammonium compound. In 1979, Bagnis et al. reported the source of the toxin to be the epiphytic coral reef dinoflagellate *Gambierdiscus toxicus* (25). In other areas, such as the Caribbean, different dinoflagellates produce structurally and chemically related toxins. These included species of *Prorocentrum*, *Gymnodinium*, and *Gonyaulax* (26). Ciguatoxin in pure form is a heat-, cold-, and acid-stable substance with a molecular weight of 1,100 and a median lethal dose (LD_{50}) for mice of 0.45 mg/kg (26). This amount is typically contained in two to five grams of ciguatoxic fish.

Actually, the clinical syndrome of ciguatera poisoning is associated with at least four more toxins. The water-soluble maitotoxin (maito is the Tahitian name for surgeon fish) has been demonstrated in G. *toxicus*, as well as from viscera and tissues of the surgeon fish *Ctenochaetus strigosus* (27,28). Moreover, a maitotoxin-associated hemolysin and a ciguatera-associated adenosine triphosphate (ATPase) inhibitor have been demonstrated to be present (28). A fifth toxin is scaritoxin, which, for uncertain reasons, has only been isolated from the parrot fish (*Scarus gibbus*) (29). Unlike ciguatoxin, its onset is delayed and produces more ataxia. Ciguatera poisoning has been observed in mackerel (*Decapterus macrosoma*); however, here the principle toxin was demonstrated to be a palytoxin (30). Palytoxins were first isolated in 1971 from coelenterates and, like ciguatoxin, are polycyclic ethers (31,32).

Similarly, ciguatoxin resembles brevetoxin C produced by the dinoflagellate *Ptychodiscus brevis*, as well as okadaic acid, which is produced by *Prorocentrum lima* (26). Clearly, the similarity of these toxins reflects the phylogeny of the dinoflagellates, but the biologic reason for their production remains obscure. Moreover, the predominance of one toxin over another or its presence in only one species of fish (e.g., scaritoxin) is also a mystery. Conjecturally, it could reflect either environmental factors or result from species-specific effects in the fish itself.

In humans, the pharmacology of the toxins is complex. Currently, ciguatoxin and related compounds are thought to competitively occupy calcium receptor sites, which increases the permeability of sodium channels in excitatory membranes (33). Hypertension and tachycardia suggest alpha-adrenergic action (34,35). Hypotension could be caused by maitotoxin, which is a cardiac depressant that acts by calcium channel activation and can be inhibited by calcium channel blockers (e.g., verapamil) (35,36,37).

The foregoing experimental data are borne out *in vitro*. Electrophysiologic studies were conducted on a rat model, as well as on 15 humans suffering from accidental acute ciguatera poisoning (38,39). Both studies demonstrated slowed nerve conduction velocities, along with lengthened absolute and relative membrane refractory periods. This was deemed indicative of delayed repolarization and thereby suggests that sodium channel activation is prolonged (34,38).

Clinical manifestations and diagnosis   As stated by Withers, "The symptom complex of ciguatera is polymorphous," and indeed symptoms are quite variable, numbering in excess of 150 (6,10). Nevertheless, they fall within confines that are gastrointestinal, neurosensory, neuromuscular, and cardiovascular. That such variability of symptoms would occur is predictable, given the multiplicity of toxins, as well as their varying concentrations in ciguatoxic fish.

Ciguatera poisoning should be suspected in any person who presents with both gastrointestinal and neurologic symptoms following a fish meal. Symptoms at presentation and during the course of illness have been tabulated in a number of reviews and are summarized in Table 12.1 (39–43). Of these, two symptoms are considered characteristic: heat-cold reversal and dental pain sometimes coupled with a spurious sensation of loose teeth. Heat-cold reversal is the sensation of burning when the skin is in contact with cold water. It occurs in two-thirds of cases, while dental pain is less common, occurring in only one-third.

Ninety percent of patients experience symptoms within 12 hours; however, their onset may be within 15 to 30 minutes. Most occur between one and three hours. Patients who experience a prolonged course often have a biphasic illness. At first, they experience typical ciguatoxic symptomatology and then improve, only to relapse in five to ten days with imbalance, ataxia, and tremor. This is characteristic of scaritoxin (29). The observation that ciguatera poisoning is more severe in those previously affected is enigmatic. This could simply reflect the accumulation or cumulative effect of the toxin. Immune sensitization has been postulated (39,42), but no antibody to any of the toxins could be demonstrated by counterimmune electrophoresis (44). Symptoms resolve with time, and most cases recover within one to four weeks. Nevertheless, with more severe poisonings, neurosensory symptoms can last six months (42).

Pruritus is especially bothersome, and, in French-speaking New Caledonia, ciguatera poisoning is known as "le gratte" or "the itch." It has been likened to the intense pruritus experienced by some people when receiving opiates. Biopsy-proven polymyositis has been reported in two patients with remote histories of severe ciguatera poisoning (45). If this were more than coincidental, one would anticipate similar reports for the huge experience in French Polynesia (42,43).

Ciguatera poisoning has also been reported to be transmitted from an affected male to an unaffected female during intercourse (46). The fetus can also be affected in a pregnant woman, with increased fetal movement noted (47,48). In one case, the infant was born with facial paralysis, which resolved, and later had dystonia. The mother experienced painful nipple paresthesias with breast feeding. Ciguatoxin may also be transferred in breast milk to the nursing infant (49).

Treatment and prevention Treatment is largely supportive. Nevertheless, with increased understanding of toxin action, clinicians may be able to base future efforts more rationally, as well as account for the success of empiric therapy.

As with any ingestion, gastric lavage, emetics, and activated charcoal can be used. Usually, nausea and vomiting are already present, so little is accomplished beyond adding to the patient's manifest misery. Volume depletion and hypotension require intravenous fluids. In otherwise healthy individuals, cardiovascular effects are well tolerated and easily managed. Bradycardia may be corrected with atropine (0.01 mg/kg). An infusion of one to three grams of calcium gluconate over 24 hours is widely recommended. If a pressor is needed, dopamine (5 to 20 mcg/kg/min) has been used. Opiates such as morphine sulfate (a cyclic ether histamine releaser) are contraindicated because they may precipitate hypotension and exacerbate pruritus (37).

Table 12.1   Common symptoms of ciguatera poisoning

Symptoms	Percentage* of cases		
	Virgin Islands	Australia	French Polynesia
Gastrointestinal			
Nausea	—	55	43
Vomiting	35	35	38
Diarrhea	91	64	71
Abdominal pain	39	52	47
Neurosensory			
Pruritus	58	76	50
Oral paresthesias	36	66	89
Dental pain	24	37	25
Hot-cold reversal	36	76	88
Perspiration	18	43	32
Headache	33	62	59
Ataxia	—	54	38
Vertigo, dizziness	21	45	42
Other			
Arthralgia	52	79	86
Myalgia	30	83	81
Fatigue/energy loss	70	90	60
Rash	9	26	21

*Nearest whole percent.
SOURCE Adapted from References 39 to 43.

Use of 20% mannitol intravenously has been advocated based on dramatic improvement in ciguatoxic patients who were mistakenly diagnosed with cerebral edema. The patients reportedly received 1 g/kg infused over one hour (50,51,52). There was rapid resolution of neurosensory symptoms and even reversal of hypotension and shock. Although the mechanism of action is obscure, the authors opined that mannitol may competitively inhibit ciguatoxin at the membrane level or somehow render it inert (50). More plausibly, the mannitol may reverse the microscopic edema of the neural tissue that has been observed histologically (51). Although these reports were not part of a controlled trial, mannitol is inexpensive, and the risk benefit ratio seems favorable.

Pruritus can be treated with hydroxyzine (20 to 50 mg P.O. q. 6 to 8 h P.R.N.) or cyproheptadine (4 mg P.O. q. 6 h P.R.N.). Antihistamines and corticosteroids are less effective (6). Headaches are usually responsive to acetaminophen, and the calcium channel blocker nifedipine (10 mg P.O. t.i.d.) has been used (52). Nonsteroidals, notably indomethacin (25 mg P.O. t.i.d.), are effective for musculoskeletal pain, possibly by blocking arachidonic acid and thromboxane A_2 (6,37). Amitriptyline (25 mg P.O. b.i.d.) may help with more persistent neuritic symptoms, presumably by blocking sodium channels, as well as by its anticholinergic effects (53). Similarly, lidocaine derivatives, which also block sodium channels, might ameliorate symptoms. Tocainide (25 mg P.O. b.i.d.) has been reported to be effective in reducing symptoms in three patients who received no benefit from amitriptyline (54).

Prevention is as simple as avoidance of ciguatoxic fish. Although these are usually larger than six pounds (2.7 kg), 18% of red snapper smaller than this were still ciguatoxic (55).

A rapid enzyme-linked immunoassay for detection of ciguatoxin has been developed and demonstrated to be superior to previously used radioimmunoassay and mouse bioassay methods (56,57,58). This assay employs a sheep-derived IgG anticiguatoxin antibody conjugated with horseradish peroxidase, which is combined with fish tissue. Hokama adapted this assay to a rapid stick method to probe fish tissue (59). This has been further refined using monoclonal antibody directed against ciguatoxin with the intent to allow fishermen immediate testing of their catch. The benefit of such testing appears obvious but as yet it is not regularly used.

Shellfish poisoning

Background   Shellfish have been widely consumed since prehistoric times and are considered in various cultures and locales as delicacies or dietary staples. Coastal middens often contain huge numbers of discarded shells, attesting to our ancestors' tastes. Demand for mussels, oysters, scallops, and clams has outstripped natural supply, giving rise to intensive aquaculture. The inherent nature of this industry carries the potential for widespread epidemic illness when "farmed" waters become contaminated. Excluding human, agricultural, and industrial effluvia, filter-feeding bivalve mollusks can accumulate biotoxins that are present either in the water or within the phytoplankton upon which they feed. As few as 15 of 1,200 species of dinoflagellates and closely related diatoms produce toxins (5–7).

Illness subsequent to eating shellfish can be allergic, infectious (either bacterial or viral), or toxic. The most common toxic forms are paralytic, neurotoxic, and diarrhetic. The most recently described amnesic shellfish poisoning will be considered separately.

Epidemiology   Outbreaks of shellfish poisoning occur throughout the world, including Europe, both coasts of Canada and the United States, as well as the Indo-Pacific (60–66). Often, these outbreaks occur in conjunction with "red tides"(60), a phenomenon that also gives the Red Sea its name. References to red tides were made as early as 1884 (67). The causative organisms can rapidly multiply from as few as 20,000 to 20,000,000 per liter of seawater. The result is a massive killing of fish and waterfowl (6,68). These red tides are frequent occurrences along the U.S. coasts during warmer months. In other waters, these "blooms," as they are called, are associated with the spring warming and autumn cooling cycles. Nevertheless serious shellfish intoxications can occur in the absence of red tides (66). Species most often involved include *Ptychodiscus brevis* (formerly *Gymnodinium*) in the case of neurotoxic shellfish poisoning and *Protogonyaulux catenella* and *tamarensis* in paralytic shellfish poisoning. Other species implicated include *Prorodinium bahamense* and species of *Gonyaulax*.

Dinophysis fortii and *acuminata* are associated with diarrhetic shellfish poisoning, with outbreaks occurring in Japan, Spain, the Netherlands, and Chile (7,69,70). Serious shellfish intoxications can occur in the absence of red tides, however, as happened in a recent outbreak in Guatemala (66).

Pathogenesis and toxinology   Animal death was associated with red tides as early as 1947 (71). A toxin was identified in 1958 (72). Two more decades of research resulted in isolation of a group of closely related polycyclic ethers, brevetoxins, A, B, and C (37,67,73). In most red tides, type B is the major toxic component. Brevetoxins are extremely potent and act through enhancement of sodium entry by binding at site 5 in the voltage-sensitive sodium channels present in the membranes of neuromuscular and neuronal cells (73). You will recall that ciguatoxin acts by the same mechanism.

The main toxin causing paralytic shellfish poisoning is saxitoxin and its hydroxy-derivative neosaxitoxin (3,5–7,67). This diguanidium purine was first isolated from the Alaskan butter clam, *Saxidomus giganteus*, which has been the source of outbreaks as recently as 1990 (65). Saxitoxin is water-soluble, heat- and acid-stable, but base-labile; hence, steaming or boiling will not destroy it. However, the process of boiling can elute the toxin from tissue into the "broth" and concentrate it by evaporation. Alcohol probably does not augment absorption from the gastrointestinal tract but may blunt early symptoms and therefore increase consumption. Maximum safe levels in shellfish are less than 80 mcg/100 g. In the recent Massachusetts outbreak, concentrations in un-eaten raw mussels were 24,400 mcg/100 g (65)! Saxitoxin is chemically related to tetro-dotoxin, and both work at site 1 of the voltage-sensitive sodium channel (37,73,74). This blocks propagation of nerve and skeletal muscle action potentials. This effect has been demonstrated repeatedly in animal experiments but also in accidental human cases with nerve conduction studies (75). Abnormalities of conduction resolved in six days and were correlated with recovery.

In diarrhetic shellfish poisoning, there are two groups of toxins. The first is okadaic acid and its derivatives dinophysistoxin 1 and 3 (69). The second comprises novel polyether lactones called pectenotoxins. A third toxin has been reported and named yessotoxin after the scallop *Pactinopecte yessoensis* (70). The exact mechanism of toxin-induced diarrhea is uncertain, possibly cytotoxicity. The minimum dose of okadaic acid causing diarrhea is 40 mcg.

Clinical manifestations   The onset of paralytic shellfish poisoning is rapid, occurring within a few minutes to hours. Neurotoxic shellfish poisoning may be viewed clinically as a milder form of paralytic shellfish poisoning. However, their respective mechanisms of action are opposite. Recall that brevetoxins stimulate sodium entry, while saxitoxin blocks it. Neurotoxic shellfish poisoning actually more closely resembles ciguatera poisoning.

In paralytic shellfish poisoning, neurologic symptoms begin within 30 minutes; gastrointestinal symptoms, though present, are not prominent. Initially, there are circum and intraoral paresthesias. These spread to the neck, then abaxially. Incoordination and weakness, associated with dysphonia, dysphagia, and ataxis, progresses to flaccid paralysis. The patient remains alert unless anoxia occurs (3–6,65–67,76). Most cases will recover without deficit within seven days if ventilation can be supported. Children may be more sensitive to saxitoxin and have a higher fatality rate (66,67).

Neurotoxic shellfish poisoning characteristically develops more slowly, usually after 30 minutes and closer to three hours. Nausea, vomiting, abdominal pain, and diarrhea are prominent. A peculiar rectal burning has been described (7,67). Paralysis has never been reported, but vertigo, ataxia, and incoordination regularly occur. Convulsions, though rare, may necessitate ventilator support (67). Symptoms and signs subside in as few as 12 hours to four days. A respiratory syndrome has been observed during red tide. Since, unlike most dinoflagellates, *Ptychodiscus brevis* lacks a rigid outer layer, toxin can be liberated and aerosolized by the pounding of the surf. This may produce cough, dyspnea, rhinorrhea, and bronchospasm in sensitive individuals (3,6,67,77).

Treatment and prevention   Treatment is supportive. In paralytic shellfish poisoning, emesis may not occur, hence gastric lavage may be warranted. Since saxitoxin is base-labile, 2% bicarbonate irrigation has been recommended. Purgatives such as absorptive charcoal slurries rarely help since most cases present after toxin absorption has occurred. Recent efforts have been directed towards developing monoclonal antibodies as antidotes against both brevetoxins and saxitoxin (78,79)

Shellfish can be screened for toxin using mouse bioassay. This is done in the United States, Europe, Australia, and Japan, so that most outbreaks involve shellfish gathered in noncommercial family or group settings. Often, warnings have been issued and shorelines posted, but they unheeded or are posted only in English and cannot be understood by non-English-speaking people. A cheap, easy, rapid assay needs to be developed.

Amnesic shellfish poisoning

Background   That there is nothing new under the sun may be a truism but does not apply to our knowledge of undersea phenomena. This is aptly demonstrated by an epidemic occurring in Canada in 1987 involving a previously undescribed intoxication following ingestion of cultured blue mussels (*Myrtilus edulis*) (80). This outbreak was later reported by the same authors in a more detailed report (81).

Two persons were hospitalized on November 22, 1987, in Moncton, New Brunswick, with gastroenteritis and mental confusion. Both had eaten mussels but from different stores (82). Two days later, two elderly men were hospitalized in Montreal with a similar symptom complex. Samples of the mussels were retrieved and traced. One day later, their source was narrowed to either Prince Edward Island or coastal Maine. The illness did not resemble paralytic or neurotoxic shellfish poisoning, which had previously been reported in Canada (83). Additional case reports ensued. By November 29, the source of the toxic mussels was pinpointed to eastern Prince Edward Island, and distribution was stopped. A national health advisory was issued on December 1, with five subsequent deaths. The two-day delay in issuing the alert, coupled with attendant confusion, touched off a national brouhaha called the "mussel mess" (84). Despite this, by December 18, the National Research Council had determined domoic acid as the cause (85). Domoic acid is a heat-stable neuroexcitatory amino acid structurally related to glutamic acid, which is a known excitatory neurotransmitter. By the time a national symposium was convened two years later in Ottawa, a story had unfolded that was every bit as fascinating as that surrounding legionnaires' disease. Amnesic shellfish poisoning is an acute illness following ingestion of mussels, characterized initially by rapid onset of nausea, vomiting, cramps, and diarrhea, followed by changing neurological symptoms, including headache, confusion, autonomic dysfunction, seizures, myoclonus, and focal deficits. Long-term sequelae include antegrade and, less frequently, retrograde amnesia (86,87).

Epidemiology   After analysis of the majority of reported cases, 98% of the implicated mussels originated from a 500-meter stretch of the Cardigan River in eastern Prince Edward Island (81,86). Oddly, no cases were reported in the United States, despite the fact that an unknown percentage of the 75,000 kg of toxic mussels harvested in November 1987 were shipped to the United States.

After domoic acid was identified in the toxic mussels, its origin was postulated to be the red alga *Chondria baileyana*, which is related to *Chondria armata*, a Japanese seaweed used in traditional folk medicine as an antihelminthic (88). However, in surrounding waters, the diatomaceous microalga *Nitzschia pungens* was the dominant species and was later confirmed as the source of the toxin (89). Diatoms are taxonomically related to dinoflagellates belonging to the division Chrysophyta rather than Pyrrophyta, but both are microalgal phytoplankton. Since this organism occurs worldwide, it seems odd that no previous outbreaks have been described. However, intense mussel aquaculture is relatively recent, having been stimulated in large part by year-round demand from regions where they are seasonally banned. Additional "blooms" of *N. pungens* occurred in 1988 and 1989, but domoic acid concentrations never reached the levels associated with development of clinical illness.

Recently, the Food and Drug Administration (FDA) issued warnings with regard to shellfish, including Dungeness crabs harvested off the coast of California, Oregon, and Washington. Crabbing was suspended in December, 1991, in Washington. Oregon banned harvesting of razor clams and mussels from November, 1991, after 11 mild cases of amnesic shellfish poisoning were reported (90).

Pathogenesis and toxinology   Mussels, like most bivalve mollusks, are extremely efficient filter feeders, processing huge volumes of seawater to extract nutritive phytoplankton. Accumulation of associated toxins within the digestive apparatus and eventually tissues results. If toxin-contaminated microalgae are not present, this same process will result in elution of the toxin from the tissues. In the case of mussels, oysters, and clams, humans eat the whole of the mollusk, including the viscera, thereby increasing the risk of intoxication. This is not true of crustaceans, such as crab, lobster, and shrimp, where the viscera are usually discarded. Domoic acid does not appear to be toxic to mollusks. However, the threshold for human toxicity appears to be 20 mcg/g (91). The level measured in the Prince Edward Island mussels reached 900 mcg/g when measured by high-pressure liquid chromatography (HPLC) (82,91,92). Thus, the severity of the outbreak appears to be directly related to the inordinately high concentration of the toxin (91). Isomers of domoic acid are created by ultraviolet light photolytically. These are much less potent, hence the intensity of sunlight may decrease toxin within the microalgae. Conversely, conditions limiting ultraviolet radiation may permit higher levels. In 1987, the "blooms" of *Nitzschia* occurred in association with thick ice (81,86).

How does domoic acid exert its toxic effects? A neuroexcitatory potential had been described previously (93). Neurotoxicity results from its effect as an agonist of glutamate, which it structurally resembles (81,93,94). It is now recognized that glutamate and aspartate are excitatory neurotransmitters. Indeed, their action may contribute to neurodegenerative disorders (94). Three glutamatergic receptor sites have been identified: one for kainic acid, a second for N-methyl-D-aspartic acid, and the third for quisqualic acid. Deleterious effects can be blocked by excitatory amino acid antagonists (e.g., ketamine, dextromethorphan) (94). Domoic acid appears experimentally to be two- to threefold more potent than kainic acid and 30- to 100-fold more potent than glutamate at respective sites. Parallel actions exist among glutamic, kainic, and domoic acid. All are potent central emetics and convulsants. All will cause neuronal damage of an acute (sodium mediated) and chronic (calcium mediated) type (95). In the case of domoic acid, greater damage occurs in older tissue, perhaps explaining increasing severity with age or chronic underlying illness.

The N-methyl-D-aspartic acid subtype receptor, when blocked, decreases long-term neuronal potentiation, a long-held electrophysiologic correlate of memory. This might explain the phenomenon of antegrade amnesia and cognitive dysfunction seen in domoic acid poisonings (94,96). Clinically, positron emission tomography (PET) performed on patients suffering domoic acid poisoning shows decreased rates of glucose metabolism in the amygdala and hippocampus, areas of the brain associated with memory and learning functions (97). Thus, in the broadest sense, the mechanism of amnesic shellfish poisoning seems to be explained.

Clinical manifestations   The acute illness follows ingestion of toxic mussels, regardless of mode of preparation. Onsets range from 15 minutes to 38 hours (median 5.5 hours) after ingestion. Gastrointestinal symptoms were present in 93% of the original 145 cases; 80% experienced nausea, 64% vomiting, 42% anorexia, and 41% abdominal cramps, along with diarrhea (86). Neurologic symptoms follow and include headache (43%) and short-term memory loss (25%), including confusion. Younger patients were more likely to have gastrointestinal symptoms, while older patients more likely had neurologic symptoms (81,86). Nineteen patients required hospitalization (4 to 101 days), 12 in the intensive care unit (ICU). Four patients less than 65 years of age had an underlying chronic illness. The ICU patients, as expected, had serious neurological dysfunction, including coma, mutism, seizures, grimacing, focal findings (alternating hemiparesis), ophthalmoplegias, hiccoughs, and emotional lability. Autonomic dysfunction, including bronchorrhea, necessitated intubation for airway protection in nine patients (81,98). Three patients died in the hospital as a direct consequence of their poisoning. Brain histology demonstrated neuronal necrosis and astrocytosis, which was most prominent in the amygdala and hippocampus (81,98,99).

Diagnosis, as with most cases of food poisoning, relies on recognition of the possibility of poisoning and thus the elicitation of the history. Rarely can toxin be shown systemically; proof comes from analysis of leftover foodstuff—in this case, mussels for domoic acid.

Perhaps the most interesting patients were those with protracted sequelae, which included memory loss and learning disorders. There was a particular problem with visuospatial recall among patients whose PET scans were abnormal (98,99).

Prevention and treatment   In Canada, Europe, the United States and Japan, there is surveillance of shellfish for important toxins, such as saxitoxin and brevetoxin. In areas where aquaculture of shellfish is economically important, stricter monitoring takes place. In Canada, mussels are examined for domoic acid. The source of each lot is labelled and batches are kept separate so that, should poisoning occur, its location can be tracked and toxic shellfish recalled. Mixing of lots by shipping cooperatives is prohibited.

Treatment of domoic acid poisoning is supportive. Usual measures are symptom and sign directed. A search for specific antidotes has shown that kynurenic acid (a neuro-excitatory amino acid) can experimentally block the gastrointestinal effect of domoic acid in animal models (100). Similarly, it has also been shown experimentally to protect mice against the neurotoxic effects of domoic acid (101). The applicability of this in clinical situations remains to be proven.

BACTERIAL TOXIN-RELATED SYNDROMES

The source of toxins for tetrodotoxin poisoning and scombroid and fish botulism (type E) is bacterial or the result of bacterial degradation of tissue components.

Tetrodotoxin or fish poisoning

Background   Poisoning from puffer fish is rare in the United States and usually inadvertent. Two cases have been reported since 1975 (102,103). This form of poisoning has been recognized for centuries (8). In Japan, puffer fish or *Fugu* are consumed as an expensive and prized delicacy, much like caviar in Europe and the United States. It, by law, must be prepared by highly trained and licensed chefs. The fugu is filleted, thinly sliced, and artfully arranged in traditional patterns (e.g., a crane). The "fugu experience" is characterized by tingling of lips and tongue, a generalized suffusion of warmth, and no doubt the psychologic exhilaration that stems from a brush with death. For many, the brush with death was too close, with death occurring in 59% of 6,386 cases reported over a period of 78 years in Japan (104). More recently, there were 372 deaths in 1,105 patients reported for the decade from 1967 to 1976 (105).

Pathogenesis and toxinology   Tetrodotoxin is a small ring molecule with elements resembling morphine and hexobarbital (37). It is heat-stable and water-soluble, with a molecular weight of 319 daltons (106). It is 50 times more potent than strychnine

(106,107). Tetrodotoxin, like saxitoxin, blocks site 1 of the voltage-sensitive sodium channels (73). Therefore, it blocks axonal transmission without affecting presynaptic release of acetylcholine or its effect upon the neuromuscular junction. Tetrodotoxin is most frequently associated with members of the puffer fish family (order Tetraodontiformes). However, the toxin has also been isolated from molas, starfish (*Astropecten polyacanthus*), the blue-ringed octopus (*Octopus maculosus* or *Hapalochlaena maculosa*), flatworms (*Planocera multitenticulata*), various crabs, and a terrestrial newt (*Taricha granulosa*), as well as other species (6,106–108). This occurrence in unrelated species implies a common source rather than convergent evolution of specialized gland or structures to produce the toxin. The weight of evidence now implicates bacterial sources (109). These are water-associated organisms and include *Listonella* (formerly *Vibrio*) *pelagia*, *Alteromonas tetraodonis*, and *Shewanella alga* (110).

Clinical manifestations   Onset of symptoms is as rapid as 10 minutes or as long as four hours. Death may occur as rapidly as 17 minutes after ingestion but usually occurs by asphyxia within 12 hours (5,6,102,107). Earliest symptoms are oral, then generalized, paresthesias, with marked nausea and vomiting. A four-stage clinical classification system is used in Japan and Asia: first degree—oral paresthesias with gastrointestinal symptoms; second degree—generalized paresthesias and motor paralysis with intact deep tendon reflexes; third degree—paralysis, aphonia, dysphagia, respiratory distress, cyanosis, and hypotension; fourth degree—respiratory paralysis, altered levels of consciousness, and shock (104,111). Two-thirds of deaths occur within six hours of ingestion. Survival past 24 hours is associated with a better prognosis (111,112). Pupils may be fixed and dilated without hypoxia and should not be used as evidence of irreversible anoxic brain damage (112).

Treatment and prevention   Intubation and ventilatory support is paramount in third- and fourth-degree stages. In earlier stages, one can monitor vital capacity and arterial blood gases. If there is a progressive reduction of vital capacity or signs of hypoventilation, then intubation can be initiated expectantly. Fluids, atropine, and pressor are used when appropriate. Recent attention has been directed to the use of anticholinesterase agents (e.g., edrophonium, neostigmine), with promising results (112,113). Ideally, these would be used early on in an attempt to prevent progression to paralysis.

Prevention is not applicable in this case since most ingestion is deliberate. As a general rule for amateur fishermen, unfamiliar species of fish should not be eaten, nor should any fish viscera be consumed.

Scombroid fish poisoning

Background   Scombroid fish poisoning is the clinical syndrome of flushing and related symptoms following ingestion of fish that has begun to spoil as a result of improper icing or refrigeration. Improper handling may occur at any time from when the fish is caught to when it is consumed (1,3). Its name derives from the family of fish most frequently associated with the syndrome, the *Scombridae*. This family comprises a number of favorite eating fish, including tuna, bonito, skipjack, wahoo, and mackerel. However, cases caused by nonscombroid fish have been widely reported and include: mahimahi (*Coryphaena hippurus*) and Atlantic bluefish (*Pomatomas saltatrix*), as well as sardines, anchovies, yellowtail, pilchard, amberjack, and black marlin (5,6,113,114). On this basis, one author has suggested changing the name to "pseudo-allergic fish poisoning" (115).

Epidemiology   Scombroid fish poisoning is probably more common than currently recognized. Nevertheless, it is widely reported throughout the United States (116–121). Since it is related to spoilage, it often occurs in areas distant from coastal waters. It has even been associated with canned tuna (122). Why it does not occur in freshwater fish has never been addressed, even theoretically.

Pathogenesis and toxinology   Histamine has long been felt to be causally related to scombroid fish poisoning. It is clear that bacteria, chiefly *Proteus morgagnii*, *Klebsiella pneumoniae*, and other water-associated, gram-negative rods produce histamine and saurine by decarboxylating L-histidine, which is present in the skin of marine fishes. Saurine, which is histamine phosphate and histamine hydrochloride, was first identified in association with a Japanese dried fish (*Cololabis saira*) called "saury" (123). Histamine levels in scombrotoxic fish exceed 20 to 50 mg/100 g of fish (6,104). Affected fish are often described as having a "peppery" or metallic taste. Red, oily fish flesh has the highest concentrations of histamine.

Whether or not histamine, along with saurine, is the sole cause of scombrotoxism is controversial. This controversy has focused on the inability to induce symptoms resembling scrombroid poisoning when either histamine or saurine are administered orally. Russell summarizes the case against histamine and saurine and argues that they are merely an index of fish deterioration (124).

Elevated urinary histamine concentrations following scombroid poisoning have recently been demonstrated in amounts exceeding those necessary for scombrotoxism (125). The histamine was not produced endogenously, as demonstrated by normal urinary levels of a mast cell secretory product (9α, 11β-dihydroxy-15-oxo-2,3,18,19-tetranoprost-5-ene 1,20 dioic acid)-PGD-M. PGD-M is the principal metabolite of prostaglandin D_2, which increases if mast cells are activated (125). The authors did not address how or in what form the histamine was absorbed; nevertheless, their study showed incontrovertibly that it was. Whether or not other substances facilitate scombrotoxism has not been demonstrated, but various amines, such as putrescine and cadaverine, are also present.

Clinical manifestation   Thus, from the above evidence, it would appear that the symptoms of scombrotoxism are those of a histamine reaction. Characteristically, there is flushing, headache, dizziness, oral and pharyngeal burning, bronchospasm, tachycardia, nausea, vomiting, cramps, and diarrhea. Pruritus and urticaria are common (3,4,5,6). Initial symptoms begin within minutes, and most have occurred within an hour. The duration of illness is one to eight hours. Few patients require hospitalization, and no direct fatalities have been reported (3,6). Symptoms may mimic monosodium glutamate poisoning. Interestingly, persons taking isoniazid may have a more severe reaction. This is attributed to blockade by the isoniazid of the gastrointestinal tract histamine (126).

Treatment and prevention   Despite arguments against histamine, clinicians are pragmatic and give antihistamines, which ameliorate most symptoms. Both diphenhydramine and hydroxyzine have been used successfully (3–6,127). Corticosteroids are not essential. Inhaled bronchodilators may be used. In general, a single treatment is all that is necessary. There are no long-term sequelae or persistent symptoms. Recently, H_2 receptor blocking agents have been tried with success. Cimetidine (300 mg IV) is commonly employed (113,128). Caution should be exercised when administering both H_1 and H_2 receptor blocking agents, as this may precipitate or aggravate hypotension.

The single most effective preventative measure against scombroid fish poisoning is prompt evisceration, followed immediately by icing or refrigeration of freshly caught fish. This refrigeration must be maintained throughout handling and transport to prevent bacterial growth (1,3,6). Such growth occurs at temperatures in excess of 20°C. Currently, the FDA is preparing guidelines for monitoring fish contamination, but no comprehensive inspection program has been initiated. Imported products undergo closer scrutiny. Clearly, this is an area for a "fresh" approach!

Fish-borne botulism

Background   Botulism is an intoxication caused by the ingestion of preformed neurotoxin produced by *Clostridium botulinum*. *C. botulinum* is an obligately anaerobic, gram-positive bacillus which forms spores (129). The organism and its spores exist in nature in soil and water (129). There are seven types of *C. botulinum*, distinguishable by the antigenic reactivities of their toxins, which are termed *C. botulinum*, types A through G. Types A, B, E, and F are the most important causes of botulism in humans (129).

C. botulinum is legitimately included in a review of poisoning caused by the ingestion of seafood because this organism is frequently found in marine sediments, is carried in the gastrointestinal contents of fish, and may contaminate fish used for food, where it may vegetate, produce toxin, be ingested, and cause disease.

C. botulinum, type E is the most prevalent of the types in marine sediments and in the guts of marine animals (129–131). It thus has been the causative agent of most episodes of botulism traced to fish products (132,133).

Epidemiology   Most outbreaks of botulism associated with fish consumption are due to *C. botulinum*, type E. The organism contaminates the surface of fish from the marine environment or resides in the gut of the animal. Methods of food preparation or preservation that encourage the spores to form vegetative organisms and elaborate toxin can result in disease in man.

During the period 1950 through 1989, the consumption of fish caused 48 (13%) of 365 food-borne botulism outbreaks in the United States (133). All but three of these outbreaks were due to *C. botulinum*, type E (133). The latter three were due to type B (133).

Most outbreaks have been due to fish that was processed. The fish may have been commercially canned, but was more likely to have been prepared in some traditional way involving fermentation or salting, often without prior removal of the viscera (133–137).

Fish-borne botulism is especially common in Alaska and Canada (136–139). In Alaska and the Canadian Arctic, hunting and fishing for subsistence are still quite common, and much food is prepared by traditional methods. These traditional methods often involve the fermentation of fish and other foods derived from the marine environment, often with the viscera and/or gills still attached to the prospective viand (136–138). Most of the victims of botulism in Canada and Alaska are Inuit, American Indians, or Aleuts (136,137).

Among 59 outbreaks of botulism studied in Canada during the period 1971 to 1984, 14 (23.7%) were associated with fish or fish products (137). Some 36 of the outbreaks were associated with the consumption of meats from marine mammals, mostly seals. Raw, parboiled, or fermented flesh was usually involved. All marine mammal outbreaks were type E. The fish-associated outbreaks were mostly type E (12), but two were type B. Outbreaks associated with the flesh of fish (7) included products that were eaten raw, parboiled, or smoked.

Half of the fish-associated outbreaks (7) reported from Canada (137) were due to the consumption of fermented salmon eggs. Such salmon eggs are fermented in their own juices, with or without added salt; they may be kneaded into a firm mass (138,139). Hauschild and Gauvreau (137) stated that adequate acid fermentation is prevented by lack of carbohydrate in the egg-juice mixture so that the eggs become putrid. They reported (137) that, in a survey of 26 lots of freshly fermented salmon eggs, the mean pH was 5.9, a pH compatible with the growth of type E and other nonproteolytic forms of *C. botulinum.*

From 1947 through 1985, 59 outbreaks of confirmed or suspected botulism were detected in Alaska (136). All 156 persons involved in the outbreaks were Alaskan natives. Some 118 (76%) were Inuits, 34 (22%) were American Indians, and four (3%) were Aleuts. Some 51% of the patients were female. There was a wide age range: from three to 77 years. The overall incidence of botulism in Alaska during the study period was 8.6 cases per 100,000 population, increasing from 1.2 cases per 100,000 in 1966 to 15.2 cases per 100,000 in 1985. Some of this increased incidence was increased ascertainment, but, as discussed in a later section, changes in methodology for the preparation of traditional native foods may have contributed to a real increased incidence.

As in Canada, the illness was associated with the consumption of traditional Inuit or Indian foods (136). Fish was a common vehicle, accounting for 37% of the confirmed laboratory outbreaks. Fermented salmon eggs were encountered in eight (44.4%) of 18 fish-caused outbreaks. These outbreaks were predominantly type E, but other types were involved more often than in the Canadian experience. Ten (44.4%) were type E, six (33.3%) were type A, and two were type B.

An unusual incident of fish-borne botulism involving fresh, unprocessed fish was reported from Hawaii in 1990 (133). Three adults from the same family suffered type B botulism. They had consumed a palani (a surgeonfish) purchased in a local market three days before the onset of illness in the first patient. Samples of leftover fish were positive for type B botulinus toxin, and cultures yielded *C. botulinum*, type B. The fish had been purchased cleaned at a local market, but, after cooking on a home grill, remnants of intestine were noted inside the fish. One patient had mild symptoms. He ate meat near the head and tail and avoided the intestinal remnants. The two severely ill patients ate the intestines and the meat around them. A fourth family member who ate meat from the back only did not become ill. Investigation showed inadequate refrigeration at the market. It is postulated that temperatures at the market allowed spores in the intestinal remnants to germinate and produce toxin. The cooking temperature on the grill was then inadequate to inactivate the toxin.

In 1987, an international epidemic of type E botulism traced to a commercially prepared ethnic food involved two persons in New York City and six others in Israel (135). All these persons consumed salted, air-dried whitefish, known as kapchunka. This food may also be called ribeyza, rostov, or betz (135). The whitefish is usually caught in the U.S. Great Lakes and, in this outbreak, was shipped on ice to New York for processing. Uneviscerated fish are stacked, approximately 275 to a tub. A coarse layer of salt is placed atop each layer of fish, and, when the tub is full, it is filled with brine. Fish are refrigerated in this solution for 23 to 28 days, then rinsed to remove all visible salt, and hung on individual hooks in a drying room for three to seven days. Following this processing, they are distributed for sale. They are eaten without further processing or cooking, although the viscera are not consumed. This processing usually results in salt (NaCl) concentrations in the flesh of the fish that are sufficiently elevated to prevent vegetation of *C. botulinum*, type E. Indeed, NaCl levels measured in the implicated product were high enough to be inhibitory for *C. botulinum*. Nevertheless, large amounts of type E botulinus toxin were found in remnants of fish consumed by the patients. It was hypothesized that the fish had *C. botulinum* spores in their guts when caught in the Great Lakes. Since the fish were not eviscerated, the gut would have been a protected low-salt environment. The spores could have vegetated and produced toxin which diffused into the flesh of the fish. As a result of this incident and two previous smaller episodes, kapchunka production has been discontinued as a commercial venture in the United States (135).

In 1982, two cases of type E botulism, one fatal, occurred in Belgium and were associated with commercially canned salmon which had been packed in a $7\frac{3}{4}$ ounce can by an Alaskan cannery (134). A "small dented in black spot and tiny hole" were found near the bottom seam of the implicated can of salmon. Investigation showed that rare tiny holes were made in the sides of the cans by processing machinery when they were reformed at the packing plant after having been shipped there in a nearly flattened form by the can manufacturer. This incident prompted a recall of approximately 60 million cans of salmon produced by nine different canneries during their 1980 to 1981 production season. As a result of this incident, industry practices have been changed in order to obviate a recurrence.

Pathogenesis and toxinology Botulism is caused by the entrance of botulinus toxin into the body. This may occur following the ingestion of spores with vegetation of the organism and subsequent absorption of the toxin from the gut; or, as in infantile botulism, by absorption of toxin produced from *C. botulinum* infecting a wound; or by the absorption of preformed toxin from a foodstuff. Only the latter mechanism is operative in fish-borne botulism.

Botulinus toxins are elaborated in culture as progenitor toxins (140). These are macromolecular complexes and are important in the pathogenesis of disease. The purified neurotoxins seem to be inactivated by passage through the stomach (132). Thus, the complexes are cleaved by digestive enzymes after passage through the stomach, yielding the absorbable neurotoxin (132). Toxigenicity in C. *botulinum* is not associated with plasmids except for type G (132). The amino acid sequences of purified botulinus neurotoxins are incompletely known (132). The known sequences of types A, B, and E light and heavy chains have considerable homology and also have homologies with tetanus toxin chains (132).

The neurotoxins of C. *botulinum* cause paralysis by recognizing a receptor on acetylcholinergic nerve endings, internalizing a portion of the toxin molecule into the nerve cell, and acting to prevent acetylcholine release from nerve endings (132,141,142). The action of the toxin is peripheral, not central; adrenergic nerves are resistant (129). Somatic efferent nerves to skeletal muscles are involved, as are efferent autonomic nerves to glands and muscles. Nerve conduction is not affected. There is a block in conduction peripheral to the site of acetylcholine release (129). Muscles are also spared (129).

Clinical manifestations and diagnosis   The primary manifestations of botulism result from the blockage imposed upon acetylcholinergic nerve endings supplying skeletal muscle. In a recent review, Wainwright et al. (136) emphasized a diagnostic pentad of clinical signs and symptoms. This pentad includes nausea and vomiting, dysphagia, diplopia or blurred vision, dry throat or mouth, and dilated and fixed pupils (136). Three or more of these manifestations were present in 38 (93%) of 41 patients studied (136). Some 38 (93%) also had one or more eye signs (diplopia or blurred vision, ptosis, or dilated and fixed pupils) (136). The nausea and vomiting are believed to be due to metabolic products of C. *botulinum* or other contaminants in food as they are not seen in wound botulism. It is important to emphasize that the diagnostic pentad results in part from the progressive descending nature of the paralysis caused by the botulinus toxin. Muscles innervated by the cranial nerves are affected first. In severe cases, paralysis descends, involves the respiratory musculature, and becomes generalized.

Confirmed botulism is defined as a person with a clinical illness compatible with botulism who has laboratory confirmation or who ate the same food as a person considered to be a laboratory-confirmed case. The laboratory investigation of a suspected case should include examination of suspected foods and the patient's serum for toxin (130,136). The detection of toxin confirms the diagnosis. Detection of toxin in vomitus is also regarded as confirmatory (136). Detection of C. *botulinum* or botulinus toxin in the stool of a person with a compatible clinical syndrome is also regarded as confirmatory (143).

Routine laboratory tests are of little help in the diagnosis of botulism. Complete blood counts, comprehensive blood chemistry panels, and cerebrospinal fluid examinations are normal unless complications supervene and cause abnormalities. Electrocardiograms are not diagnostic, but nonspecific S-T and T wave changes have been noted (144,145). Electromyography may be helpful. The muscle action potential in botulism is diminished after a single supramaximal nerve stimulus. On the other hand, paired stimuli at intervals of 2.5 milliseconds and repetitive supramaximal stimulation at rates of 20 to 50 per second result in the facilitation (augmentation) of action potentials in experimental animals (146) and man (130,147,148). These changes are not pathognomonic, may not be present in all muscle groups, and may not be present early in illness. Similar facilitation during rapid repetitive stimulation may occur in the Eaton-Lambert syndrome, a variant of myasthenia gravis (149).

Treatment and prevention   One case of suspected botulism is a public health emergency. Immediate efforts should be made to delineate the suspected food source. *Public health authorities should be notified immediately by telephone and informed of suspected cases* so they can interview others who may have ingested the suspect foodstuff and interdict the sale of the material if it was obtained commercially.

Close medical supervision is advised for persons potentially exposed to botulinus toxin, even if they are asymptomatic. Elimination of unabsorbed toxin should be facilitated by induction of vomiting, gastric lavage, and administration of laxatives (130). The administration of antitoxin to asymptomatic individuals is controversial. The material is of equine origin, and serum sickness and anaphylaxis are possibilities.

Individuals who are clinically diagnosed as having botulism should receive the above measures to eliminate unabsorbed toxin. Appropriate diagnostic laboratory tests should be done. Trivalent antitoxin directed against types A, B, and E toxin, produced by Connaught, Ltd., is available from the Centers for Disease Control (CDC) on a round-the-clock basis (130). Physicians needing antitoxin should call the CDC switchboard at (404) 639-311 from 0800 to 1630 Eastern time weekdays. After hours and on weekends and holidays, call the CDC duty officer at (404) 639-2888 and ask for the physician on call to answer questions about botulism. The antitoxin should be given as soon as possible (130). However, it may be beneficial even if given late. Circulating toxin has been demonstrated 30 days after ingestion of contaminated food (150).

A major portion of the management of the patient with botulism is providing good supportive care. That care includes respiratory support, if necessary. Prevention of aspiration and phlebothrombosis are major goals.

A recent report from Alaska (151) examined the effect of administering antimicrobial agents to eliminate persistent C. *botulinum* in the gut of botulism patients. It was concluded that the antibiotic administration correlated with an unacceptably high incidence of nosocomial pneumonia (151).

Prevention of botulism is preferable to the treatment of the disease. Proper home canning practices and continued vigilance directed at commercial food suppliers have made botulism a rare disease from those sources. Nevertheless, type E botulism from traditional foods remains a real problem in Alaska and the Canadian Arctic.

Recent changes have occurred in traditional methods of preparing fermented foods in the Arctic that predispose to the production of botulinus toxin (152). Containers set above ground have replaced traditional covered pits. Temperatures may be higher in the above-ground containers. Sealed jars or other plastic containers may be used (136,137,152). Slow, low-temperature fermentation seems to be a safer process (152). Fermentation in plastic bags is especially hazardous (136,152).

It is possible to produce immunogenic botulinus toxoids for active immunization. The immunization of populations at risk in the Arctic has been rejected because of the large number of persons involved, coupled with the relative rarity of the disease (136). The public health authorities in Alaska and Canada have stressed education of health care providers and persons at risk about botulism (136,137). They have mounted programs that include an alert surveillance system, widespread availability of antitoxin, prompt supportive medical care, and rapid exhaustive investigation of every outbreak (136,137). These programs have resulted in a marked reduction in the case fatality ratios (136,137). It is hoped that further educational efforts will reduce the hazards associated with the consumption of traditional foods in this region.

REFERENCES

1 **Consumers Union.** Is our fish fit to eat? *Consumer Reports* 1992;103–120.

2 **Svensson BG, Nilsson A, Hansson M, et al.** Exposure to dioxins and dibenzofurans through consumption of fish. *N Engl J Med* 1991; 324:9–12.

3 **Hughes JM, Merson MH.** Fish and shellfish poisoning. *N Engl J Med* 1976;295:1117–1120.

4 **Sanders WE.** Intoxications from the seas; ciguatera, scombroid, and paralytic shellfish poisoning. *Infect Dis Clin NA* 1987;1:665–676.

5 **Eastbaugh J, Shepard S.** Infectious and toxic syndromes from fish and shellfish consumption; a review. *Arch Intern Med* 1989;149: 1735–1740.

6 **Auerbach PS, Halstead BW.** Hazardous aquatic life. In: Auerbach PS, Geehr EC, eds. *Management of Wilderness and Environmental Emergencies.* St. Louis: CV Mosby, 1989;987–1002.

7 **Ragelis EP, ed.** *Seafood Toxins.* ACS Symposium Series, 242, Washington, DC: American Chemical Society, 1984.

8 **Mills AR, Passmore R.** Pelagic paralysis. *Lancet* 1988;1:161–164.

9 **Gudger EW.** Poisonous fishes and fish poisoning with special reference to ciguatera in the West Indies. *Amer J Trop Med* 1930;10:43–55.

10 **Withers NW.** Ciguatera fish poisoning. *Ann Rev Med* 1982;33:97–111.

11 **Halstead BW.** Poisonous and venomous marine animals of the world. Washington, DC: U.S. Government Printing Office, 1970:328–402.

12 **Ruff TA.** Ciguatera in the Pacific: a link with military activities. *Lancet* 1989;1:201–204.

13 **Lawrence DN, Enriquez MB, Lumish RM, et al.** Ciguatera fish poisoning in Miami. *JAMA* 1980;244:254–258,272–274.

14 **Morris JG, Lewin P, Smith CW, et al.** Ciguatera fish poisoning: epidemiology of the disease on St. Thomas, U.S., Virgin Islands. *Amer J Trop Med Hyg* 1982;31:574–578.

15 **Holt RJ, Miro G, Del Valle A.** An analysis of poison control center reports of ciguatera toxicity in Puerto Rico for one year. *J Toxicol Clin Toxicol* 1984;22:177–185.

16 **Morris PD, Campbell DS, Freeman JI.** Ciguatera fish poisoning: an outbreak associated with fish caught from North Carolina coastal waters. *South Med J* 1990;83:379–382.

17 **CDC.** Ciguatera fish poisoning—Vermont. *MMWR* 1986;35:263.

18 **Johnson R, Jong EC.** Ciguatera: Caribbean and Indo-Pacific fish poisoning. *West J Med* 1982;138:872–874.

19 **Ho AMH, Fraser IM, Ewen CDT.** Ciguatera poisoning: a report of three cases. *Ann Emerg Med* 1986;15:1225–1228.

20 **Frenette C, MacLean JD, Gyorros W.** A large common-source outbreak of ciguatera fish poisoning. *J Infect Dis* 1988;158:1128–1130.

21 **Helfrich P.** Fish poisoning in Hawaii. *Hawaii Med J* 1964;22:361–372.

22 **Bogart J, Perorotta D.** Ciguatera intoxication from Texas gulf coast (Letter). *Texas Med* 1989;85:15.

23 **Swift AEB, Swift TR.** Ciguatera. *J Med Assoc GA* 1990;79:313–318.

24 **Scheuer PJ, Takahashi W, Tsutsumi J, et al.** Ciguatoxin: isolation and chemical nature. *Science* 1967;155:1267–1268.

25 **Bagnis R, Chanteau S, Chungue E, et al.** Origins of ciguatera fish poisoning; a new dinoflagellate, *Gambierdisous toxicus,* Adachi and Fukuyo, definitely involved as a causal agent. *Toxicon* 1980;18:199–208.

26 **Ragelis EP.** Ciguatera seafood poisoning—overview. In: Ragelis EP, ed. *Seafood Toxins.* ACS Symposium Series 262. Washington, DC: American Chemical Society, 1984:25–36.

27 **Yasumoto T, Bagnis RA, Venoux JP.** Toxicity of the surgeon fishes II: properties of the principle water soluble toxin. *Bull Jpn Soc Scient Fish* 1976;43:359–365.

28 **Campbell B, Nakagawa K, Kobayashi N, et al.** *Gambierdiscus toxicus* in gut content of the surgeon fish *Ctenochaetus strigosus* (herbivore) and its relationship to toxicity. *Toxicon* 1987;25: 1125–1127.

29 **Chungue E, Bagnis RA.** Isolation of two toxins from a parrotfish *Scarus gibbus. Toxicon* 1977; 15:89–93.

30 **Kodama AM, Hokama Y, Yasumoto T, et al.** Clinical and laboratory findings implicating palytoxin as a cause of ciguatera poisoning due to *Decapterus macrosoma* (mackeral). *Toxicon* 1989;27:1051–1053.

31 **Moore RE, Scheuer PJ.** Palytoxin a new marine toxin from a coelenterate. *Science* 1971;172:495–498.

32 **Noguchi T, Hwang DF, Arakawa O, et al.** Palytoxin as the causative agent in the parrotfish poisoning. In: Gopalkrishnakone P, Tan CK, eds. *Progress in Venom and Toxin Research: Proceedings of the First Asia-Pacific Congress on Animal, Plant, and Microbial Toxins.* Singapore: June 24–27, 1987:372–384.

33 **Legrand AM, Galonnier M, Bagnis R.** Studies on the mode of action of ciguateric toxins. *Toxicon* 1982;20:311–315.

34 **Benoit E, Legrand AM, Dubois JM.** Effects of ciguatoxin on current and voltage clamped frog myelinated nerve fibres. *Toxicon* 1987;24: 357–364.

35 **Miyahara JT, Akau OK, Yasumoto T.** Effects of ciguatoxin and maitotoxin on the isolated guinea pig atrium. *Res Commun Chem Pathol Pharmacol* 1979;25:177–180.

36 **Takahashi M, Okizumi Y, Yasumoto T.** Maitotoxin a calcium channel activator candidate. *J Biol Chem* 1982;257:7287.

37 **Sims JK.** A theoretical discourse on the pharmacology of toxic marine ingestion. *Ann Emerg Med* 1987;16:1006–1015.

38 **Cameron J, Flowers AE, Capra MF.** Effects of ciguatoxin on nerve excitability in rats (Part 1); electrophysiological studies on ciguatera poisoning in man (Part II). *J Neurol Sciences* 1987;101,87–97.

39 **Morris JG, Lewin P, Hargett NT, et al.** Clinical features of ciguatera poisoning—a study of the disease in the U.S. Virgin Islands. *Arch Intern Med* 1982;142:1090–1092.

40 **Gillespie NC, Lewis RJ, Pearn JH, et al.** Ciguatera in Australia. *Med J Austral* 1986; 145:584–590.

41 **Narayan Y.** Fish poisoning in Fiji. *Fiji Med* 1980;8:567–574.

42 **Bagnis R, Kuberski T, Laugier S.** Clinical observations on 3009 cases of ciguatera (fish poisoning) in the South Pacific. *Amer J Trop Med Hyg* 1979;28:1067–1073.

43 **Bagnis RA, Legrand AM.** Clinical features in 12,820 cases of ciguatera (fish poisoning) in French Polynesia. In: Gopalakrishmakone P, Tan CK, eds. *Progress in Venom and Toxin Research: Proceedings of the First Asia-Pacific Congress on Animal, Plant, and Microbial Toxins.* Singapore: June 24–27, 1987:372–384.

44 **Emerson DL, Galbraith RM, McMillan JP, et al.** Preliminary immunologic studies of ciguatera poisoning. *Arch Intern Med* 1983;143: 1931–1933.

45 **Stommel EW, Parsonnet J, Jenkyns LR.** Polymyositis after ciguatera toxin exposure. *Arch Neurol* 1991;48:874–877.

46 **Lange WR, Lipkin KM, Yang GC.** Can ciguatera be a sexually transmitted disease. *Clin Toxicol* 1989;27:193–197.

47 **Pearn JH, Harvey P, DeAmbrose W.** Ciguatera and pregnancy. *Med J Austral* 1982;1:57–58.

48 **Senecal PE, Osterloh JD.** Normal fetal outcome after maternal ciguatera toxin exposure in the second trimester. *Clin Toxicol* 1991;29: 473–478.

49 **Blythe DG, DeSylva D.** Mother's milk turns toxic following fish feast (Letter). *JAMA* 1990; 264:2074.

50 **Palafox NA, Jain LG, Pinano AZ.** Successful treatment of ciguatera fish poisoning with intravenous mannitol. *JAMA* 1988;259:2740–2742.

51 **Pearn JH, Lewis RJ, Ruff T, et al.** Ciguatera and mannitol. *Med J Austral* 1989;151:77–80.

52 **Williams RK, Palafox NA.** Treatment of pediatric ciguatera fish poisoning. *Amer J Dis Child* 1990;144:747–748.

53 **Calvert GM, Hryhorczuk DO, Leiken JB.** Treatment of ciguatera fish poisoning with amitriptyline and nefedepine. *Clin Toxicol* 1987;25:423–428.

54 **Lange WR, Krieder SD, Hattwick M, et al.** Potential benefit of tocainide in the treatment of ciguatera: report of three cases. *Amer J Med* 1988;84:87–88.

55 **Lang WR.** Ciguatera toxicity. *Amer Fam Phys* 1987;35;177–182.

56 Hokama Y, Abad MA, Kimura LH. A rapid enzyme-immunoassay for the detection of ciguatoxin in contaminated fish tissue. *Toxicon* 1983;21:817–824.

57 Kimura LH, Hokama Y, Abad MA, et al. Comparison of three different assays for the assessment of ciguatoxin in fish tissues; radioimmunoassay, mouse bioassay and *in vitro* guinea pig atrium assay. *Toxicon* 1982;20:907–912.

58 Hokama Y. A rapid, simplified enzyme immunoassay stick test for the detection of ciguatoxin and related polyethers from fish tissue. *Toxicon* 1985;23:939–946.

59 Hokama Y, Osugi AM, Honda SA, et al. Monoclonal antibody in the detection of ciguatoxin and other toxic polyether in fish by a rapid poke test. In: Gabrie C, Salvat B, eds. *Proceedings of the 5th International Coral Reef Congress Tahiti.* Vol 4, Moorea Antenne Museumephe 1985;449–455.

60 Hughes JM, Horwitz MA, Merson MH, et al. Foodborne disease outbreak of chemical etiology in the United States, 1970–1974. *Amer J Epidemiol* 1977;105:133–144.

61 Rhodes RA, Mills GCG, Popei K. Paralytic shellfish poisoning in Papua, New Guinea. *Papua New Guinea Med J* 1975;18:197–202.

62 Roy RN. Red tide and outbreak of paralytic shellfish poisoning in Sabah. *Med J Malaysia* 1977;31:247–251.

63 McCollum JPK, Pearson RCM, Ingham HR, et al. An epidemic of mussel poisoning in north-east England. *Lancet* 1968;2:767–770.

64 Anderson DM, Sullivan JJ, Reguera B. Paralytic shellfish poisoning in northwest Spain: the toxicity of the dinoflagellate *Gymnodinium catenatum. Toxicon* 1989;27:667–689.

65 CDC. Paralytic shellfish poisoning, Massachusetts and Alaska, 1990. *MMWR* 1991;40:157–161.

66 Rodrigue DC, Etzel RA, Hall S, et al. Lethal paralytic shellfish poisoning in Guatemala. *Amer J Trop Med Hyg* 1990;42:267–271.

67 Sakamoto Y, Lockey RF, Krzanowski JJ. Shellfish and fish poisoning related to the toxic dinoflagellates. *South Med J* 1987;80:866–871.

68 Clarke RB. Biologic causes and effects of paralytic shellfish poisoning. *Lancet* 1968;2:770–771.

69 Murata M, Shimitani B, Sugatani H, et al. Isolation and structural elucidation of the causative toxin of diarrhetic shellfish poisoning. *Bull Jpn Soc Sci Fish* 1982;48:549–552.

70 Murata M, Kumagai M, Yanagi T, et al. New aspects of diarrhetic shellfish poisoning. In: Gopalkrishnakone P, Tan CK, eds. *Progress in*

Venom Research: Proceedings of the First Asia-Pacific Congress on Animal, Plant, and Microbial Toxins. Singapore: June 24–27, 1987: 433–437.

71 Davis CG. *Gymnodinium breve,* a cause of discolored water and animal mortality in the Gulf of Mexico. *Bot Gaz* 1947;109:358–360.

72 Starr TJ. Notes on a toxin from *Gymnodinium breve. Texas Rep Biol Med* 1958;16:500–507.

73 Baden DG. Brevetoxins: unique polyether dinoflagellate toxins. *FASEB J* 1989;3:1807–1817.

74 Kao CY. Pharmacology of tetrodotoxin and saxitoxin. *Fed Pro* 1972;31:117–123.

75 Long RR, Sargent JC, Hammer K. Paralytic shellfish poisoning: a case report and serial electrophysiologic observations. *Neurology* 1990;40: 1310–1311.

76 Acres J, Gray J. Paralytic shellfish poisoning. *Can Med Assoc J* 1978;119:1195–1197.

77 Woodcock AH. Note concerning human respiratory irritation associated with high concentrations of plankton and mass mortality of marine organisms. *J Marine Dis* 1948;7:56–62.

78 Davis SR. Neutralization of saxitoxin in rabbit serum. *Toxicon* 1985;23:669–675.

79 Templeton CR, Poli MA, Solon R. Prophylactic and therapeutic use of an anti-brevetoxin (PbTx) antibody in conscious rats. *Toxicon* 1989;27:1389–1395.

80 Perl TM, Bedard L, Remis S, et al. Intoxication following mussel ingestion in Montreal. *Can Dis Wkly Rep* 1987;13:224–226.

81 Perl TM, Bedard L, Kosatsky T, et al. An outbreak of toxic encephalopathy caused by eating mussels contaminated with domoic acid. *New Engl J Med* 1990;322:1775–1780.

82 Todd ECD. Chronology of the toxic mussel outbreak. *Can Dis Wkly Rep* 1990;16(Suppl 1E):3–4.

83 Todd ECD. Shellfish and fish poisoning in Canada, 1972–1983. *Can Dis Wkly Rep* 1984;10:21–24.

84 Gray C. Mussel mystery: the more you know, the more you don't know (Editorial). *Can Med Assoc J* 1988;350–351.

85 Wright JLC, Boyd RK, DeFreitas ASW, et al. Identification of domoic acid, a neuroexcitatory amino acid in toxic mussels from east Prince Edward Island. *Can J Chem* 1989;67:481–490.

86 Perl TM, Bedard L, Kosatsky T, et al. Amnesic shellfish poisoning; a new clinical syndrome due to domoic acid. *Can Dis Wkly Rep* 1990;16(Suppl 1E):41–45.

87 Perl FM, Teitlebaum J, Hockin J, et al. Definition of the syndrome (panel). *Can Dis Wkly Rep* 1990;16 (Suppl 1E):41–45.

88 Takemoto T, Daigo K. Constituents of *Chondria armata*. *Chem Pharm Bull* 1958;6: 578–580.

89 Subba-Rao DV, Quillam MA, Pockington R. Domoic acid a neurotoxic amino acid produced by the marine diatom *Nitzschia pungens* in culture. *Can J Fish Aquatic Sci* 1988;45: 2076–2079.

90 Associated Press. FDA warns against eating organs of Dungeness crab. *Los Angeles Times* 1991; December 28, p A19.

91 Wright JLC, Bird CJ, DeFreitas ASW, et al. Chemistry, biology and toxicology of domoic acid and its isomers. *Can Dis Wkly Rep* 1990;16(Suppl 1E):21–25.

92 Lawrence JF. Determination of domoic acid in seafoods and in biologic tissues and fluids. *Can Dis Wkly Rep* 1990;16(Suppl 1E):27–31.

93 Zaczek R, Coye JT. Excitatory amino acid analogues; neurotoxicity and seizures. *Neuropharmacol* 1982;21:15–26.

94 Olney JW. Excitotoxicity: an overview. *Can Dis Wkly Rep* 1990;16(Suppl 1E):47–57.

95 Coyle JT. Neurotoxic action of kainic acid. *J Neurochem* 1983;41:1–11.

96 Biscoe TJ, Evans RH, Headly PM, et al. Domoic acid and quisqualic acid as potent amino acid excitants of frog and rat spinal neurons. *Nature* 1975;255:166–167.

97 Gjedde A, Evans AC. PET studies of domoic acid poisoning in humans: excitotoxic destruction of brain glutamatergic pathways, revealed in measurement of glucose metabolism by positron emission tomography. *Can Dis Wkly Rep* 1990;16(Suppl 1E):111–114.

98 Teitlebaum JS, Zatorre RJ, Carpenter S, et al. Neurological sequelae of domoic acid intoxication due to the ingestion of contaminated mussels. *N Engl J Med* 1990;322: 1781–1787.

99 Carpenter S. The human neuropathology of encephalopathic mussel toxin poisoning. *Can Dis Wkly Rep* 1990;73–75.

100 Glavin GB, Pinsky C, Bose R. Gastrointestinal effects of contaminated mussels and putative antidotes thereof. *Can Dis Wkly Rep* 1990;16(Suppl 1E):111–114.

101 Pinsky C, Glavin GB, Bose R. Kynurenic acid protects against neurotoxicity and lethality of toxic extract from contaminate Atlantic coast mussels. *Prog Neuropsychopharmacol Biol Psychiatry* 1989;13:569–572.

102 Sims JK, Ostman DC. Pufferfish poisoning: emergency diagnosis and management of mild human tetrodointoxication. *Ann Emerg Med* 1986;15:1094–1098.

103 CDC. Puffer fish poisoning—Florida. *MMWR* 1975;24:68.

104 Halstead BW. Poisonous and venomous marine animals of the world. Princeton, N.J. *Darwin* 1978;4373–4548.

105 Tsuenari S, Uchimura Y, Kanda M. Pufferfish poisoning in Japan—a case report. *J Forensic Sci* 1980;25:240–245.

106 Mosher HS, Fuhrman FA, Buckwald HD, et al. Tarichotoxin—tetrodotoxin, a potent neurotoxin. *Science* 1964;1100–1110.

107 Lange WR. Puffer fish poisoning. *Amer Fam Physician* 1990;42:1029–1033.

108 Bradley B, Klika L. A fatal poisoning from the Oregon rough skinned newt. *JAMA* 1981;246:247.

109 Yotsu M, Yamazaki T, Meguro Y, et al. Production of tetrodotoxin and its derivatives by *Pseudomonas* sp isolated from the skin of a pufferfish. *Toxicon* 1987;25:225–228.

110 Simidu U, Kita-Tsukamoto K, Yasumoto T, et al. *Int J Syst Bacteriol* 1990;40:331–336.

110 Halstead BW. Poisonous and venomous marine animals of the world. Princeton, N.J. *Darwin* 1978;4373–4548.

111 Kai CS. Therapeutics in pufferfish (tetrodotoxin) poisoning—the Singapore experience. In: Gopalakrishnakone P, Tan CK, eds. *Progress in Venom and Toxin Research: Proceeding of the First Asia-Pacific Congress on Animal, Plant, and Micobial Toxins.* Singapore: June 24–27, 1987:307–309.

112 Tibbals J. Severe tetrodotoxin fish poisoning. *Anaesthes Intensive Care* 1988;16:215–217.

113 Kim R. Flushing syndrome due to mahi-mahi (scromboid) fish poisoning. *Arch Dermatol* 1979;115:963–965.

114 Etkind P, Wilson ME, Gallagher K, et al. Bluefish-associated scombroid poisoning: an example of the expanding spectrum of food poisoning from seafood. *JAMA* 1987;258: 3409–3410.

115 Prescott BD. Scombroid poisoning and bluefish: the Connecticut connection. *Conn Med* 1984;48:105–110.

116 CDC. Scombroid poisoning—New Jersey. *MMWR* 1980;29:106–107.

117 CDC. Scombroid poisoning—Illinois, Michigan. *MMWR* 1980;29:167–168.

118 CDC. Restaurant-associated scombroid fish poisoning—Alabama, Tennessee. *MMWR* 1986;35:264–265.

119 CDC. Scombroid fish poisoning—New Mexico, 1987. *MMWR* 1988;37:451.

120 CDC. Scombroid fish poisoning—Illinois, South Carolina. *MMWR* 1980;38:140–142, 147.

121 Bartholomew BA, Berry PR, Rodehouse JC, et al. Scombrotoxic fish poisoning in Britain: features of over 250 suspected incidents from 1976–1986. *Epidemiol Infect* 1987;99:775–782.

122 Merson MH, Baine WB, Gangarosa EJ, et al. Scombroid fish poisoning: outbreak traced to commercially canned tuna fish. *JAMA* 1974; 220:1268–1269.

123 Foo LY. Scombroid: isolation and identification of "saurine." *J Food Agric Sci* 1976;27: 807–810.

124 Russell FE, Maretic Z. Scombroid poisoning: mini-review with case histories. *Toxicon* 1986; 24:967–973.

125 Morrow JD, Margolis GR, Rowland J. Evidence that histamine is the causative toxin of scombroid-fish poisoning. *N Engl J Med* 1991;324:716–719.

126 Uragoda CG. Histamine poisoning in tuberculous patients after ingestion of tuna fish. *Amer Rev Resp Dis* 1980;121:157–159.

127 Dickinson G. Scombroid fish poisoning syndrome. *Ann Emerg Med* 1982;11:487–489.

128 Blakesley ML. Scombroid poisoning: prompt resolution of symptoms with cimetidine. *Ann Emerg Med* 1983;12:104–106.

129 Gilbert RJ, Roberts D, Smith G. Foodborne diseases and botulism. In: Smith GR, ed. *Topley and Wilson's Principles of Bacteriology, Virology and Immunity.* Seventh Edition in 4 volumes. Baltimore, MD: Williams and Wilkins, 1983–84;3:477–514.

130 CDC. *Botulism in the United States, 1899–1977: Handbook for Epidemiologists, Clinicians, and Laboratory Workers.* Atlanta: US Department of Health, Education and Welfare, Public Health Service, 1979;10–13.

131 Ward BQ, Carroll BJ, Garrett ES, Reese GB. Survey of the US Gulf Coast for the presence of *Clostridium botulinum. Appl Microbiol* 1967;15:629–636.

132 Hatheway CE. Toxigenic clostridia. *Clin Microbiol Rev* 1990;3:66–98.

133 CDC. Fish botulism—Hawaii, 1990. *MMWR* 1991;40(24):412–414.

134 Hayes AH. The Food and Drug Administration's role in the canned salmon recalls of 1982. *Pub Health Rep* 1983;98:412–415.

135 Tezak EE, Bell EP, Kautter DA, et al. An internal outbreak of type E botulism due to uneviscerated fish. *J Infect Dis* 1990; 161:340–342.

136 Wainwright RB, Heyward WL, Midduagh JP, Hatheway CL, Harpster AP, Bender TR. Foodborne botulism in Alaska, 1947–1985: epidemiology and clinical findings. *J Infect Dis* 1988;157:1158–1162.

137 Hauschild AHW, Gauvreau L. Foodborne botulism in Canada, 1971–84. *Can Med Assoc J* 1985;133:1141–1146.

138 Dolman CE. Further outbreaks of botulism in Canada. *Can Med Assoc J* 1961;84:191–200.

139 Dolman CE, Iida H. Type E botulism: its epidemiology, prevention and specific treatment. *Can J Public Health* 1963;54:293–308.

140 Sakaguchi G. *Clostridium botulinum* toxins. *Pharmacol Ther* 1983;19:165–194.

141 Simpson LL. Molecular pharmacology of botulinum toxin and tetanus toxin. *Ann Rev Pharmacol Toxicol* 1986;26:427–453.

142 Simpson LL. The origin, structure, and pharmacological activity of botulinum toxin. *Pharmacol Rev* 1981;33:155–188.

143 Dowell VR Jr, McCroskey LM, Hatheway CL, Lombard GL, Hughes JM, Merson MH. Coproexamination for botulinal toxin and *Clostridium botulinum:* a new procedure for laboratory diagnosis of botulism. *JAMA* 1977; 238:1829–1832.

144 Koenig MG, Spickard A, Cardella MA, et al. Clinical and laboratory observations of type E botulism in man. *Med* 1964;43:517–545.

145 Koenig MG, Drutz DJ, Mushlin AI, et al. Type B botulism in man. *Amer J Med* 1967;42:208–219.

146 Mosland RL, Gammon GD. The effect of botulinus toxin on the electromyogram. *J Pharm Exp Ther* 1949;97:499–506.

147 Cheringon M, Ryan DW. Treatment of botulism with guanidine: early neurophysiologic studies. *N Engl J Med* 1970;282:195–197.

148 Cherington M, Ginsberg S. Type B botulism: neurophysiologic studies. *Neurology* 1971;21: 43–46.

149 Lambert EH, Rooke ED, Eaton LM, et al. Myasthenic syndrome occasionally associated with bronchial neoplasm: neurophysiologic studies in myasthenia gravis. In: Viets HR, ed. *The Second International Symposium Proceedings.* Charles C. Thomas, 1961.

150 Merson MH, Hughes JM, Dowell VR Jr, Taylor A, Barker WH, Gangarosa EJ. Current trends in botulism. *JAMA* 1974;229: 1305–1308.

151 Barrett D. Endemic foodborne botulism: clinical experience, 1973–1986 at Alaska Nature Medical Center. *Alaska Med* 1991;33: 101–108.

Management of infectious complications following liver transplantation

MICHAEL R. KEATING
MARK P. WILHELM

INTRODUCTION

Remarkable progress has been made in the field of hepatic allotransplantation since the first human liver transplant was performed by Starzl in 1963 (1). Refinement of surgical technique, improved organ preservation, the use of veno-venous bypass, more effective immunosuppressive agents, and improved techniques to diagnose, treat, and prevent rejection have transformed liver transplantation from an experimental procedure to a widely accepted therapeutic modality for end-stage hepatobiliary disease due to multiple causes (2). During 1991, 2,935 cadaveric liver transplants were performed at approximately 90 centers in the United States (3). One-year survival of liver transplant recipients has risen from approximately 30% in the early 1970s to the current level of about 80% (4). Despite these successes, however, infection remains a significant obstacle, particularly during the first few months following transplantation. Serious infection occurs in approximately two-thirds of liver transplant recipients. Death was attributable to infection in 37% of liver transplant recipients from 1988 to 1990 (4). A lessening of the risk of infection in these patients awaits further refinement of surgical technique, narrower spectrum immunosuppressive agents, and an enhanced ability to prevent infectious complications.

BACKGROUND

The liver can be transplanted either as an extra (auxiliary) organ placed usually in the right paravertebral space or in an orthotopic location following host hepatectomy. Although auxiliary liver transplantation continues to be performed sporadically (5), the vast majority of liver transplants currently being performed are orthotopic.

The risk for and incidence of opportunistic infection in hepatic allograft recipients roughly parallels that seen with other commonly performed solid organ transplants. The higher rate of infection encountered in liver transplantation is attributable largely to the technical aspects of the transplant operation. Orthotopic liver transplantation

226

(OLT) is a technically demanding procedure involving the construction of complex vascular and biliary anastomoses. At the time of transplantation, patients are often severely ill with coagulopathy, ascites, encephalopathy, and other effects of end-stage liver disease. The transplant surgical procedure is usually prolonged (mean duration 6.5 hours) (6) and involves large-volume blood component replacement, large fluid shifts, enterotomy (with choledochojejunostomy), and frequent postoperative bleeding with hematoma formation.

For hepatic diseases that spare the large bile ducts (e.g., postnecrotic cirrhosis,

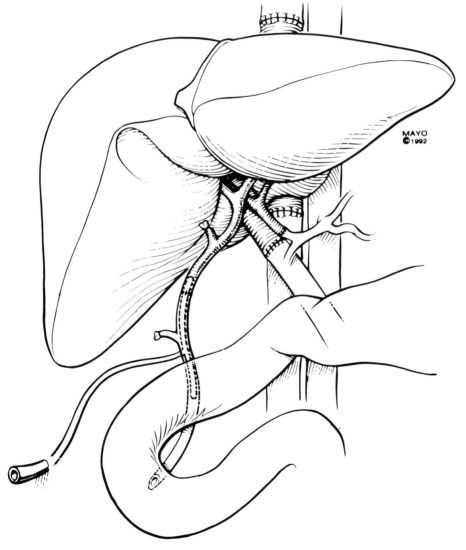

Figure 13.1   Duct-to-duct biliary anastomosis (choledochocholedochostomy).

chronic active hepatitis), a donor-to-recipient ductal anastomosis (choledochocho-ledochostomy) is usually performed (Figure 13.1). With diseases such as sclerosing cholangitis that involve the entire recipient biliary tree, the common duct of the allograft is connected to a limb of jejunum in a Roux anastomosis (choledocho-jejunostomy) (Figure 13.2). The main complication of choledochocholedochostomy is obstruction at the anastomosis, while choledochojejunostomy is more commonly associated with reflux of microorganisms into the biliary tree. A T-tube stent is placed intraoperatively across the biliary anastomosis to allow visualization of the biliary tree following transplantation. This allows for an assessment of the contribution of potential anatomical bile duct problems to postoperative graft dysfunction.

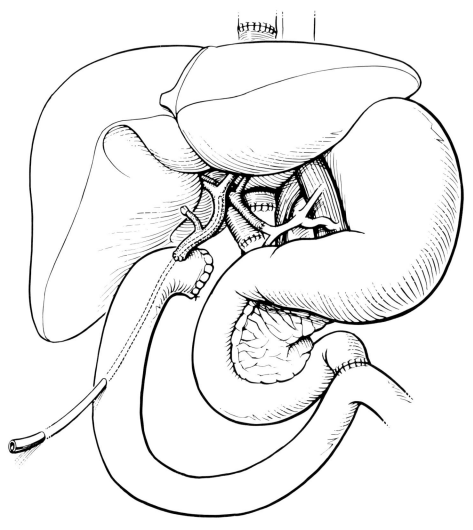

Figure 13.2 Roux-en-Y biliary anastomosis (choledochojejunostomy).

Following implantation of the allograft, immunosuppression is initiated to prevent graft rejection. The immunosuppressive agent cyclosporine A (7), which ushered in the modern era of organ transplantation in the early 1980s, is largely responsible for the improved survival of recipients of hepatic allografts. Most liver transplant programs currently employ a three-drug immunosuppressive regimen, including cyclosporine A, prednisone, and azathioprine. Acute rejection is typically treated either with augmented steroid doses or with an antilymphocyte-globulin preparation, either polyclonal (e.g., ATG) or a murine monoclonal preparation (e.g., OKT-3).

Although hyperacute rejection, as occasionally occurs in renal or cardiac transplantation, is very rarely encountered in liver transplantation, acute cellular rejection may occur at any time posttransplantation and cause various degrees of cholestasis, impaired hepatic synthetic function, and elevation of hepatic enzymes. Chronic rejection, which is a more insidious and often irreversible process, is typically associated with occlusive arterial lesions, graft fibrosis, and the destruction of intrahepatic bile ducts (8). Those patients who require frequent and/or intense, acute antirejection therapy or who must be maintained at a higher level of baseline maintenance immunosuppressive therapy are at increased risk for the development of infectious complications. In addition, the net state of immunosuppression may be augmented by the presence of chronic infection with an immune modulating virus such as cytomegalovirus or hepatitis B or C viruses (9).

In contrast to the situation with kidney transplantation, no salvage therapy exists for hepatic graft failure. There is no hepatic equivalent of dialysis. Therefore, the option of drastically lessening or discontinuing exogenous immune suppression in the treatment of serious infection would not be compatible with patient survival.

SPECTRUM AND CHRONOLOGY OF INFECTIONS

Although infections due to a wide variety of microorganisms may occur at any point following transplantation, they do not occur entirely at random but are to a significant extent chronologically predictable. To arrive at a meaningful differential diagnosis for a potential infectious disease syndrome posttransplantation, several factors need to be considered:

1 The presence of any preexisting or latent infection in the allograft recipient.

2 Possible transmission of infection via the donor graft.

3 Knowledge of anatomic/technical complexities in each individual patient.

4 The actual dosage of immunosuppressive agents and, even more importantly, the duration of immunosuppression.

5 The patient's history of acute rejection episodes or the presence of chronic rejection.

6 A knowledge of donor and recipient serostatus, particularly with respect to cytomegalovirus infection risk.

The occurrence of infection following liver transplantation can perhaps best be conceptualized, as suggested by Rubin (9), by considering three separate periods of risk posttransplantation: the early period (first month), the middle period (one to six months), and the late period (beyond six months). The occurrence of specific infection syndromes and their relevant differential diagnostic possibilities vary during each of these periods. It must be kept in mind that overlap may occur, particularly when rejection is encountered in the late period or when surgical complications confer an ongoing risk for certain bacterial and candidal infections beyond the initial postoperative month.

Infection in the early post transplant period (first month)

During the first month posttransplantation, organisms usually encountered include aerobic and anaerobic bacteria, *Candida* sp, and reactivation mucocutaneous syndromes due to herpes simplex virus. Although the actual doses of immunosuppressive agents administered during this period are usually higher than during subsequent months, the duration of immunosuppression is usually not sufficient to render the recipient susceptible to infection syndromes due to opportunistic agents such as cytomegalovirus or pneumocystis. During the first several weeks posttransplantation, the patient is at risk to develop postoperative and nosocomial infectious problems such as wound infection, pneumonia, catheter-related infection, and urinary tract infection, as well as intraabdominal infections, including peritonitis, intrahepatic or intraperitoneal abscess, and cholangitis. Risk factors for the development of early postoperative intraabdominal infections include biliary leaks, presence of hematomas, and vascular insults to the allograft such as with hepatic artery thrombosis. Ischemia of bile duct epithelial cells can result in the development of biliary strictures with subsequent cholangitis and intrahepatic abscess formation. Organisms typically encountered include enterococci, streptococci, staphylococci, *Enterobacteriaceae*, and *Candida* sp.

Early infection in the transplant recipient may arise from the allograft itself, such as bacterial infection which may have occurred during the preterminal period prior to organ harvesting. In addition, the allograft itself may have become contaminated with bacteria or *Candida* sp at some point between harvest and implantation in the recipient. It is during this early period that the hyperinfection syndrome due to *Strongyloides stercoralis* may potentially occur in susceptible recipients.

Infections in the middle posttransplant period (one to six months)

This middle period represents the time of greatest risk for the development of life-threatening opportunistic infection. By this point in the posttransplantation period, the duration of immunosuppressive therapy has been prolonged enough to cause marked depression of cell-mediated immunity. It is during this period that disease syndromes due to cytomegalovirus are most commonly encountered, including pneumonitis, hepatitis, or involvement of the gastrointestinal tract. Dermatomal reactivation of varicella-zoster virus is first encountered during this period, but may also occur during the late period. Infections due to *Pneumocystis carinii*, *Cryptococcus neoformans*, and filamentous fungi, primarily *Aspergillus* sp, occur during this period. The diagnosis of infection due to *Aspergillus* sp during the first month posttransplantation should prompt a search for an unusual epidemiologic/nosocomial hazard (10). Bacteremia and/or meningitis due to *Listeria monocytogenes* is typically first seen during this period.

During the middle period, reactivation disease syndromes are occasionally encountered due to organisms present in the recipient prior to transplantation. The introduction of high-dose immunosuppression may result in clinical illness due to reactivation of *Mycobacterium tuberculosis*, an occult focus of bacterial infection, viral hepatitis, or one of the dimorphic fungi (e.g., *Histoplasma capsulatum*, *Coccidioides immitis*). Chronic or latent infection of the donor that involves the liver may be transmitted to the immunosuppressed recipient and become clinically apparent during this period. Organisms that may be transmitted in this manner include human immunodeficiency virus (11), hepatitis B or C viruses, and latent mycobacterial or fungal organisms.

Various lymphoproliferative syndromes associated with the Epstein-Barr virus are occasionally seen during this period and beyond. Those patients that have sustained graft, particularly biliary, injury may continue to present with associated infection during this time period, usually due to bacteria or *Candida* sp. A patient presenting with an infiltrative pulmonary disease during this time period is more likely to have infection due to an opportunistic organism such as cytomegalovirus or *Pneumocystis carinii* than pneumonia during the first month, which is more likely to be caused by bacterial organisms.

Infection in the late posttransplant period (beyond six months)

Patients who have reached this point in their posttransplant course with good allograft function maintained at a low baseline level of immunosuppression have a considerably lessened risk for the development of serious infection. Infection due to opportunistic organisms is quite rare during this period. Patients remain susceptible, however, to community-acquired infections such as influenza, pneumococcal pneumonia, and simple urinary tract infection. Although organ-specific cytomegalovirus (CMV) syndromes involving the lung, gastrointestinal tract, and liver are not frequently encountered, CMV retinitis may occur during this late period.

Patients who have had frequent episodes of acute rejection requiring augmented immunosuppressive therapy or those with chronic rejection who are maintained at a higher baseline level of immunosuppression continue to be at risk for the development of serious opportunistic infections that are otherwise encountered more commonly during the middle posttransplant period.

BACTERIAL INFECTION

Infections caused by bacteria constitute the most common group of infections encountered following orthotopic liver transplantation. These occur most frequently during the first month following transplantation but may recur at any time. In a report of 103

OLT operations, 68% developed bacterial infection, and 13% died as a result of the infection (12). Fifty-three percent of these infections occurred within the first two weeks following OLT. Similarly, in a report from the University of Pittsburgh, 59% of all patients developed bacterial infection (13). Others have reported rates ranging from 53% to more than 70% (14,15).

The biliary anastomosis plays an important role in the risk for infection. During the transplant operation, external biliary drainage is secured via a T-tube at the duct-to-duct anastomosis or a tube through the roux-en-Y loop with the choledochojejunostomy anastomosis. Postoperatively, cultures of bile frequently yield coagulase-negative staphylococci, enterococci, or occasionally other streptococci. These positive cultures rarely reflect infection in the absence of clinical signs or symptoms. The choledochojejunostomy appears to be more prone to colonization with enteric pathogens that have refluxed up the roux-en-Y loop.

There are some data to suggest that the type of anastomosis influences the frequency of posttransplant infection. Overall, the frequency of bacterial infection in patients with a choledochojejunostomy is higher than in those with a choledochocholedochostomy (13). When subgroup analysis was performed on these data, the frequency of infection between the two anastomoses was very similar among patients with a single transplant operation. In contrast, in those patients who had more than one transplantation, the frequency of infection was significantly higher than in those with a choledochojejunoshymy. Buback et al. reported that 12.5% of patients with a choledochojejunostomy had one or more liver biopsies complicated by infection, while only 1% of patients with a choledochocholedochostomy anastomosis developed infection after biopsy (16). Pseudomonas bacteremia has been reported to occur more frequently in patients with a roux-en-Y anastomosis than in patients with a duct-to-duct anastomosis (17). These reports support the hypothesis that the choledochojejunostomy more readily allows reflux of bowel flora into the biliary tree.

Other risk factors for early bacterial infection have been delineated by a number of investigators. Of 19 potential risk factors examined by univariate analysis, George et al. found that, among patients surviving and not requiring retransplantation in the first two postoperative weeks, the duration of transplant surgery was the only significant risk factor for infection (12). Using logistic regression analysis, the duration of transplant surgery and a pretransplant serum bilirubin level of greater than or equal to 12 mg/dL were significant risk factors. If both factors were present, the risk of infection was 70%; with increased duration of surgery alone, the risk was 49%; with an elevated level of bilirubin alone, the risk was 36%; and if neither variable was present, the risk was 18%.

These findings corroborate those reported by Kusne et al. who found that infection rates increased steadily as surgical time increased (13). Moreover, these investigators noted that patients requiring more than one abdominal operation had increased frequency of infection compared with those who had only one; however, this influence was more significant among patients having severe fungal or viral infections than in those with bacterial infections alone.

While many organ transplant centers routinely obtain surveillance cultures from blood, urine, bile, and other sites, the utility of this practice has never been analyzed in a critical manner. Nevertheless, on theoretical grounds, there is some justification for this practice. Considering the frequency of serious bacterial infections following transplantation, a knowledge of the bacterial flora may help guide empiric therapy in the event of infection. As emergence of resistance has increasingly become a problem among bacteria, surveillance cultures with susceptibility testing may help identify multiresistant organisms. A well-designed study evaluating the role of this practice in liver transplantation is needed.

In the first month following transplantation, bacterial infections are generally those that are recognized to occur following major abdominal surgery. These include intraabdominal abscess, pneumonia, wound infection, cholangitis, peritonitis, urinary tract infection, line-associated sepsis, primary bacteremia, and others.

Intraabdominal infections are the most common and account for over 50% of bacterial infections (14). These include hepatic abscess, extrahepatic abscess, and cholangitis. Intraabdominal infection may occur within the allograft itself or as an infected intraabdominal fluid collection. The latter poses a challenging problem in posttransplant management. Fluid collections in the surgical bed are common following transplantation and are seen frequently with routine ultrasonography. In the absence of signs or symptoms, these collections are usually simply observed; however, in the presence of unexplained fever or other signs and symptoms of infection in the early post transplant period, aspiration and culture are warranted.

Cholangitis may occur at any time following transplantation. In a report of nine episodes of cholangitis, one occurred within three days of surgery and another occurred 18 months posttransplant and was associated with biliary duct strictures (13).

Similarly, bacterial pneumonia may occur as both an early and late infectious complication. Of 15 episodes of bacterial pneumonia from the University of Pittsburgh, ten were nosocomial (13). Seven occurred while the patient was still intubated, and three followed early postoperative aspiration. These 15 episodes were associated with a 40% mortality. Transplant recipients are also at risk for late community-acquired pneumonia due to *Streptococcus pneumoniae, Staphylococcus aureus*, and other bacterial pathogens.

Bacteremia may arise from either a known or unknown source. Among 16 cases of bacteremia reported by Paya et al., eight had a demonstrable underlying focus of infection (14). Similarly, in another report, 27 of 58 cases of bacteremia arose from an identifiable infected site (12). Primary or secondary bacteremia is often associated with a poor outcome. Thirty-six percent of bacteremic liver transplant recipients at the University of Pittsburgh died (13).

There is considerable variation in the microbiology of bacterial infection. Most centers report aerobic gram-negative bacilli as the most common pathogens causing infection following liver transplantation. Among 115 infection episodes reported by the University of Chicago, 37% were polymicrobial and 16% were due to gram-negative bacilli (see Table 13.1) (12). Of the bacteremias in this report, 25 were due to aerobic gram-negative bacilli, and 12 were due to gram-positive cocci. In contrast, in a report from the Mayo Clinic, gram-negative isolates were rarely encountered (14). Of 16 bacteremias, only one was caused by an aerobic gram-negative organism. Although unproven due to the absence of a control group, this low incidence of gram-negative infection has been attributed to the use of prophylactic selective bowel decontamination.

Table 13.1 Bacterial isolates causing infection at two different liver transplant centers

Organism	University of Chicago* (115 infection episodes)‡	Mayo Clinic† (27 infection episodes)
Aerobic gram-positive cocci	73 (63%)	25 (64%)
Staphylococcus aureus	18	5
Staphylococcus coagulase negative	11	9
Streptococcus Group D	34	4
Other streptococci	10	7
Aerobic gram-negative bacilli	103 (89%)	6 (15%)
Enterobacter	34	1
Pseudomonas	22	3
Escherichia coli	24	1
Other gram-negative bacilli	23	1
Anaerobic bacteria	14 (12%)	8 (21%)

*Data from Reference 12.
†Data from Reference 14.
‡Many infections were polymicrobial.

Studies utilizing this regimen in other patient populations have demonstrated a reduced incidence of gram-negative infection and an increased frequency of gram-positive infection (18,19). Empirical antimicrobial therapy for suspected bacterial infection must, therefore, be guided by the prevailing isolates and antimicrobial susceptibility profiles encountered at each center.

FUNGAL INFECTIONS

Infections caused by fungi are a particularly devastating complication of liver transplantation. While fungal infections may be less common than bacterial or viral infections, the associated mortality is considerably higher. In one series of 18 fungal infections following liver transplantation, 78% of patients died. Fungal infections account for 13% to 24% of infection episodes (13).

Fungal infections may be classified as either reactivation of latent or occult infection present in the transplant recipient or primary acquisition of an endemic or opportunistic fungal pathogen. Reactivation syndromes following immunosuppression may be seen with *Histoplasma*, *Blastomyces*, or *Coccidioides* in the appropriate epidemiologic setting. Primary exposure and subsequent disease may occur due to opportunistic pathogens such as *Aspergillus*, *Candida* species, *Trichophyton*, or the endemic mycoses in patients who are immunosuppressed following transplantation. Fungal infection may be focal, as in the case of an intraabdominal fluid collection infected with *Candida* sp or invasive pulmonary aspergillosis. Disseminated mycoses may be caused by *Candida* sp, *Aspergillus* sp, the endemic mycoses, or other opportunistic fungi.

In a retrospective review of 72 patients with fungal infection among 303 liver transplant recipients, discriminant risk factor analysis identified retransplantation, reintubation, bacterial infections, intraoperative blood transfusions, urgent status before transplantation, number of steriod boluses, vascular complications, prolonged antibiotic use, method of biliary reconstruction, and risk score as significant risk factors for fungal infection (20). The two most important variables were retransplantation and reintubation. When reanalyzed with the exclusion of retransplantation and reintubation, bacterial infections, transfusion requirements, urgent status, steroid dose, vascular complications, and antibiotic use remained highly significant risk factors. Fulminant hepatic failure, an only recently recognized indication for liver transplantation, may also be a risk factor for fungal infection (21).

Since fungi, in particular *Candida* sp, may colonize postsurgical and transplant patients, the diagnosis of fungal infection may be difficult. The diagnosis of fungal infection should be based on histological evidence of tissue invasion on biopsy or a positive culture from a normally sterile body fluid or deep tissue specimen. Moreover, repeatedly positive cultures from multiple sites (e.g., bile, urine, respiratory tract, etc.) and a positive stain or culture from a bronchoalveolar lavage specimen in the setting of suspected clinical infection with no alternative pathogen recovered may indicate fungal infection. Aggressive diagnosis and early initiation of therapy are critical factors in successful treatment.

The spectrum of infection with fungi may range from peritonitis, infected fluid collections, or urinary tract infection with or without associated fungemia to widely disseminated infection involving multiple organs. While infection with *Candida* sp is most common overall, disseminated disease is more common when *Aspergillus* is involved. Of 13 cases of *Aspergillus* infection reported by Castaldo, 62% were disseminated (20). In contrast, only 16% of *Candida* infections were disseminated. Although these two pathogens account for most of the fungal infections following liver transplantation, infection with *Trichosporon beigelii*, *Pseudallescheria boydii*, *Cryptococcus neoformans*, and other pathogens have been reported (20,22–24).

Amphotericin B remains the mainstay of therapy for fungal infections following transplantation. Treatment is greatly complicated by the fact that most immunosuppressive regimens for liver transplantation are cyclosporine based and result in an accelerated rate of renal toxicity when amphotericin is administered simultaneously. Reducing cyclosporine to the lowest acceptable level should be attempted. Other efforts to reduce nephrotoxicity, such as saline loading, may be of some benefit (25). Pentoxifylline has been reported to reduce the nephrotoxicity of both cyclosporine and amphotericin B (26). Although promising, a randomized, placebo-controlled trial should be performed before this agent is routinely administered to prevent nephrotoxicity in this patient population.

Due to the high frequency of nephrotoxicity with amphotericin B, the use of azole antifungal agents for treating fungal infections is attractive. Ketoconazole should not generally be used in transplant patients due to a low level of efficacy against the pathogens commonly encountered, poor efficacy in immunocompromised hosts, and a significant interaction with cyclosporine A. Fluconazole has been used successfully for treatment of fungal infections due to both *Candida* sp and *Cryptococcus neoformans* in organ transplant recipients (27). The minimal pharmacokinetic interaction with cyclosporine, low incidence of major toxicity, and ease of administration are particularly favorable features of this agent. Until more efficacy data are available, however, amphotericin B remains the drug of choice for most life-threatening infections due to these agents. Itraconazole has been used successfully in the treatment of *Aspergillus* infection in organ transplant recipients (28). Although an appealing potential alternative, amphotericin B, with or without concomitant flucytosine, remains the drug of choice for *Aspergillus* infection until more data become available (29).

VIRAL INFECTIONS

CMV infection

Cytomegalovirus is the most common cause of infection following liver transplantation (13). Active CMV infection most commonly occurs from four to 10 weeks following transplantation. CMV infection is defined as direct or indirect laboratory evidence of active viral replication. This includes a fourfold or higher increase in CMV antibody titer, seroconversion from the seronegative to seropositive state, positive viral cultures from clinical specimens, or direct detection of CMV antigen. Many patients with CMV infection will remain asymptomatic. In contrast, CMV disease is defined as clinical signs and symptoms attributable to the virus.

CMV infection and disease may take three forms. Primary infection occurs in transplant recipients who are CMV seronegative (R−) pretransplant and who subsequently show evidence of infection in the posttransplant period. This most commonly occurs when the donor is CMV seropositive (D+) and the virus is transmitted with the allograft. Primary infection may also occur following blood transfusion, but the risk of this can be diminished by using blood from CMV seronegative donors or by using filtered blood products (30). Reactivation CMV infection occurs when latent virus replicates following initiation of immunosuppression. This will only occur with seropositive recipients (R+). In a seropositive patient who receives an organ from a seronegative donor (D−), viral replication implies reactivation. In contrast, CMV infection in a seropositive recipient of an allograft from a seropositive donor represents either reactivation or superinfection with a donor-transmitted viral strain. Under the usual clinical circumstances, it is not possible to distinguish superinfection from reactivation, and this distinction probably has little clinical importance.

CMV infection may occur in as many as 59% of patients following transplantation and is frequently asymptomatic (31). Of 30 episodes of CMV infection in a series of 53 patients reported by Paya et al., only 18 were symptomatic (14). Similarly, of 93 assessable patients from the University of Pittsburgh, 55 patients had infection, but only 27 of these were symptomatic (31).

Several factors have been identified that contribute to the frequency and severity of CMV infection. Immunosuppression is probably the most important factor contributing to morbidity. While prednisone alone will infrequently cause reactivation of CMV in seropositive patients, the addition of cytotoxic agents, such as cyclophosphamide or azathioprine, is more likely to be associated with infection and disease (32). Moreover, antilymphocyte therapy, such as with OKT-3 antibodies, appears to be a potent enhancer of CMV infection and disease (31). The serologic status of the recipient and donor are also of critical importance. The serologic status and incidence of infection in 218 evaluable patients from the Mayo Clinic is found in Table 13.2 (33). The patient at highest risk for developing CMV infection is the seronegative recipient of a seropositive organ. Seventy-seven percent of patients in this risk category developed CMV infection. In contrast, infection occurred in 66% of seropositive recipients of a seropositive allograft and 49% of seropositive recipients of a seronegative allograft. Ten percent of seronegative recipients of a seronegative organ developed infection. Similar findings have been reported by other investigators. In a multivariate analysis of risk factors performed at the Cleveland Clinic, a positive donor CMV serology was the single most important risk factor for the subsequent development of cytomegalovirus infection, irrespective of recipient CMV serostatus (34).

These factors also contribute to the incidence of symptomatic CMV disease. In the Mayo Clinic study, 61% of the D+R− patients were symptomatic, whereas only 23% of the D+R+, 10% of the D−R+, and 10% of D−R− patients had symptomatic disease (33). The use of OKT-3 antibodies has been shown to be associated with disseminated disease only in patients with primary infection and not with reactivation (31).

Symptomatic CMV infection exhibits a wide range of clinical manifestations. Mild disease usually includes simple fever and malaise without additional signs or symptoms. These patients may develop leukopenia with or without thrombocytopenia. The mononucleosis syndrome seen in immunocompetent hosts and characterized by atypical lymphocytosis is rarely seen in transplant patients. With both reactivation and primary CMV infection after transplantation, myalgias, arthralgias, and at times frank arthritis may occur. Most CMV disease after transplantation is of mild to moderate severity and is rarely fatal (32). Severe organ-specific CMV disease may manifest as pneumonitis, hepatitis, gastrointestinal disease, retinitis, disseminated disease, and, on rare occasions, direct involvement of other organs.

In a study of CMV pneumonitis in liver transplant recipients involving 29 episodes

Table 13.2   Association between the CMV serological status of donor and recipient and the frequency of CMV infection, disease, and hepatitis in liver transplant recipients

		Patients with					
		CMV infection		CMV disease		CMV hepatitis	
CMV serologic status at transplantation*	N	N	(%)	N	(%)	N	(%)
D+/R−	44	34	(77)	27	(61)	21	(48)
D+/R+	73	43	(66)	17	(23)	10	(14)
D−/R+	72	35	(49)	7	(10)	5	(7)
D−/R−	29	3	(10)	3	(10)	2	(7)
Total	218	115	(53)	54	(25)	38	(17)

*D+ = CMV seropositive donor; R+ = CMV seropositive recipient; D− = CMV seronegative donor; R− = CMV seronegative recipient.
SOURCE Data from Reference 33.

of pneumonitis, 13 cases occurred in which CMV was recovered with another pulmonary pathogen (35). These included pneumocystis (7 cases), bacteria (4), and fungi (2). Bilateral interstitial infiltrative disease was the most frequent radiographic presentation described, although a unilateral lobar infiltrative process was seen in ten cases and a nodular infiltrate in four cases.

CMV hepatitis is the most common organ-specific manifestation of CMV disease in liver transplant recipients, and it is most likely to occur in the D+R− patient. In a recent report from the Mayo Clinic, 48% of seronegative recipients of a seropositive allograft developed hepatitis (33). Paya et al. reported a mean time to diagnosis of 40 days after transplantation (range 20 to 52 days) (36). No characteristic biochemical profile has been associated with CMV hepatitis, and it rarely leads directly to serious acute graft dysfunction.

Cytomegalovirus infection has been associated with a number of secondary effects. It has been shown to depress neutrophil function which may predispose to secondary bacterial infections (37). Natural killer cell activity and T-cell proliferation may also be depressed (38). Superinfection with opportunistic pathogens has been observed to occur more frequently in patients with active CMV infection (39). In vitro studies have demonstrated that CMV infection results in enhanced expression of class I human leukocyte antigens (HLA) which may increase the likelihood of graft rejection (40).

The diagnosis of CMV infection has traditionally been based on the recognition of cytomegalic inclusion bodies in tissue specimens. CMV will exhibit cytopathic effect in standard cell culture after seven to 14 days of incubation. Several recent rapid diagnostic techniques have dramatically increased the ability of the virology laboratory to recognize viral replication and allow an early diagnosis of CMV infection. The rapid shell vial culture technique can detect the presence of CMV after 16 hours of incubation by an indirect immunofluorescence test using a monoclonal antibody directed at an early antigen of the virus (41). This technique has been shown to be as effective as standard tube culture. More recently, detection of CMV antigenemia has been found to offer a more rapid laboratory result, enhanced sensitivity, and earlier detection of infection (42). The level of antigenemia using this technique seems to correlate with severity of disease. Polymerase chain reaction (PCR) has also been shown to be a sensitive and effective detector of active CMV infection (43). No studies comparing PCR with other viral detection techniques have thus far been performed.

Serologic responses to CMV disease have been regarded as sensitive indicators of active infection. Recent reports suggest that the newer culture and antigen detection techniques represent a considerable advancement over viral serologic testing (44). In one report, CMV serology alone reduced the detection of CMV disease by 21% when compared with the shell vial culture (45).

While no controlled studies have been performed, several reports suggest the efficacy of ganciclovir in the treatment of severe CMV infection (36,46). One hundred eight episodes of CMV disease in 81 patients were treated with ganciclovir at the University of Nebraska over a 54-month period (46). Seventy-four percent of patients experienced prompt and sustained improvement of CMV disease manifestations. Twenty-one percent developed recurrent CMV disease after stopping ganciclovir, but most were successfully retreated. Of 17 deaths among the study patients, five had autopsy evidence of

CMV infection. Ganciclovir is well tolerated in liver transplant patients and appears to have a lower incidence of side effects than that seen in HIV-infected patients.

There is less experience with the use of foscarnet for treatment of severe CMV infection in transplant patients (47). Until more data are available, foscarnet should be reserved for patients who are intolerant of ganciclovir or have failed ganciclovir therapy.

OTHER HERPES VIRUSES

Epstein-Barr virus (EBV) has been recognized as a cause of several posttransplant infection syndromes. Since EBV infection and seropositivity is so common and isolation of EBV in the virology laboratory so difficult, the spectrum of infection due to Epstein-Barr virus following transplantation has thus far been incompletely defined and remains an evolving area of investigation. EBV has been associated with asymptomatic elevation in antibody titers to EBV viral capsid antigen (VCA), a mononucleosis syndrome, acute hepatitis, chronic hepatitis, and posttransplantation lymphoproliferative disorders (46,48–51).

Of 85 evaluable patients among 119 EBV seropositive transplant recipients, 24% developed fourfold or greater rise in EBV VCA antibody titers (31). In this study, only one patient had evidence of symptoms attributable to EBV manifested as lymphoproliferative disease. In another study of six cases of primary EBV infection, all patients had EBV hepatitis, and, in three cases, this was closely linked to a lymphoproliferative disorder (46). All six patients had received OKT-3 therapy prior to developing EBV hepatitis. Telenti et al. reported EBV in association with chronic hepatitis and persistent graft dysfunction (50). In situ hybridization studies and PCR analysis confirmed the presence of high levels of EBV in the liver. Moreover, in these cases, augmented immunosuppression resulted in worsening of graft function, whereas reduced immunosuppression was associated with improved graft function.

Lymphoproliferative disease associated with Epstein-Barr virus following liver transplantation has been recognized with increased frequency in recent years. Among heart transplant patients, the risk of lymphoproliferative disease appears to be increased in patients that have received high doses of OKT-3 monoclonal antibody therapy (52). Anecdotal reports suggest a similar association in liver transplantation (46). This problem appears to be more significant among pediatric liver transplant recipients due to a lower incidence of EBV seropositivity and an increased risk of primary infection in this population. Among 132 pediatric liver transplant recipients from the University of Pittsburgh, 12 cases of lymphoproliferative disease were reported, with a lethal outcome in five patients (49). There are no consistent data that confirm the efficacy of antiviral therapy for EBV-associated lymphoproliferative disorders; nevertheless, antiviral therapy and reduction of immunosuppression are currently recommended for treatment (53–55).

Herpes simplex virus (HSV) is most commonly seen as reactivation orolabial or genital disease. Singh et al. noted that symptomatic reactivation occurred more frequently in HSV seropositive recipients who were treated with OKT-3 (53%) than in seropositive recipients who were not (31%) (31). Disseminated HSV disease has been reported but is uncommon (56). Varicella-zoster infection occurring after transplantation is typically characterized by localized dermatomal disease occurring more than six months after transplantation. Primary varicella in the immunosuppressed organ transplant recipient is a rare but life-threatening infection.

HEPATITIS VIRUSES

The problem of hepatitis due to hepatitis B and C viruses presents a difficult challenge. From 1988 to 1990, 8% of patients undergoing liver transplantation in the United States had hepatitis B infection (4). Reinfection of the allograft is common in HBsAg-positive patients after liver transplantation. Recovery and long-term survival are substantially reduced in patients with posttransplantation recurrence. Similarly, hepatitis C virus (HCV) has been recognized in recent years as a common cause of chronic liver disease in patients requiring transplantation. A recent retrospective study found that 50% of patients previously transplanted with non-A, non-B chronic hepatitis were anti-HCV positive, using an enzyme-linked immunosorbent assay (ELISA) and confirmatory testing (57). In this retrospective cohort, HCV infection developed in the graft in 17% of all patients; however, the incidence of posttransplantation HCV hepatitis was not significantly different between anti-HCV negative and anti-HCV positive patients. Further study is needed to establish the exact role of HCV in posttransplantation hepatitis.

With hepatitis B, recent efforts have focused on preventing recurrent disease in the allograft. Rakela et al. reported the failure of recombinant human leukocyte A interferon (rIFN-A) to prevent recurrent viral replication in the allograft (58). Others have reported using immunoprophylaxis with human anti-HBs hyperimmune globulin (HBIG). While no controlled studies utilizing either immunoprophylaxis, rIFN-A, or the combination have been performed, several reports suggest efficacy (59,60,61). Mueller et al. reported that, among 34 HBsAg positive allograft recipients, the rate of recurrent infection was less than 20% in patients receiving long-term HBIG prophylaxis, whereas 11 graft recipients with only short-term HBIG or no prophylaxis were reinfected within 15 months (62). While promising, the precise role of passive immunization and other modalities in the prevention of hepatitis B virus infection following transplantation needs further clarification.

OTHER INFECTIONS

Pneumonia caused by *Pneumocystis carinii* occurs in 6% to 11% of liver transplant patients if prophylaxis is not given (13,14). Most cases tend to occur within the first six months following transplantation, but sporadic late cases have also been reported (63). Of 18 cases of *P. carinii* pneumonia (PCP) following liver transplantation reported by Lomboy et al., the median time interval between transplantation and diagnosis was 83 days, with a range of 36 to 744 days (63). Eighty-nine percent of these patients received an allograft from a CMV seropositive donor, and 56% were seronegative before transplantation. *Pneumocystis carinii* pneumonia is frequently associated with coinfection with cytomegalovirus. In a series of 11 patients from the University of Pittsburgh, all of three fatalities were associated with concurrent CMV pneumonitis (13). Risk factors for developing PCP after liver transplantation include CMV D+/R− serostatus and a CD4 count of less than 250 (63).

As with human immunodeficiency virus (HIV)-infected patients, the primary regimen for treatment of PCP in the organ transplant recipient is trimethoprim-sulfamethoxazole. Those who fail this regimen may be considered candidates for parenteral pentamidine or investigational regimens. Considering the frequency of this very serious infection and how well tolerated prophylactic trimethoprim-sulfamethoxazole treatment is, PCP should be a completely preventable infection (see below).

Mycobacterial infection is a relatively infrequent cause of serious infection following liver transplantation. Almost all reported cases of mycobacterial infection in this setting have been due to *Mycobacterium tuberculosis* (64). As in other organ transplant recipients and immunosuppressed patients, disseminated disease is more common than in the nonimmunosuppressed patient population. Risk factors for developing mycobacterial infection include exposure in an endemic area, severe pretransplantation illness, rejection episodes requiring augmented immunosuppression, and HIV infection (65).

To identify patients at risk, all potential transplant candidates should have a tuberculin test performed. Due to the possibility of cutaneous anergy from the underlying liver disease, a negative test does not exclude the possibility of previous tuberculosis exposure. The American Thoracic Society recommends prophylactic isoniazich (INH) for those patients who require prolonged immunosuppression, which would include organ transplant recipients (66). This recommendation is complicated in liver transplant patients because of the problem of distinguishing INH toxicity from rejection. Among kidney transplant recipients, the incidence of hepatocellular enzyme elevation has been calculated to be higher than the incidence of tuberculosis in patients at risk (67). A reasonable approach is to identify patients at increased risk for reactivation tuberculosis. Patients with radiographic evidence of pulmonary disease or recently documented conversion of the tuberculin skin test should be considered for INH prophylaxis. Other patients should be monitored carefully for evidence of reactivation.

Nocardiosis and toxoplasmosis have both been reported in liver transplantation but are rare (68,69). Recently, primary infection with human herpes virus 6 (HHV-6) has been reported in liver transplant recipients (70). This appears to be a donor-transmitted virus, but reactivation infection has also been described (71). The complete spectrum of clinical illness due to HHV-6 has not been fully characterized. Papovaviruses have been commonly recovered from transplant patients. Utilizing the polymerase chain reaction, polyomaviruses (JC and BK) have been detected in 50% of liver transplant recipients (72). This appears to be asymptomatic viral shedding and not associated with signs or symptoms of infection. The JC virus has, however, been found to cause progressive multifocal leukoencephalopathy in immunosuppressed patients (73). Adenovirus can cause severe allograft hepatitis in children (74).

PREVENTION OF INFECTION

Despite considerable improvement in organ procurement and preservation, surgical technique, and immunosuppressive therapy, infection continues to be a source of considerable morbidity and mortality among liver transplant recipients. As the knowledge of the timing and spectrum of infection following transplantation has improved, the emphasis in the field of transplant infectious diseases has shifted from the diagnosis and management of established infection to prevention of infection. Most of the studies conducted in transplant patients have involved recipients of renal allografts or bone marrow transplant patients. Nevertheless, there are sufficient data for recommending a similar treatment strategy for prevention of infection in liver transplant patients.

With an integrated multispecialty approach to liver transplantation, the prevention of posttransplantation infection begins with a detailed and comprehensive pretransplant medical evaluation. Transplant candidates should be questioned regarding their history of severe or recurrent infections and screened for the presence of indolent infection. As noted previously, it is important to document a history of a positive tuberculin test or a significant tuberculosis exposure. Moreover, the travel history should be reviewed to determine the possibility of past exposure to endemic mycoses, *Strongyloides stercoralis*, or other organisms. Efforts should be made to update immunizations prior to transplantation and immunosuppression as the response following transplantation is often suboptimal.

Pretransplant serologic testing should be performed for cytomegalovirus, Epstein-Barr virus, varicella-zoster virus, herpes simplex virus, hepatitis B virus, hepatitis C virus, and human immunodeficiency virus (Table 13.3). In patients with significant exposure to the endemic mycoses, fungal serologies may also be warranted. Stool specimens should be examined for ova and parasites and cultured for enteric bacterial pathogens. Unless there is a known history of tuberculin reactivity, a tuberculin test should be performed.

No prospective studies to determine the most appropriate perioperative antibiotic prophylaxis have been performed. Numerous regimens have been reported in the literature including cefoxitin, cefotaxime, ceftriaxone, ampicillin, and aminoglycosides (12–15). In the absence of precise data, general principles of surgical antimicrobial prophylaxis should be observed. Prophylaxis should be given for no more than 24 to 48 hours, with doses given in the operating room to ensure adequate tissue levels at the time of surgery. Moreover, prophylaxis should be adjusted to reflect the spectrum of infections typically encountered in patients in a particular transplant center.

Table 13.3 Pre-liver transplantation serological evaluation at the Mayo Clinic

Cytomegalovirus
Herpes simplex virus
Varicella-zoster virus
Epstein-Barr virus
Hepatitis A virus
Hepatitis B virus
Hepatitis C virus
Human immunodeficiency virus (HIV)
Toxoplasma
Fungal survey (endemic mycoses)

Considerable interest has been focused on the use of selective bowel decontamination to prevent postoperative infections. While no randomized prospective studies have been done in this patient population, several reports have noted a low level of serious gram-negative infections when this approach is utilized (75–77). Wiesner et al. reported only five infections caused by gram-negative bacteria in 145 patients undergoing initial transplantation and experiencing 45 major bacterial infections (78). Moreover, only one patient experienced a systemic *Candida* infection. These findings suggest that selective bowel decontamination reduces the incidence of gram-negative and candidal infection and has led many liver transplant centers to adopt a similar strategy.

The regimen used at the Mayo Clinic is a suspension of oral nonabsorbable antibiotics—polymixin E, gentamicin, and nystatin—administered four times daily from the time of activation for liver transplantation until 21 days posttransplantation. Patients are also maintained on a low bacterial diet. Surveillance cultures before and after selective bowel decontamination using this regimen typically show eradication of aerobic gram-negative bacilli and *Candida* sp from the rectum, throat, and other sites (78). The oral selective bowel decontamination regimen has no impact on the anaerobic flora.

While emergence of resistant gram-negative bacteria has not been reported using this regimen, this remains a serious consideration. In addition, the optimal initiation of prophylaxis, duration of prophylaxis, and optimal agents are issues that require further clarification.

Apart from the apparent impact of selective bowel decontamination on the prevention of *Candida* infection, no published studies have demonstrated an effective means of reducing the incidence of fungal infection in this population. Both clotrimazole troches and oral nystatin suspension have been shown to be effective in preventing oropharyngeal candidiasis in renal transplant patients (79). A similar effect would be expected in liver transplant patients. Due to the risk of liver toxicity and a possible confounding factor in evaluating allograft dysfunction and rejection, clotrimazole should best be avoided in liver transplant recipients. Preliminary results from a randomized study comparing prophylactic oral fluconazole 100 mg daily with oral nystatin in liver transplant recipients indicate that fluconazole is well tolerated and reduces the incidence of *Candida* colonization and minor infection (CV Paya, personal communication). Too few major infections were encountered to note any difference. A report from Baylor University Medical Center suggests that prophylactic amphotericin B given to patients at high risk for developing fungal infection may reduce the incidence and severity of fungal infections (80). Further well-designed studies in this area are needed.

Since cytomegalovirus infection is so common following transplantation, prevention of this infection has generated intense interest. Successful regimens and strategies have been described for renal, heart, and bone marrow transplantation. These have included the use of high-dose oral acyclovir in kidney transplant recipients, the use of CMV hyperimmune globulin in kidney transplant patients, ganciclovir prophylaxis in heart transplant recipients and in selected bone marrow transplant recipients, and pretransplant immunization for CMV in kidney transplant candidates (39,81–84). Extrapolation from findings in one organ transplant group to another, however, may not be valid.

Intravenous immunoglobulin has had mixed results in the prevention of CMV infection in liver transplant recipients (85). A randomized, double-blind, placebo-controlled trial of CMV hyperimmune globulin in liver transplant patients is currently being conducted (86). The combination of intravenous immunoglobulin at weekly intervals for six weeks and acyclovir for three months significantly reduced the incidence of CMV disease in high-risk patients (87). In a recent report comparing two weeks of ganciclovir followed by high-dose oral acyclovir with high-dose oral acyclovir and utilizing a cohort of historical controls, the ganciclovir-containing regimen was found to significantly reduce the incidence of CMV infection and viremia but did not result in a significant reduction of symptomatic CMV infection (88). Further investigation into the optimal regimens and strategies for preventing CMV infection is needed.

Low-dose oral acyclovir (200 mg three times daily) has been shown to be effective in preventing reactivation herpes simplex stomatitis in kidney transplant recipients (89). No studies have been performed in liver transplant recipients, but efficacy has been demonstrated in other immunosuppressed hosts. Among liver transplant centers utilizing an acyclovir prophylactic regimen, the incidence of HSV infection is very low (14). In contrast, when no prophylaxis is used, the incidence may be as high as 53% (31). At this dosage, acyclovir is extremely well tolerated and is not associated with significant adverse effects. There is no apparent prophylactic efficacy against cytomegalovirus at this low dose.

Data from leukemic and acquired immunodeficiency syndrome (AIDS) patients indicate that prophylaxis of *Pneumocystis carinii* pneumonia is highly effective. PCP should be regarded as a completely preventable illness among liver transplant recipients if prophylaxis is given. Trimethoprim-sulfamethoxazole (TMP/SMX) is the most widely studied agent, and a variety of regimens, including one double-strength tablet daily, twice daily three days per week, or twice daily every day, are effective in preventing infection (91,92,93,94). This is well tolerated in organ transplant recipients and is not associated with significant interactions with cyclosporine or other agents used for immunosuppression. Moreover, there may be other benefits of trimethoprim-sulfamethoxazole prophylaxis. In studies performed in renal transplant recipients, there was a significantly reduced frequency of bacterial infection in patients receiving TMP/SMX compared with controls (94). The effect was most prominent in preventing urinary tract infections, but it also reduced bacteremias. Infections caused by *Nocardia* and *Listeria* may also be prevented with TMP/SMX prophylaxis.

For patients who are sulfa allergic or who cannot tolerate TMP/SMX, aerosolized pentamidine may be used, although breakthrough infections may occur, particularly in the upper lobes (59). Dapsone is also effective in preventing PCP. There are few data regarding the use of this agent in organ transplant recipients. Side effects such as anemia and methemoglobinemia may be limiting factors.

FUTURE CONSIDERATIONS

The management of infectious complications following liver transplantation is certain to remain a challenging and evolving area of endeavor in the future. In the last ten years, tremendous advances have been made in the definition of the spectrum and timing of infection, the identification of patients at risk for infection, the rapidity of diagnosis, new approaches to treatment, and strategies for prevention of infection. Nevertheless, considerable challenges remain. Cytomegalovirus remains the most frequently encountered pathogen. While ganciclovir appears to be effective in treating established infection, a prophylactic regimen with low toxicity that is easy to administer and inexpensive is needed. Similarly, progress has been made in identifying risk factors for fungal infection, but noninvasive diagnostic tests and nontoxic treatment options are desperately needed. Selective bowel decontamination appears to offer a safe and inexpensive means of reducing the incidence of gram-negative bacterial and candidal infections. Further study is needed to define the optimal timing and duration of prophylaxis.

As new immunosuppressive regimens are introduced and studied and strategies for diagnosing, managing, and preventing infections following transplantation evolve, an integrated multispecialty approach offers the greatest promise for maximizing survival and quality of life in these very challenging patients.

REFERENCES

1   Starzl TE, Marchioro TL, von Kaulla KN, Hermann G, Britain RS, Waddell WR. Homotransplantation of the liver in humans. *Surg Gynecol Obstet* 1963;117:659–676.

2   National Institutes of Health Consensus Development Conference Statement: liver transplantation—June 20–23, 1983. *Hepatology* 1983;Suppl:107S–110S.

3   Glascock F, UNOS Research Department, Richmond, Virginia (personal communication).

4   Belle SH, Beringer KC, Murphy JB, et al. Liver transplantation in the United States: 1988 to 1990. In: Terasaki P, ed. *Clinical Transplants*. Los Angeles: UCLA Tissue Typing Laboratory, 1991.

5   Terpstra OT, Schalm SW, Weimar W, et al. Auxilliary partial liver transplantation for end-stage chronic liver disease. *N Engl J Med* 1988;319:1507–1511.

6   Krom RAF. Liver transplantation at the Mayo Clinic. *Mayo Clin Proc* 1986;61:278–282.

7   Kahan SD. Cyclosporine: the agent and its actions. *Transplant Proc* 1985;17 Suppl 1:5–18.

8   Starzl TE, Demetris AJ, Van Thiel D. Liver transplantation (second of two parts). *N Engl J Med* 1989;321:1092–1099.

9   Rubin RH. Infectious disease problems. In: Maddrey WC, ed. *Transplantation of the Liver.* New York: Elsevier, 1988:279–308.

10 Tolkoff-Rubin NE, Rubin RH. Infections in the organ transplant recipient. In: Cerilli GJ,

ed. *Organ Transplantation and Replacement.* Philadelphia: JB Lippincott, 1988:445–461.

11 Dummer JS, Erb S, Breinig MK, et al. Infection with human immunodeficiency virus in the Pittsburgh transplant population. *Transplantation* 1989;47:134–139.

12 George DL, Arnow PM, Fox AS, et al. Bacterial infection as a complication of liver transplantation: epidemiology and risk factors. *Rev Infect Dis* 1991;13:387–396.

13 Kusne S, Dummer JS, Singh N, et al. Infection after liver transplantation: an analysis of 101 consecutive cases. *Medicine* 1988;67:132–143.

14 Paya CV, Hermans PE, Washington JA II, et al. Incidence, distribution, and outcome of episodes of infection in 100 orthotopic liver transplantations. *Mayo Clin Proc* 1989;64:555–564.

15 Corti A, Sabbadini D, Pannacciulli E, et al. Early severe infections after orthotopic liver transplantation. *Transplant Proc* 1991;23:1964.

16 Bubak ME, Porayko MK, Krom RAF, Wiesner RH. Complications of liver biopsy in liver transplant patients: increased sepsis associated with choledochojejunostomy. *Hepatology* 1991;14:1063–1065.

17 Korvick JA, Marsh JW, Starzl TE, Yu VL. *Pseudomonas aeruginosa* bacteremia in patients undergoing liver transplantation: an emerging problem. *Surgery* 1991;109:62–68.

18 Cockerill FR III, Muller SM, Anhalt JP, et al. Selective decontamination of the digestive tract

for prevention of infection in critically ill patients. *Ann Intern Med.* 1992;117:545–553.

19 Gastinne H, Wolff M, Delatour F, Faurisson F, Chevret S. A controlled trial in intensive care units of selective decontamination of the digestive tract with nonabsorbable antibiotics. *N Engl J Med* 1992;326:594–599.

20 Castaldo P, Stratta RJ, Wood RP, et al. Clinical spectrum of fungal infections after orthotopic liver transplantation. *Arch Surg* 1991;126:149–156.

21 Brems JJ, Hiatt JR, Klein AS, et al. Disseminated aspergillosis complicating orthotopic liver transplantation for fulminant hepatic failure refractory to corticosteroid therapy. *Transplantation* 1988;46:479–481.

22 Ness MJ, Markin RS, Wood RP, Shaw BW, Woods GL. Disseminated *Trichosporon beigelii* infection after orthotopic liver transplantation. *Am J Clin Pathol* 1989;92:119–123.

23 Patterson TF, Andriole VT, Zervos MJ, Therasse D, Kauffman CA. The epidemiology of pseudallescheriasis complicating transplantation: nosocomial and community-acquired infection. *Mycoses* 1990;33:297–302.

24 Aldape KD, Fox HS, Roberts JP, Ascher NL, Lake JR, Rowley HA. *Cladosporium trichoides* cerebral phaeohyphomycosis in a liver transplant recipient: report of a case. *Am J Clin Pathol* 1991;95:499–502.

25 Llanos A, Cieza J, Bernardo J, et al. Effect of salt supplementation on amphotericin B nephrotoxicity. *Kid Int* 1991;40:302–308.

26 Bianco JA, Almgren J, Kern DL, et al. Evidence that oral pentoxifylline reverses acute renal dysfunction in bone marrow transplant recipients receiving amphotericin B and cyclosporine: results of a pilot study. *Transplantation* 1991;51:925–927.

27 Conti DJ, Tolkoff-Rubin NE, Baker GP Jr, et al. Successful treatment of invasive fungal infection with fluconazole in organ transplant recipients. *Transplantation* 1989;48:692–695.

28 Gamba A, Fiocchi R, Ferrazzi P, et al. Pulmonary and disseminated aspergillosis in cardiac transplanted patients: itraconazole as a first choice therapy? *J Heart Transplant* 1991; 10:189.

29 Denning DW, Stevens DA. Antifungal and surgical treatment of invasive aspergillosis: review of 2121 published cases. *Rev Infect Dis* 1990;12:1147–1201.

30 Sayers MH, Anderson KC, Goodnough LT, et al. Reducing the risk for transfusion-transmitted cytomegalovirus infection. *Ann Intern Med* 1992;116:55–62.

31 Singh N, Dummer JS, Kusne S, et al. Infections with cytomegalovirus and other herpesviruses in 121 liver transplant recipients: transmission by donated organ and the effect of OKT3 antibodies. *J Infect Dis* 1988; 158:124–131.

32 Ho M. Observations from transplantation contributing to the understanding of pathogenesis of CMV infection. *Transplant Proc* 1991;23: 104–109.

33 Marin E, Wiesner RH, Porayko MK, Keating MR, Wahlstrom E, Krom RAF. Cytomegalovirus infection following liver transplantation: incidence, timing, and predictors of disease severity. American Society of Transplant Physicians 10th Annual Scientific Meeting, Chicago, Illinois, May 28–29, 1991.

34 Gorensek MJ, Carey WD, Vogt D, Goormastic M. A multivariate analysis of risk factors for cytomegalovirus infection in liver-transplant recipients. *Gastroenterology* 1990;98:1326–1332.

35 Marshall WF, Walker RC. Pulmonary cytomegalovirus infections after orthotopic liver transplantation. The International Symposium of Infections in the Immunocompromised Host, Peebles, Scotland, 1990.

36 Paya CV, Hermans PE, Wiesner RH, et al. Cytomegalovirus hepatitis in liver transplantation: prospective analysis of 93 consecutive orthotopic liver transplantations. *J Infect Dis* 1989;160:752–758.

37 Abramson JS, Mills EL. Depression of neutrophil function induced by viruses and its role in secondary microbial infections. *Rev Infect Dis* 1988;10:326–341.

38 Rinaldo CR Jr, Ho M, Hamoudi WH, Gui Z, DeBiasio RL. Lymphocyte subsets and natural killer cell responses during cytomegalovirus mononucleosis. *Infect Immun* 1983;40: 472–477.

39 Balfour HH Jr, Chace BA, Stapleton JT, Simmons RL, Fryd DS. A randomized, placebo-controlled trial of oral acyclovir for the prevention of cytomegalovirus disease in recipients of renal allografts. *N Engl J Med* 1989;320: 1381–1387.

40 Grundy JE, Ayles HM, McKeating JA, Butcher RG, Griffiths PD, Poulter LW. Enhancement of class I HLA antigen expression by cytomegalovirus: role in amplification of virus infection. *J Med Virol* 1988;25:483–495.

41 Shuster EA, Beneke JS, Tegtmeier GE, et al. Monoclonal antibody for rapid laboratory detection of cytomegalovirus infections: characterization and diagnostic application. *Mayo Clin Proc* 1985;60:577–585.

42 van den Berg AP, Klompmaker IJ, Haagsma EB, et al. Antigenemia in the diagnosis and monitoring of active cytomegalovirus infection after liver transplantation. *J Infect Dis* 1991; 164:265–270.

43 Einsele H, Ehninger G, Steidle M, et al. Polymerase chain reaction to evaluate antiviral therapy for cytomegalovirus disease. *Lancet* 1991;338:1170–1172.

44 Marsano L, Perrillo RP, Flye MW, et al. Comparison of culture and serology for the diagnosis of cytomegalovirus infection in kidney and liver transplant recipients. *J Infect Dis* 1990;161:454–461.

45 Paya CV, Smith TF, Hermans PE. Rapid shell vial culture and tissue histology compared with serology for the rapid diagnosis of cytomegalovirus infection in liver transplantation. *Mayo Clin Proc* 1989;64:670–675.

46 Stratta R, Shaefer M, Markin R, et al. Ganciclovir therapy for viral disease in liver transplant recipients. *Transplant Proc* 1991; 23:1968.

47 Klintmalm G, Lönnqvist B, Öberg B, et al. Intravenous foscarnet for the treatment of severe cytomegalovirus infection in allograft recipients. *Scand J Infect Dis* 1985;17:157–163.

48 Lamy ME, Favart AM, Cornu C, et al. Epstein-Barr virus infection in 59 orthotopic liver transplant patients. *Med Microbiol Immunol* 1990;179:137–144.

49 Malatack JJ, Gartner JC, Urbach AH, Zitelli BJ. Orthotopic liver transplantation, Epstein-Barr virus, cyclosporine, and lymphoproliferative disease: a growing concern. *J Pediatr* 1991;118:667–675.

50 Telenti A, Smith TF, Ludwig J, Keating MR, Krom RAF, Wiesner RH. Epstein-Barr virus and persistent graft dysfunction after liver transplantation. *Hepatology* 1991;14:282–286.

51 Billiar TR, Hanto DW, Simmons RL. Inclusion of uncomplicated infectious mononucleosis in the spectrum of Epstein-Barr virus infections in transplant recipients. *Transplantation* 1988;46:159–161.

52 Swinnen LJ, Costanzo-Nordin MR, Fisher SG, et al. Increased incidence of lymphoproliferative disorder after immunosuppression with the monoclonal antibody OKT3 in cardiac transplant recipients. *N Engl J Med* 1990;323:1723–1728.

53 Hanto DW, Frizzera G, Gajl-Peczalska KJ, et al. Epstein-Barr virus-induced B-cell lymphoma after renal transplantation: acyclovir therapy and transition from polyclonal to monoclonal B-cell proliferation. *N Engl J Med* 1982;306:913–918.

54 Hanto DW, Frizzera G, Gajl-Peczalska KJ, Simmons RL. Epstein-Barr virus, immunodeficiency, and B cell lymphoproliferation. *Transplantation* 1985;39:461–472.

55 Pirsch JD, Stratta RJ, Sollinger HW, et al. Treatment of severe Epstein-Barr virus-induced lymphoproliferative syndrome with ganciclovir: two cases after solid organ transplantation. *Am J Med* 1989;86:241–244.

56 Markin RS, Langnas AN, Donovan JP, Zetterman RK, Stratta RJ. Opportunistic viral hepatitis in liver transplant recipients. *Transplant Proc* 1991;23:1520–1521.

57 Read AE, Donegan E, Lake J, et al. Hepatitis C in patients undergoing liver transplantation. *Ann Intern Med* 1991;114:282–284.

58 Rakela J, Wooten RS, Batts KP, Perkins JD, Taswell HF, Krom RAF. Failure of interferon to prevent recurrent hepatitis B infection in hepatic allograft. *Mayo Clin Proc* 1989;64: 429–432.

59 Samuel D, Bismuth A, Mathieu D, et al. Passive immunoprophylaxis after liver transplantation in HBsAg-positive patients. *Lancet* 1991;337:813–815.

60 Rossi G, Grendele, Colledan M, et al. Prevention of hepatitis B virus reinfection after liver transplantation. *Transplant Proc* 1991; 23:1969.

61 Neuhaus P, Steffen R, Blumhardt G, et al. Experience with immunoprophylaxis and interferon therapy after liver transplantation in HBsAg positive patients. *Transplant Proc* 1991; 23:1522–1524.

62 Müller R, Gubernatis G, Farle M, et al. Liver transplantation in HBs antigen (HBsAg) carriers: prevention of hepatitis B virus (HBV) recurrence by passive immunization. *J Hepatol* 1991;13:90–96.

63 Lomboy CT, Wiesner RH, Hermans PE, Krom RAF. Risk factors for the development of *Pneumocystis carinii* pneumonia following liver transplantation. *Hepatology* 1990;12:82.

64 Sterneck M, Ferrell L, Ascher N, Roberts F, Lake J. Mycobacterial infection after liver transplantation: a report of three cases and review of the literature. *Clin Transplant* 1992; 6:55–61.

65 Higgins RSD, Kusne S, Reyes J, et al. *Mycobacterium tuberculosis* after transplantation: management and guidelines for prevention. *Clin Transplant* 1992;6:70–81.

66 American Thoracic Society. Treatment of tuberculosis and tuberculosis infection in adults and children. *Am Rev Respir Dis* 1986;134: 355–363.

67 Thomas P, Mozes M, Jonasson O. Hepatic dysfunction during isoniazid chemoprophylaxis in renal allograft recipients. *Arch Surg* 1979; 114:597.

68 Raby N, Forbes G, Williams R. *Nocardia* infection in patients with liver transplants or chronic liver disease: radiologic findings. *Radiology* 1990;174:713–716.

69 Forbes GM, Harvey FAH, Philpott-Howard JN, et al. Nocardiosis in liver transplantation: variation in presentation, diagnosis and therapy. *J Infect* 1990;20:11–19.

70 Sutherland S, Christofinis G, O'Grady J, Williams R. A serological investigation of human herpesvirus 6 infections in liver transplant recipients and the detection of cross-reacting antibodies to cytomegalovirus. *J Med Virol* 1991;33:172–176.

71 Ward KN, Gray JJ, Efstathiou S. Brief report: primary human herpesvirus 6 infection in a patient following liver transplantation from a sero-positive donor. *J Med Virol* 1989;28:69–72.

72 Marshall WF, Telenti A, Proper J, Aksamit AJ, Smith TF. Survey of urine from transplant recipients for polyomaviruses JC and BK using the polymerase chain reaction. *Molecular Cell Probes* 1991;5:125–128.

73 Walker DL. Progressive multifocal leukoencephalopathy. In: Vinken PJ, Bruyn GW, Klawans HL, eds. *Handbook of Clinical Neurology.* Vol. 47. Vinken PJ, Bruyn GW, Klawans HL, Koetsier JC, eds. Demyelinating diseases. Amsterdam: Elsevier Press, 1985:503–524.

74 Koneru B, Jaffe R, Esquivel CO, et al. Adenoviral infections in pediatric liver transplant recipients. *JAMA* 1987;258:489–492.

75 Wiesner RH, Hermans PE, Rakela J, et al. Selective bowel decontamination to decrease gram-negative aerobic bacterial and *Candida* colonization and prevent infection after orthotopic liver transplantation. *Transplantation* 1988;45:570–574.

76 Raakow R, Steffen R, Lefèbre B, Bechstein WO, Blumhardt G, Neuhaus P. Selective bowel decontamination effectively prevents gram-negative bacterial infections after liver transplantation. *Transplant Proc* 1990;22:1556–1557.

77 Rosman C, Klompmaker IJ, Bonsel GJ, Bleichrodt RP, Arends JP, Slooff MJH. The efficacy of selective bowel decontamination as infection prevention after liver transplantation. *Transplant Proc* 1990;22:1554–1555.

78 Wiesner RH. The incidence of gram-negative bacterial and fungal infections in liver transplant patients treated with selective decontamination. *Infection* 1990;18(Suppl 1):19S–21S.

79 Gombert ME, duBouchet L, Aulicino TM, Butt KMH. A comparative trial of clotrimazole troches and oral nystatin suspension in recipients of renal transplants. *JAMA* 1987;258: 2553–2555.

80 Mora NP, Klintmalm G, Solomon H, Goldstein RM, Gonwa TA, Husberg BS. Selective amphotericin B prophylaxis in the reduction of fungal infections after liver transplant. *Transplant Proc* 1992;24:154–155.

81 Snydman DR, Werner BG, Heinze-Lacey B, et al. Use of cytomegalovirus immune globulin to prevent cytomegalovirus disease in renal transplant recipients. *N Engl J Med* 1987;317: 1049–1054.

82 Merigan TC, Renlund DG, Keay S, et al. A controlled trial of ganciclovir to prevent cytomegalovirus disease after heart transplantation. *N Engl J Med* 1992;326:1182–1186.

83 Schmidt GM, JHorak DA, Niland JC, et al. A randomized controlled trial of prophylactic ganciclovir for cytomegalovirus pulmonary infection in recipients of allogeneic bone marrow transplants. *N Engl J Med* 1991;324: 1005–1011.

84 Plotkin SA, Starr SE, Friedman HM, et al. Effect of towne live virus vaccine on cytomegalovirus disease after renal transplant. *Ann Intern Med* 1991;114:525–531.

85 Cofer JB, Morris CA, Sutker WL, et al. A randomized double-blind study of the effect of prophylactic immune globulin on the incidence and severity of CMV infection in the liver transplant recipient. *Transplant Proc* 1991; 23:1525–1527.

86 Snydman DR. Prevention of cytomegalovirus-associated diseases with immunoglobulin. *Transplant Proc* 1991;23:131–135.

87 Stratta RJ, Shaefer MS, Cushing KA, et al. Successful prophylaxis of cytomegalovirus disease after primary CMV exposure in liver transplant recipients. *Transplantation* 1991;51:90–97.

88 Dickson RC, Porayko MK, Keating MR, et al. Antiviral drug prophylaxis of cytomegalovirus (CMV) infections following liver transplantation. American Gastroenterological Association, American Association for the Study of Liver Diseases, San Francisco, May 10–13, 1992.

89 Gold D, Corey L. Acyclovir prophylaxis for herpes simplex virus infection. *Antimicrob Agents Chemother* 1987;31:361–367.

90 Fischl MA, Dickinson GM, La Voie L. Safety and efficacy of sulfamethoxazole and trimethoprim chemoprophylaxis for *Pneumocystis carinii* pneumonia in AIDS. *JAMA* 1988;259: 1185–1189.

91 Hughes WT, Rivera GK, Schell MJ, Thornton D, Lott L. Successful intermittent chemoprophylaxis for *Pneumocystis carinii* pneumonitis. N Engl J Med 1987;316:1627–1632.

92 Morgan A, Grayiani A, MacGregor RR. Daily vs intermittent trimethoprim sulfamethoxazole for *Pneumocystis carinii* pneumonia prophylaxis. Program and Abstracts of the 1990 Interscience Conference on Antimicrobial Agents and Chemotherapy, Atlanta, 1990.

93 Wormser GP, Horowitz HW, Duncanson FP, et al. Low dose intermittent trimethoprim-sulfamethoxazole for prevention of *Pneumocystis carinii* pneumonia in patients with human immunodeficiency virus infection. *Arch Intern Med* 1991;151:688–692.

94 Fox BC, Sallinger HW, Belzer FO, Maki DG. A prospective, randomized, double-blind study of trimethoprim-sulfamethoxazole for prophylaxis of infection in renal transplantation: clinical efficacy, absorption of trimethoprim-sulfamethoxazole, effects on the microflora and the cost benefit of prophylaxis. Am J Med 1990;89:255–274.

95 Jules-Elysee KM, Stover DE, Zaman MB, Bernard EM, White DA. Aerosolized pentamidine: effect on diagnosis and presentation of *Pneumocystis carinii* pneumonia. Ann Intern Med 1990;112:750–757.

The management of cryptococcal disease in patients with AIDS

SAMUEL A. BOZZETTE

INTRODUCTION

Cryptococcus neoformans is a common serious pathogen in persons with advanced human immunodeficiency virus (HIV) infection. (1). Five to 10% of persons with acquired immunodeficiency syndrome (AIDS) will contract cryptococcal infection, and cryptococcal disease accounts for a similar proportion of both AIDS-related hospital admissions and acute HIV-associated neurologic dysfunction (2–8). Furthermore, unless effective primary prevention or immune restoration supervene, improved survival for advanced HIV disease and the more widespread use of primary prophylaxis for *Pneumocystis carinii* pneumonia make it likely that HIV-related cryptococcal disease will be increasingly common.

C. *neoformans* is a round or occasionally oval encapsulated yeast which reproduces by budding. Four serotypes have been identified according to the antigenicity of the capsular polysaccharide. Serotypes A and D have been classified as var *neoformans*. This strain is widely distributed in soil and pigeon droppings worldwide and can exist as a perfect (sexual) form known as *Filobasidiella neoformans* var *neoformans* (9). Cryptococcal disease in persons with AIDS is almost always caused by A/D serotypes, even on the west coast of the United States where serotypes B/C, classified as var *gattii*, have accounted for up to 40% of clinical isolates (10–14). Interestingly, the first and only identified natural reservoir of serotype B/C organisms are eucalyptus trees, which, in the United States, are common only on the west coast (15). C. *neoformans* var *gattii* also has a perfect (sexual) form known as *Filobasidiella neoformans* var *bacillispora* (16).

Cryptococcal infection is acquired via inhalation of the small, unencapsulated or poorly encapsulated form of the yeast that is found in the environment or possibly by inhalation of the basidiospore of the hyphal form (17,18). Depending upon the degree of host immunity, infection may be cleared, remain limited to the lungs, or disseminate (19). Host defenses against the cryptococcus are primarily mediated by neutrophils and mononuclear cells, but antibody, complement, and cytokines play an important role via opsinization by mediating chemoattraction and activation of cellular elements

(20–22). In patients with AIDS, general quantitative and qualitative defects in immunity, as well as possible specific defects, combine to create a state of high vulnerability to infection and a high propensity to disseminate.

The most common manifestations of disseminated disease are spread to the central nervous system (CNS) and fungemia. The reason for the central nervous system predilection is unknown, but it has been suggested that the cerebrospinal fluid (CSF), which lacks complement, may be a protected site for multiplication or that local factors may promote growth of the organism (23,24). After dissemination has occurred, a high burden of capsular polysaccharide may exacerbate a patient's vulnerability to further progression of disease via depletion of complement, specific impairment of antibody response, and inhibition of phagocytosis and cell migration (25–27).

CLINICAL MANIFESTATIONS

Cryptococcosis is the presenting manifestation of HIV infection in 15% to 40% of cases and is the AIDS-defining event in 40% to 60% of cases (28,29). Characteristically, the disease strikes individuals with very advanced immune depletion; CD4 counts of 50 cells/mm^3 or less are usual. Although isolated focal infection is occasionally seen, the infection is usually characterized by potentially lethal dissemination with a heavy burden of organisms at the time of initial presentation. The central nervous system is almost universally involved in disseminated disease, but up to 75% of patients will also have fungemia, and many will have other local sites of infection such as the skin, prostate, and the organs of the gastrointestinal tract. Accordingly, a presumptive diagnosis should be made as soon as possible in suspected cases, and institution of therapy should normally not wait for cultural confirmation.

Central nervous system infection

Cryptococcal disease accounts for up to 11% of acute HIV-associated neurologic disease, and meningitis is found in greater than 80% of HIV-associated cryptococcal disease (30). Headache and fever occur in 70% to 90% of patients and nausea in about half of the patients. Less common are the more specific manifestations of central infection such as meningismus and photophobia each of which occurs in only 20% to 30% of patients. Thus, cryptococcal disease is among the many complications of HIV infection that usually present with symptoms that are very common in this population. A timely diagnosis therefore depends on detecting changes in the severity or chronicity of symptoms, a high index of suspicion, and a low threshold for initiating a laboratory evaluation.

HIV-associated cryptococcal meningitis may occasionally present as a new neurologic disorder. The most common of these, altered mental status, is an ominous prognostic sign which is found in 10% to 20% of patients (31). Other neurologic manifestations are less common, but cryptococcal disease should be suspected when they occur, as this infection accounts for up to 13% of new-onset seizures, 16% of cerebral infarction, and 30% of extraocular muscle dysfunction in AIDS patients (32).

The serum cryptococcal antigen is positive in 75% to 100% of AIDS patients with meningitis and therefore, unlike in non-HIV-infected patients, it may be useful for screening when there is a low suspicion of infection (33). However, an immediate lumbar puncture is the diagnostic procedure of choice for rapid diagnosis whenever suspicion of a central nervous system process is even moderate. Opening pressure should always be performed when evaluating for cryptococcal meningitis, as intracranial hypertension is not uncommon, and early detection will alert the clinician of its possible contribution to a deteriorating course (34).

The cerebrospinal fluid usually shows a combination of both heavy infection and poor host response, which is reminiscent of that found in poor-prognosis, non-HIV-infected patients (35,36). The India ink preparation is positive for cryptococci in 70% to 90% of patients and is of great value because it offers the possibility of immediate diagnosis. The cerebrospinal fluid cryptococcal antigen is also highly specific when properly performed and is positive in 90% to 100% of infected persons.

Other tests immediately available to the clinician may be less helpful, as the cerebrospinal fluid findings show pleocytosis in only 10% to 35% of cases, elevated cerebrospinal fluid protein in 50% of cases, and a low glucose in less than 25% of cases. Culture of the cerebrospinal fluid is highly sensitive. A negative culture of a specimen obtained at the initiation of therapy in the presence of symptoms and a repeatedly positive cerebrospinal antigen titer raises the unusual possibility of isolated basilar meningitis or cryptococcoma.

The computed tomography (CT) scan of the head is abnormal in a majority of patients, but the most common finding, atrophy, is most likely related to the HIV rather than cryptococcal infection (37). Abnormalities more likely related to cryptococcus are found in 20% to 30% of patients. Mass lesions with or without enhancement account for 10% to 15% of the abnormalities, while hydrocephalus, edema, and occasionally infarcts or focal hypodense lesions of the basal ganglia compose the rest (38). Abnormalities on magnetic resonance imaging (MRI) may be more common (39). Mass lesions and clusters of small abnormal foci in the basal ganglia, which are hyperintense on T-2 weighted images, may be seen more easily. These lesions and the hypodense lesions in the basal ganglia seen on CT apparently represent the Virchow-Robin spaces of the penetrating arteries being distended by cryptococci (40). Additionally, a striking milliary-like pattern of multiple small enhancing lesions scattered throughout the parenchymal and meninges may be seen on MRI.

Eye

Neuroophthalmic abnormalities may occur in up to one-third of persons with cryptococcal meningitis (41). Arachnoiditis may lead to optic neuropathy with atrophy and visual field loss which may be partially reversible (42–44). Limitation of eye movement may also occur, presumably via a similar mechanism. Additionally, infection of the optic nerve, uvea, vitreous, and retina have been documented (45). The chorioretinitis appears as bilateral, multifocal, creamy choroidal infiltrates with retinal hemorrhage.

Pulmonary infection

The lungs are the portal of entry for the cryptococcus, and cryptococcosis is the most common cause of mycotic pulmonary disease in AIDS patients (46). Pulmonary involvement may be found in 25% to 45% of patients with HIV-associated cryptococcal disease, and the lungs are the site of initial diagnosis in up to 25% of patients at some institutions (47–50). Pulmonary cryptococcosis in severely immunocompromised patients with AIDS has usually already disseminated by the time of clinical presentation. Seventy to 100% of patients reportedly have extrapulmonary dissemination with meningitis and/or fungemia at the time that pulmonary disease is discovered (51). In addition, up to 50% of patients with pulmonary cryptococcosis may have a second infectious complication of HIV disease such as *Mycobacterium avium* or *Pneumocystis carinii*.

Symptomatic patients present acutely or subacutely. Fever occurs in 85% and cough in 60% to 80%. Other localizing complaints and signs such as dyspnea, pleuritis, or hypoxemia are less common. The most common radiographic pattern seen is an interstitial infiltrate which is often somewhat nodular. However, focal nodulelike infiltrates, cavitation, and hilar adenopathy may be seen (52). Uncommonly, chest disease may present as a mediastinal mass, a pleural effusion, or as pulmonary opacification and respiratory distress syndrome (53–58). Since the presentation of pulmonary cryptococcosis may be indistinguishable from other HIV-related atypical pulmonary syndromes, the diagnosis should be considered, and, at a minimum, a serum antigen should be obtained in all such patients. This is particularly true if the planned management is for presumptive treatment of *Pneumocystis carinii* pneumonia rather than for pursuit of a definitive diagnosis. Furthermore, as the presence of disseminated disease has prognostic and therapeutic implications, a presumptive or confirmed diagnosis of pulmonary cryptococcosis mandates a full evaluation, including a lumbar puncture.

As in other immunocompromised hosts, the serum cryptococcal antigen is positive in over 90% of HIV-infected patients with pulmonary cryptococcosis and is therefore a reasonable screening test (59). A rapid and definitive diagnosis of pulmonary cryptococcosis can often be made by direct examination of pulmonary secretions. Examination of expectorated or preferably induced sputum is worthwhile, but examination of bronchioalveolar lavage fluid using special stains has a much higher sensitivity of up to 80% or greater (60,61). Histologic examination of bronchoscopic biopsies of intrabronchial plaques, ulcers, or "pearly" granulomas is also reliable. Cultural confirmation of infection is easily obtained from bronchoscopic specimens and, in 50% to 80% of cases, sputum. However, the performance of a full evaluation and the institution of full-dose therapy should not await confirmation if a suspicious organism is seen or if antigenemia is found.

Prostate

Symptomatic prostatic cryptococcal infection is unusual, and other documented sites of urinary tract infection are rare in both HIV-infected and other patients (62–65). However, postprostatic massage urine cultures are positive in 20% to 30% of HIV-infected patients after otherwise successful treatment of disseminated cryptococcal infection (66). Additionally, foci of infection likely persist in the prostates of some patients despite negative end-of-therapy urine cultures as up to 30% of such patients will develop culture-positive prostatic disease unless given maintenance therapy (67). It is unclear if the prostate serves as a reservoir from which recurrent dissemination may occur or as a marker for incompletely treated disease elsewhere, but clinical experience and extrapolation from the case of isolated pulmonary foci in immunocompromised patients suggest that dissemination is likely in untreated cases of persistent prostatic cryptococcosis.

Prostatic infection is best documented by examination of India ink preparations and cultures of expressed prostatic secretions or centrifuged first-void, postprostatic massage urine. Of interest, isolates obtained from patients completing combination therapy with amphotericin B and flucytosine have been uniformly flucytosine resistant, suggesting that poor penetration of amphotericin B has a role in the failure to clear infection at this site (unpublished observation).

Mucocutaneous

Cutaneous lesions of cryptococcal disease may be quite varied. Skin lesions include pustules, nodules, papules resembling molluscum contagiosum, and ulcers which may appear herpetic (68–71). Lingual, palatal, anal, and endobronchial mucosal lesions reportedly include ulcers and papules which often have a "pearly" appearance (72–75). Biopsy of any of these lesions reliably yields material diagnostic of disseminated disease and should be undertaken when suspicious lesions arise. The differential diagnosis of such lesions is wide and, depending on location, includes molluscum contagiosum, herpes simplex, cytomegalovirus, histoplasma, *Candida* sp, aphthous ulcers, inflammatory bowel disease, amebiasis, cancer, lymphoma, and other conditions, as well as cryptococcosis.

Fungemia

Cryptococci represent up to one-fourth of isolates from blood in HIV-infected patients (76). In non-AIDS patients, cryptococcemia is a relatively unusual manifestation of cryptococcal disease and carries a poor prognosis (77). Cryptococcemia is much more common in AIDS, occurring in 10% to 50% of patients with meningitis, but it appears to have little prognostic significance. Isolated fungemia appears to account for less than 10% of HIV-related cryptococcosis. Isolation of cryptococci from the blood always mandates aggressive therapy and performance of a lumbar puncture. Although the presence of meningitis has possible implications for the duration of intensive therapy, lifetime maintenance therapy after HIV-associated crytococcemia is prudent even if meningitis is not found.

Antigenemia

Isolated high-titer antigenemia with negative cultures reportedly occurs in 1% to 3% of patients thought to have cryptococcal disease. However, it is unclear from the literature how extensive a search for disease was performed in the reported cases, and it seems likely that bronchoscopy, postprostatic massage urine culture, cranial imaging, and perhaps cisternal puncture would have uncovered a source of antigenemia in at least some patients. One report indicated that a positive culture from the site can be obtained from all patients with an antigenemia titer of greater than 1:2 (33).

Nonetheless, high titers on repeated serum samples from a reliable laboratory will be obtained from some patients in whom a source cannot be found. Prudence dictates that such instances must be managed as indicative of true occult disease and treated. The implications of lower titers found on single determinations are less clear. For example, one report indicated that only one of seven untreated patients with isolated cerebrospinal fluid titer of less than 1:32 developed meningitis (78). A reasonable practice would be to customize management according to the indication for obtaining the specimen in question. Low titers (i.e. 1:2) simply might be repeated if discovered in a screen of asymptomatic individuals, but should be fully investigated if obtained in patients with symptoms. Similarly, a titer of 1:4 should be investigated further in asymptomatic individuals, but such persons could be followed carefully with repeated determinations rather than treated if the evaluation is negative. Azole therapy should be considered even after a negative evaluation in a symptomatic individual with such a titer. The availability of a nontoxic azole, which may be effective for primary prophylaxis eases the difficulty of managing this situation. Clinical benefit may accrue (or at least clinical harm is unlikely) even if the antigen titer being treated for the use of such an agent were in fact a false-positive result.

Other anatomical sites

Disseminated disease in HIV-infected patients with cryptococcosis can involve multiple sites throughout the body. In the gastrointestinal tract, invasive disease of the stomach, duodenum, colon, pancreas, and liver has been reported, and, rarely, clinical hepatitis may be seen. Both myocarditis and pericarditis have been seen. Additionally, involvement of the bone marrow, adrenal glands, kidneys, and placenta has been reported, and one suspects that, in carefully performed autopsies, nearly every organ of the body may be found to be affected. Although infection at these uncommon sites is usually part of obvious systemic disease, it can be essentially asymptomatic or without distinguishing clinical characteristics.

LABORATORY DIAGNOSIS

Once considered, the diagnosis of cryptococcal disease is usually easily confirmed. Discussion of direct examination of specimens, culture, and antigen detection follows.

Direct examination of specimens

Typical organisms may be identified in biopsy material and body fluids, including cerebrospinal fluid, urine, and occasionally pulmonary secretions or even blood. In tissue, special stains such as periodic acid-Schiff (PAS), Gomori's methenamine silver

(GMS), or other silver stain must be used to identify fungi reliably as the organisms take up routine hematoxylin-eosin (HE) stain poorly. Additionally, mucicarmine stain, which is taken up by the capsule of the cryptococcus, is often quite helpful in distinguishing the cryptococcus from other yeast, but may be misleading if capsule-deficient or partially autolysed organisms are present.

The India ink preparation is by far the most important means of identifying the organism by direct examination because it is immediately accessible to all clinicians. The sensitivity of the technique is good in patients with HIV infection and may be improved by centrifuging the fluid to be examined. However, the test may be less than completely specific in some situations. Inexperienced observers may misidentify lymphocytes or other particulate material; all observers should guard against this by looking carefully for definite capsules and budding. Consideration should be given to confirming positives with a gram stain. Additionally, clinicians should be aware that the presence of correctly identified cryptococci in the cerebrospinal fluid of patients may not indicate active disease when the question is one of recurrence. Twenty-five to 40% of patients who are culture negative at the completion of therapy will have persistently positive India ink preparations.

Culture

C. neoformans is easily grown, but false-negative cultures do occur. All clinicians who see significant numbers of AIDS patients occasionally encounter patients with sustained cryptococcal antigenemia, a compatible syndrome, and a response to specific therapy despite negative cultures (79). Reasons for false-negative cultures vary. When only blood and cerebrospinal fluid are cultured, infection confined to another site, such as the lungs or urinary tract, may be missed. Mishandling of a specimen from an infected site, a low number of organisms (particularly in urine specimens), or the presence of inhibitory substances such as antibody or leukocytes all may lead to false-negative results but may be counteracted by appropriate maneuvers (80,81). Reliance on radiometric detection systems may lead to a failure to detect growth when it occurs (82,83). Atypical properties of organisms isolated from some patients with AIDS such as urease negativity or poor encapsulation with dry (as opposed to the usual mucoid) primary colonies may lead to misidentification (84–88). However, false-negative cultures from any cause are the exception and usually have minimal clinical implications, as a well-justified presumptive diagnosis mandates acute treatment and lifetime maintenance in most circumstances.

Antigen detection

The latex agglutination test for the presence of cryptococcal capsular polysaccharide in body fluids is rapidly performed, widely available, 90% to 100% sensitive, and 90% to 100% specific (89,90). False-positive results can be due to rheumatoid factors or other antibodies, cross-reactivity with other fungal or bacterial products, and nonspecific agglutination of the latex particles attributable to drugs such as pentamidine (91–94). Clinically, false-negative results may be the result of poor production of capsular polysaccharide associated with rapid growth or, more likely, minimal shedding of capsular polysaccharide into fluids in early or localized infection (95,96). More commonly, in patients with AIDS, very large amounts of antigen (the prozone effect) or interfering substances may saturate the binding sites for capsular polysaccharide on the latex beads, leading to failure to agglutinate or to observe a clear end point. Maneuvers such as diluting all specimens from patients with AIDS, boiling, ethylenediaminetetraacetic acid (EDTA)-heat extraction, or treatment with pronase will mitigate these difficulties (97,98). The latter may be particularly important in this setting, since observed titers in most specimens from AIDS patients increase after pronase treatment (99). As most good laboratories have adopted these maneuvers and a heavy burden of organisms is usual in HIV-associated cryptococcal disease, complete false-negative results are seldom a practical problem.

TREATMENT AND PROGNOSIS

There has been a great deal of activity in research on treatment for cryptococcal disease because of the increased caseload and the development of new, potent triazole antifungals. Studies in HIV-associated disease have demonstrated that amphotericin B treatment with or without flucytosine is unlikely to lead to true cure, that maintenance therapy is mandatory after the completion of primary treatment, and that a new oral triazole is effective in both primary therapy for some patients and maintenance therapy for most. However, these studies have not clearly identified the optimal forms of therapy for various classes of patients and have created new uncertainty about when, how, and how long amphotericin B should be used. Furthermore, all of the prospective treatment studies have focused on meningitis. Although lessons learned in that setting are clearly relevant to cases of fungemia or widespread dissemination, they are of less help in localized disease, and little in the way of data-derived guidance is available for the management of such cases.

Primary treatment

Seventy percent or more of patients in most series survive the acute episode if treated; most deaths occur in the first two weeks of therapy. Injection drug users and patients who already have AIDS at presentation do less well. However, complete response rates for all patients, generally defined as clinical response plus sterilization of cerebrospinal fluid and blood, are disappointingly low and are less than 50% in most series. Furthermore, occult sites of infection clearly persist even among "complete responders." The organism can be cultured from a single postprostatic massage urine in more than 20% of such patients, and, in the absence of maintenance therapy, recrudescence occurs in up to 50% by six months. Thus, although regimens producing high sterilization rates are preferred, primary therapy in HIV-infected patients must be viewed as part of a lifelong strategy of control rather than an attempt at cure.

The mainstay of traditional therapy remains the polyene antibiotic amphotericin B (100). Optimal outcomes using this agent for meningitis require prolonged therapy, with at six least weeks being clinically superior to four weeks in immunocompromised but non-HIV-infected patients and with the median HIV-infected patient requiring seven weeks before conversion of cerebrospinal fluid cultures to negative (101). Although amphotericin B is effective in certain local sites such as the lungs, poor pharmacokinetics and penetration make it minimally effective in the prostate and probably other sites where the fungus might be sequestered. Additionally, prolonged amphotericin B treatment is often difficult to administer to these patients. Renal compromise is common in HIV disease, particularly in injection drug users. Amphotericin B nephrotoxicity, which may become dose limiting during prolonged therapy or repeated courses, is manifest as reduced creatinine clearance and/or distal tubule defects which frequently complicate management with other medications and perturb electrolytes such as potassium, magnesium, and bicarbonate (102,103). Amphotericin B-associated hematotoxicity may also be significant in patients with HIV infection, especially those receiving zidovudine. Finally, a full course of therapy usually requires placement of an indwelling intravenous line. The use of such indwelling catheters in HIV-infected patients is associated with a risk of infectious complication which is, at 0.25 to 0.5 per 100 catheter days, approximately five times higher than that seen in other patient populations (104,105).

Flucytosine is a fluorinated cytosine analog which is 100% absorbed from the gastrointestinal tract and 90% excreted unchanged in the urine (106). It has a half-life of approximately four hours in normal individuals, but this may be prolonged to greater than 24 hours in patients with renal failure, with rapid accumulation of the drug to toxic levels unless dosing is reduced. The frequent emergence of secondary resistance limits the usefulness of flucytosine in monotherapy of cryptococcosis. However, combination therapy with amphotericin B and oral flucytosine is preferred to monotherapy with either agent in non–HIV-infected patients because of the amphotericin-sparing effect and the more rapid sterilization of cerebrospinal fluid that it provides (107).

In HIV-infected patients, the use of flucytosine is controversial. Some retrospective reports have indicated no survival benefit, and many report toxicity rates greater than 50% in AIDS patients compared with the 30% to 40% that had been reported prior to the HIV epidemic (108). Vulnerability to both myelosuppression and gastrointestinal distress seems to be increased, even in individuals with normal serum creatinine. However, other series report longer survival or better sterilization rates for individuals given combination therapy, and some centers report that most of their patients can tolerate at least several weeks of combination therapy, which may be sufficient to assist in gaining control of the infection. However, all of these studies are flawed by selection bias, the "hearty survivor effect," and/or the failure to use drug level monitoring to adjust flucytosine doses. Fortunately, a cooperative randomized controlled trial to examine the role of flucytosine is underway by the ACTG/MSG.

In another attempt to increase its potency, intrathecal amphotericin B is sometimes administered via cisternal punctures or placement of a subcutaneous intraventrical reservoir (109). However, others have not observed improvement in outcomes due to high complication rates, and, at most centers, the practice is seldom employed for this infection (110).

Fluconazole is a new triazole antifungal agent which is licensed for use in candidal and cryptococcal infection (111,112). It acts by inhibition of the fungal cytochrome P450 enzyme ergosterol synthetase and, as opposed to early generation azoles, has a 10,000-fold lower affinity for the human cytochrome P450 enzymes necessary for steroid synthesis. It is an orally active, water-soluble compound with a half-life of 22 hours and excellent penetration into the body fluids, including cerebrospinal fluid, and tissues (113). The drug is effective against cryptococcus in a variety of animal models.

A large, uncontrolled experience in humans with cryptococcal meningitis has indicated that fluconazole is active but that rapid sterilization of the cerebrospinal fluid is uncommon (114,115). Recently, the results of two randomized trials of fluconazole as primary therapy for meningitis became available. Both defined complete response as clinical responses plus sterilization of the cerebrospinal fluid and blood. The first was a small, single-center trial performed in a county-hospital population (116). In this trial, zero of six patients treated with amphotericin B plus flucytosine failed, whereas eight of fourteen treated with 400 milligrams per day of fluconazole failed. Failures on fluconazole included three deaths, three cases of severe neurologic deterioration, and two cases of persistently positive cerebrospinal fluid cultures. The second study was a large, pivotal, multicenter trial with a broader range of patients. In this trial, amphotericin B was not shown to be clearly superior to fluconazole with respect to 12-week outcome. Twenty-five of 63 (40%) patients treated with amphotericin B and 44 of 131 (34%) initially treated with 200 milligrams per day of fluconazole were complete responders. (*Note:* nine amphotericin B patients also received flucytosine, and 48 fluconazole patients had dose escalation to 400 milligrams per day for poor response.) Clinical failures on amphotericin B included a 14% death rate, with 8% of the patients dying during the first two weeks of therapy, while failures on fluconazole included a 18% death rate, with 15% of the deaths occurring in the first two weeks. Also of note, the median patient had culture conversion at day 42 in the amphotericin B group and day 64 in the fluconazole group.

The latter study demonstrated that fluconazole is active and effective for some patients. Although better outcomes were still observed with amphotericin B in both treatment groups, mortality was less than 5% among patients with good prognosis (good prognosis was defined as having a normal mental status and cerebrospinal fluid cryptococcal antigen titer of less than 1:1024 and a white cell count of 20/mm^3). The difference in outcomes between the treatment regimens was greater in the group of more severely ill patients. The increase in unfavorable outcomes among the sicker patients, the high early death rate, and the longer time to sterilization in the fluconazole group, coupled with the results of the previously cited study, lead most investigators to reserve primary fluconazole therapy for the most mildly ill patients or to start all except those with serious contraindications on amphotericin B for at least the initial weeks of therapy.

It should be noted that the results of this latter study are not definitive but rather are somewhat contradictory and may not be directly applicable to the management of difficult cases today. It has been hypothesized that the overall disappointing outcomes were related to low dosages of the study drugs. This is particularly true for fluconazole since 400 mg daily has become the standard dose for persons with serious active infection, and unapproved doses of 600 mg daily or higher have become routine at some centers. The pivotal study cannot address the dose-efficacy relationship for fluconazole, as the high dose of 400 mg may have been most important for the patients who expired in the first two weeks of the study when fluconazole dose escalation was not allowed. With respect to amphotericin B dosing, one can only note that most patients actually received well above the minimal amount required by the protocol (0.3 mg/kg) and that outcomes were not related to dosing. It has also been hypothesized that the excess early deterioration among fluconazole-treated patients is related to a less vigorous antifungal effect in sicker patients. However, the results of the study were not entirely consistent with this hypothesis since the observed *relative* risk for death with fluconazole treatment was actually a bit smaller for the poor-prognosis group than for the good-prognosis group at 0.049/0.026 or 1.9 versus 0.40/0.33 or 1.2.

Development of regimens that contain these drugs is ongoing. In a pilot study, 600 mg daily of fluconazole resulted in response in five of eight patients who had failed one to several forms of previous therapy (117). The combination of fluconazole at 400 mg daily and flucytosine at standard doses resulted in a cumulative cerebrospinal fluid sterilization rate of 84% in a pilot study of 32 patients (118; Bozzette et al., unpublished).

Less well studied agents include another triazole antifungal agent, itraconazole. It is well absorbed and has a half-life of 17 hours, but its penetration into cerebrospinal fluid is very poor (119). Nonetheless, it is effective in animal models of cryptococcal meningitis, suggesting that intrameningeal or intracerebral drug levels may be important in the control of infection (120). Ten of 14 patients with HIV-associated cryptococcal meningitis had complete microbiologic (CSF) and clinical responses in one series (121). In a small randomized trial, 10 of 10 patients given amphotericin B plus flucytosine, but only five of fourteen given itraconazole had complete responses, and recrudescence despite maintenance was common in the latter group (122). Various preparations of liposomal or lipid-associated amphotericin B have been used in patients with HIV-associated cryptococcal meningitis, but experience has been too limited to draw any conclusions about the merits of these preparations relative to Fungizone, which is the standard commercially available amphotericin B preparation (123–127).

As has been mentioned, although the optimal primary treatment regimen has not been defined, treatment decisions must be made. The frequency of significant co-morbidity and the limited life expectancy of AIDS patients make the desirability of nontoxic oral treatment for cryptococcal disease obvious. In certain circumstances, a patient and physician may believe that these advantages outweigh a higher relative risk of treatment failure. Such circumstances may include severe comorbidity, severe renal compromise, absolute refusal of amphotericin B, or local or mild illness, in which the prognosis with treatment is good regardless of the specific regimen selected. In these circumstances, fluconazole should be used at doses of 400 to 600 mg daily for 10 weeks or until sterilization of cultures. Thereafter, dosing may be reduced to maintenance levels of 100 to 200 mg daily.

Most investigators, including the author, continue to prefer amphotericin B for initial therapy in most patients. Although the optimal regimen is not clear, it does not appear that amphotericin B must be continued for the traditional full course of six weeks or two grams because the goal of initial parenteral therapy is control rather than cure of the acute infection. Operational definitions of "short-course" amphotericin B therapy vary, but, as short-term management in reaction to culture results is impractical, therapy is generally continued until there is clinical improvement and two weeks or a total of 500 mg of amphotericin B has been delivered. The use of flucytosine is favored by many investigators, including the author, since the majority of patients will easily tolerate two to four weeks when careful dosing is employed. Anemia, leukopenia, renal insufficiency, or gastrointestinal distress are relative contraindications. Tolerance is improved by initiation of flucytosine at 100 mg/kg/day rather than the traditional 150 mg/kg/day and, most importantly, by monitoring blood levels to maintain peaks of 50 to 75 micrograms per deciliter. Finally, placement of indwelling intravenous lines may be avoided in patients who do well with initial therapy, as early crossover to oral treatment can be anticipated. If shorter courses of amphotericin B are used, initial oral treatment should be with therapeutic doses of fluconazole to complete 10 weeks of therapy or more if persistently positive cultures are found from any site, including the urine. Thereafter, maintenance doses may be used.

If a traditional full course of amphotericin B is elected, the author still prefers to add flucytosine for as long as it is tolerated. Flucytosine is dosed as above, and blood levels are obtained weekly or biweekly. Using this approach, more than 50% of patients can tolerate at least four weeks of combination therapy. The amphotericin B-sparing effect of the combination facilitates home or clinic dosing. A dose of 0.7 to 0.8 milligrams per kilogram of amphotericin B thrice weekly is usually adequate. Patients who cannot tolerate combination therapy should receive more intensive amphotericin B four to six times a week, with an average dose of 0.6 to 0.9 mg/kg/day. Blood chemistries and hematology studies are obtained weekly or twice weekly during prolonged therapy. Saline infusions are used to mitigate amphotericin B nephrotoxicity, and parenteral and oral electrolyte replacement therapy is often necessary. At the completion of therapy, maintenance doses of oral suppressive therapy are mandatory.

Regardless of the regimen selected, clinicians must be alert to the possibility that the patient may deteriorate while on therapy. Such individuals should be examined for a complication of cryptococcal disease or a second complication of HIV disease. Complicating conditions commonly include other opportunistic infections or malignancies or secondary bacterial infections, including indwelling vascular line-associated bacteremia, intracranial mass lesions, or intracranial hypertension. Mass lesions, depending on location, rarely require excision. Intracranial hypertension may be intractable but is often treated successfully with daily repeated lumbar punctures using large bore needles or shunting. If complications are not found, intensification of therapy should be considered, including adding flucytosine, increasing amphotericin B dosage, or even adding intrathecal amphotericin B in selected cases. In individuals receiving oral therapy, deterioration may be considered a relative indication for switching to parenteral therapy regardless of whether noncompliance is suspected.

Data to guide the management of other forms of cryptococcal disease are inadequate in both HIV-infected and other patients, but inferences can be made from the experience with meningitis. All forms present a risk for dissemination and require a lifelong management strategy. Fungemia or dissemination to abdominal organs should be managed aggressively and similarly to meningitis. Localized pulmonary infection can probably be managed effectively with fluconazole, but, in the absence of specific data, some clinicians continue to prefer amphotericin B. Sustained antigenemia without a focus can probably also be managed with fluconazole, but it is prudent to manage patients with symptoms or high antigen titers as though they had fungemia until cultures mature. Additional amphotericin B is ineffective in the treatment of persistent prostatic cryptococcosis, but fluconazole treatment results in sustained suppression in about one-half of patients (128). Itraconazole has also been used for this indication with perhaps somewhat less success (129; Denning D, personal communication).

Maintenance therapy

Long-term survival was limited to less than 20% of patients at six months in early series (10). Much of the mortality was late and attributable to highly lethal relapses which occur in 50% or more of patients surviving an acute episode. Adoption of prolonged maintenance therapy with weekly amphotericin B was associated with reductions in the relapse rate to less than 10% and apparent increases in survival to 60% or more (130,131). When it became clear that cultures of both cerebrospinal fluid and extraneural sites were frequently positive at the completion of standard therapy, suspicion was that many "relapses" were in fact recrudescences of incompletely treated culture-positive disease. However, in one trial, patients receiving placebo and careful monitoring after a diligent negative search for persistent infection at the end of therapy still had an overall relapse rate of 37% with extraneural relapses (26%), outnumbering meningeal relapses (11%) (67).

This same trial also confirmed previous suggestions of the effectiveness of fluconazole in preventing both urinary and meningeal recurrence (67). A larger trial demonstrated the superiority of fluconazole at 200 mg daily to amphotericin B at 1 mg/kg weekly in maintenance therapy, as 2% of the fluconazole group (2/111) and 12% of the amphotericin B group (14/78) had recurrence of symptomatic disease (132). Of note, all meningeal relapses in both studies presented symptomatically, and none were detected on routine follow-up lumbar punctures. Additionally, in the second study, adverse events occurred in 67% of amphotericin B-treated patients and only 38% of fluconazole-treated patients. Of particular concern, bacteremia, presumably associated with the presence of a chronic indwelling venous line, occurred in 18% of the former group but only 4% of the latter. Fluconazole is thus globally superior to amphotericin B for this indication. Furthermore, the high complication and relapse rates on amphotericin B, coupled with the possibility that prolonged exposure to the drug limits therapeutic dosing should relapse occur, suggest that careful monitoring of serum antigen and extraneural sites, combined with prompt resumption of therapy for recrudescence, may be superior to weekly amphotericin B in patients unable to receive fluconazole.

Other agents may also have activity. Itraconazole appears to have activity in small series of patients and is being evaluated further (133). In other series, ketoconazole, an azole with both limited penetration into cerebrospinal fluid and limited anticryptococcal activity, has been associated with benefit similar to that seen with amphotericin B (134). The mechanism for such an effect is unclear, but it may act via suppression of extraneural disease prior to dissemination.

Prophylaxis

As has been noted, cryptococcal disease is prevalent in advanced HIV disease. Natural history data on the risk of cryptococcosis in this population are incomplete, but suggest that the one-year incidence of infection is probably greater than 3% in symptomatic HIV-infected patients with <200 CD4 cells and 6% in those with <100 CD4 cells (135; Phair J, Northwestern University, personal communication). Success in the prevention of *Pneumocystis carinii* pneumonia and the availability of agents active against *C. neoformans* and other fungi that frequently cause disease in HIV-infected patients, such as *Histoplasma capsulatum* and *Candida* sp, make the possibility of primary chemoprophylaxis attractive.

A large retrospective study has suggested that fluconazole may prevent the development of cryptococcal meningitis, while a report of a smaller study suggests that ketoconazole may also have an effect, presumably via suppression of spread from the lungs (136). While provocative, recommendations regarding the routine use of prophylaxis must await confirmation of efficacy and an assessment of the practical impact of such an intervention. For example, if the true effect of fluconazole is as estimated by the former report, the expected number of cases of serious fungal disease would be reduced from 7.5 to 1.9 per hundred patients treated. Thus, a total of 36,500 doses of fluconazole would have to be administered in order to prevent five to six cases per year. Given that individuals with advanced HIV disease already may be suffering from ill effects due to polypharmacy, the overall benefit provided by such a strategy, even given mycological efficacy, is an empiric question which should be addressed in clinical trials.

REFERENCES

1 Bozzette SA, Waskin HA. Cryptococcal disease in AIDS. In: Voldberding P, Jacobsen MN, eds. *AIDS Clinical Review 1990* New York and Basal: Dekker 1990.

2 Eng RHK, Bishburg E, Smith SM, Kapila R. Cryptococcal infections in patients with acquired immunodeficiency syndrome. *Am J Med* 1986;81:19–23.

3 Zuger A, Louie E, Holzman RS, Simberkoff MS, Rahal JJ. Cryptococcal disease in patients with acquired immunodeficiency syndrome. *Ann Intern Med* 1986;104:234–240.

4 Wilkes MS, Felix JC, Fortin AH, Godwin TA, Thompson WG. Value of necropsy in acquired immunodeficiency syndrome. *Lancet* 1988; ii:85–88.

5 Levy RM, Janssen RS, Bush TJ, Rosenblum ML. Neuroepidemiology of acquired immunodeficiency syndrome. *J Acquir Immune Def Syndr* 1988;1:31–40.

6 Dismukes WE. Cryptococcal meningitis in patients with AIDS. *J Infect Dis* 1988;157: 624–628.

7 Holtzman D, Kaku DA, So Y. New onset seizures associated with human immunodeficiency virus infections: causation and clinical features in 100 cases. *Am J Med* 1989; 87:173–177.

8 Clark RA, Greer D, Atkinson W, Valainis GT, Hyslop N. Spectrum of *Cryptococcus neoformans* infection in 68 patients infected with human immunodeficiency virus. *Rev Infect Dis* 1990;12:768–777.

9 Kwon-Chung KJ. A new genus, Filobasidiella, the perfect state of *Cryptococcus neoformans*. *Mycologia* 1975;67:1197–2000.

10 Kwon-Chung KH, Bennett JE. Epidemlogic differences among serotypes of *Cryptococcus neoformans*. *Am J Epidem* 1984;120:123–130.

11 Shimizu RY, Howard DH, Clancy MN. The variety of *Cryptococcus neoformans* in patients with AIDS. *J Infect Dis* 1986;154:1042.

12 Bottone EJ, Salkin IF, Hurd NJ, Wormser GP. Serogroup distribution of *Cryptococcus neoformans* in patients with AIDS. *J Infect Dis* 1987;156:242.

13 Clancy MN, Fleischmann J, Howard DH, Kwon-Chung KJ, Shimizu RY. Isolation of *Cryptococcus neoformans* var *gatti* from a patient with AIDS in Southern California. *J Infect Dis* 1990;161:809.

14 Levitz SM. The ecology of *Cryptococcus neoformans* and the epidemiology of cryptococcosis. *Rev Infect Dis* 1991;13:1163–1169.

15 Ellis DH, Pfeiffer TJ. Ecology, life cycle, and infectious propagule of *Cryptococcus neoformans*. *Lancet* 1990;336:923–925.

16 Kwon-Chung KJ. A new species of Filobasidiella, the sexual form of *Cryptococcus neoformans* B and C serotypes. *Mycologia* 1976;68:942–946.

17 Dimond RD. *Cryptococcus neoformans*. In: Mandel GL, Douglas RG Jr, Bennett JE, eds. *Principles and Practice of Infectious Diseases*. 3rd ed. New York: Churchhill Livingstone, 1990;1980–1989.

18 Perfect JR. Cryptococcosis. *Infect Dis Clin North Am* 1989;3:77–102.

19 Weinberg RB, Becker S, Granger DL, et al. Growth inhibition of *Cryptococcus neoformans* by human alveolar macrophages. *Am Rev Resp Dis* 1987;136:1242–1247.

20 Graybill JR, Alford RH. Cell-mediated immunity in cryptococcosis. *Cell Immunol* 1974;14:12–21.

21 Diamond RD, Allison AC. Nature of the effector cells responsible for antibody-dependent cell-mediated killing of *Cryptococcus neoformans*. *Infect Immun* 1976;14:716–720.

22 Perfect JR, Granger DL, Durack DT. Effects of antifungal agents and gamma-interferon on macrophage activity of murine macrophages. *J Clin Invest* 1988;81:1129–1136.

23 Igel JH, Bolande RP. Humoral defense mechanisms in cryptococcosis: substances in normal human serum, saliva and cerebrospinal fluid affecting the growth of *Cryptococcus neoformans*. *J Infect Dis* 1966;116:75–83.

24 Kwon-Chung KJ, Rhodes JC. Encapsulation and melanin formation as indicators of virulence in *Cryptococcus neoformans*. *Infect Immun* 1986;41:218–223.

25 Macher A, Bennett J, Gadek J, et al. Complement depletion in cryptococcal sepsis. *J Immunol* 1978;120:1686–1690.

26 Henderson DK, Bennett JE, Huber MA. Long-lasting specific immunologic unresponsiveness associated with cryptococcal meningitis. *J Clin Invest* 1982;69:1185–1190.

27 Laxit KA, Kozel TR. Chemotaxigenesis and activation of the alternative complement pathway by encapsulated and nonencapsulated *Cryptococcus neoformans*. *Infect Immun* 1979;26:435–440.

28 Kovacs JA, Kovacs AA, Polis M, et al. Cryptococcosis in the acquired immunodeficiency syndrome. 1985;103:533–538.

29 Chuck SL, Sande MA. Infections with *Cryptococcus neoformans* in the acquired immunodeficiency syndrome. *New Eng J Med* 1989;321:794–799.

30 Waskin H, Bartlett JA, Gallis H. Cryptococcal disease and HIV infection in North Carolina. V International Conference on AIDS 1989; Abstract WBP 15.

31 Saag MS, Powderly WG, Cloud GA, et al. Comparison of amphotericin B with fluconazole in the treatment of acute AIDS-associated cryptococcal meningitis. *N Engl J Med* 1992;326:83–89.

32 Keane JR. Neuro-ophthalmologic signs of AIDS: 50 patients. *Neurology* 1991;41:841–845.

33 Gal AA, Evans S, Meyer PR. The clinical laboratory evaluation of cryptococcal infections in the acquired immunodeficiency syndrome. *Diag Microbiol Infect Dis* 1987;7:249–254.

34 Denning DW, Armstrong RW, Lewis BH, Stevens DA. Elevated cerebrospinal fluid pressures in patients with cryptococcal meningitis and acquired immunodeficiency syndrome. *Am J Med* 1991;91:267–272.

35 Butler WT, Alling DW, Spickard A, Utz JP. Diagnostic and prognostic value of clinical and laboratory finding in cryptococcal meningitis. *N Engl J Med* 1964;270:59–67.

36 Diamond RD, Bennett JE. Prognostic factors in cryptococcal meningitis. A study in 111 cases. *Ann Intern Med* 1974;80:176–181.

37 Tien RD, Chu PK, Hesselink JR, Duberg A, Wiley C. Intracranial cryptococcosis in immunocompromised patients: CT and MR findings in 29 cases. *Am J Neuroradiol* 1991;12:283–289.

38 Popovich MJ, Arthur RH, Helmer E. CT of intracranial cryptococcosis. *Am J Roentgenol* 1990;154:603–606.

39 Takasu A, Taneda M, Otuki H, Okamoto Y, Oku K. Gd-DTPA-enhanced MR imaging of cryptococcal meningoencephalitis. *Neuroradiology* 1991;33:443–446.

40 Wehn SM, Heinz ER, Burger PC, Boyko OB. Dilated Virchow-Robin spaces in cryptococcal meningitis associated with AIDS: CT and MR findings. *J Comput Assist Tomogr* 1989;13:756–762.

41 Jabs DA, Green WR, Fox R, Polk BF, Bartlett JG. Ocular manifestations of acquired immu-

nodeficiency syndrome. *Ophthalmol* 1989;96: 1092–1099.

42 Lipson BK, Freeman WR, Beniz J, Goldbaum MH, Hesselink JR, Weinreb RN, Sadun AA. Optic neuropathy associated with cryptococcal arachnoiditis in AIDS patients. *Am J Ophth* 1989;107:523–527.

43 Golnik KC, Newman SA, Wispelway B. Cryptococcal optic neuropathy in the acquired immunodeficiency syndrome. *J Clin Neuro Ophthalmol* 1991;11:96–103.

44 Winward KE, Hamed LM, Glaser JS. The spectrum of optic nerve disease in human immunodeficiency virus infection. *Am J Ophthal* 1989;107:373–380.

45 Holland GN. Endogenous fungal infections of the retina and choroid. In: Ryan SJ, ed. *Retina, Volume 2.* St. Louis: CV Mosby, 1989;625–636.

46 Hopewell PC, Luce JM. Pulmonary involvement in the acquired immunodeficiency syndrome. *Chest* 1985;87:104–112.

47 Wasser L, Talavera W. Pulmonary cryptococcosis in AIDS. *Chest* 1987;92:692–695.

48 Cameron M, Bartlett J, Waskin H, Gallis H. Manifestations of pulmonary cryptococcosis in patients with acquired immunodeficiency syndrome. *Rev Infect Dis* 1991;13:64–67.

49 Clark RA, Greer D, Atkinson W, Valainis GT, Hyslop N. *Cryptococcus neoformans* pulmonary infection in HIV-1-infected patients. *J Acquir Immune Defic Syndr* 1990;3:480–484.

50 Chechani V, Kamholz SL. Pulmonary manifestations of disseminated cryptococcosis in patients with AIDS. *Chest* 1990;98:1060–1066.

51 Kerkering TM, Dumbar RJ, Shadomy S. The evolution of pulmonary cryptococcosis in the immunocompromised host. *Ann Intern Med* 1981;94:611–616.

52 Miller WT Jr, Edelman JM, Miller WT. Cryptococcal pulmonary infection in patients with AIDS: radiographic appearance. *Radiology* 1990;175:725–728.

53 Witt D, McKay, Schwam L, Goldstein D, Gold J. Acquired immune deficiency syndrome presenting as bone marrow and mediastinal cryptococcosis. *Amer J Med* 1987;82:149–150.

54 Perla EN, Maayan S, Miller SN, Ramaswamy G, Eisenberg H. Disseminated cryptococcosis presenting as the adult respiratory distress syndrome. *NY State J Med* 1985;85:704–706.

55 Murray RJ, Becker P, Furth P, Criner GJ. Recovery from cryptococcemia and the adult respiratory distress syndrome in the acquired immunodeficiency syndrome. *Chest* 1988;93: 1304–1306.

56 Katz AS, Niesenbaum L, Mass B. Pleural effusion as the initial manifestation of disseminated cryptococcosis in the acquired immunodeficiency syndrome. *Chest* 1989;96:440–441.

57 Grum EE, Schwab R, Margolis ML. Cryptococcal pleural effusion preceding cryptococcal meningitis in AIDS. *Am J Med Sci* 1991; 301(5):329–330.

58 Newman TG, Soni A, Acaron S, Huang CT. Pleural cryptococcosis in the acquired immunodeficiency syndrome. *Chest* 1987;91:459–461.

59 Fisher BD, Armstrong D. Cryptococcal interstitial pneumonia. Value of antigen determination. *New Engl J Med* 1977;297:1440–1441.

60 Malabonga VM, Basti J, Kamholz SL. Utility of bronchoscopic sampling techniques for cryptococcal disease in AIDS. *Chest* 1991;99: 370–372.

61 Gal AA, Koss MN, Hawkins J, Evans S, Einstein H. The pathology of pulmonary cryptococcal infections in the acquired immunodeficiency syndrome. *Arch Pathol Lab Med* 1986;110:502–507.

62 Hinchey WW, Someren A. Cryptococcal prostatitis. *Am J Clin Pathol* 1981;75:257–260.

63 Huynh MT, Reyes CV. Prostatic cryptococcosis. *Urology* 1982;20:622–623.

64 Lee M, Sarfarazi F. Prostatic cryptococcosis in acquired immunodeficiency syndrome. *Urology* 1986;28:318–319.

65 Staib F, Seibold M, L'age M, Heise W, Skorde J, Grosse G, Nurnberger F, Bauer G. *Cryptococcus neoformans* in the seminal fluid of an AIDS patient. *Mycosis* 1989;32:171–180.

66 Larsen RA, Bozzette S, McCutchan JA, et al. Persistent *Cryptococcus neoformans* infection of the prostate after successful treatment of meningitis. *Ann Intern Med* 1989;111:125–128.

67 Bozzette SA, Larsen RA, Chiu J, et al. A placebo-controlled trial of maintenance therapy with fluconazole after treatment of cryptococcal meningitis in the acquired immunodeficiency syndrome. *N Engl J Med* 1991;324: 580–584.

68 Miller SJ. Cutaneous cryptococcus resembling molluscum contagiosum in a patient with acquired immunodeficiency syndrome. *Cutis* 1988;41:411–412.

69 Rico MJ, Penneys NS. Cutaneous cryptococcosis resembling molluscum contagiosum in a patient with AIDS. *Arch Dermatol* 1985; 121:901–902.

70 Jimenez-Acosta F, Casado M, Borbujo J. Cutaneous cryptococcosis mimicking molluscum contagiosum in a haemophiliac with AIDS. *Clin Exp Dermatol* 1987;12:446–450.

71 Borton LK, Wintroub BU. Disseminated cryptococcosis presenting as herpetiform lesions in a homosexual man with acquired immunodeficiency syndrome. *J Am Acad Dermatol* 1984;10:387–390.

72 Lynch DP, Naftolin LZ. Oral *Cryptococcus neoformans* infections in AIDS. *Oral Surf Oral Med Oral Pathol* 1987;64:449–453.

73 Lynch DP. Oral Cryptococcus in AIDS patients (letter). *J Oral Maxillofa Surg* 1990;48:329.

74 Glick M, Cohen SG, Cheney RT, Crooks GW, Greenberg MS. Oral manifestations of disseminated *Cryptococcus neoformans* in a patient with acquired immunodeficiency syndrome. *Oral Surg Oral Med Oral Pathol* 1987;64:454–459.

75 Van Calck M, Motte S, Rickaert F, Serruys E, Adler M, Wybran J. Cryptococcal anal ulceration in a patient with AIDS. *Am J Gastroenterol* 1988;83:1306–1308.

76 Whimbey E, Gold JW, Polsky B, et al. Bacteremia and fungemia in patients with the acquired immunodeficiency syndrome. *Ann Intern Med* 1986;104:511–514.

77 Perfect JR, Durack DT, Gallis HA. Cryptococcemia. *Medicine* 1983;2:98–109.

78 Gurtman A, Masci J, Pierone G, Nicholas P. The significance of isolated positive cerebrospinal fluid cryptococcal antigen in HIV-infected patients. *Int Conf AIDS.* 1990;6:236 (abstract no. Th.B.457).

79 Lewis JL, Rabinovic S. The wide spectrum of cryptococcal infections. *Am J Med* 1972;53:315–332.

80 Brannon P, Kiehn TE. Large scale clinical comparison of the lysis centrifugation and radiometric systems for blood culture. *J Clin Microbiol* 1985;22:951–954.

81 Staib F, Seibold M. Use of the membrane filtration technique and Staib agar for the detection of *Cryptococcus neoformans* in the urine of AIDS patients. *Mycoses* 1989;32:63–72.

82 Robinson PG, Sulita MJ, Matthews E, Warren JR. Failure of the Bactec 460 radiometer to detect *Cryptococcus neoformans* fungemia in an AIDS patient. *Am J Clin Pathol* 1987;87:783–786.

83 Love GL, Boyd GD, Leblanc EJ. Cryptococcemia and the Bactec 460 blood culture system (letter). *Ann Intern Med* 1987;106:633–634.

84 Farhi F, Bulmer GS, Tacker JR. *Cryptococcus neoformans.* IV. The not-so-encapsulated yeast. *Infect Immun* 1970;1:526–531.

85 Bottone EJ, Toma M, Johansson BE, Wormser GP. Capsule-deficient *Cryptococcus neoformans* in AIDS patients (letter). *Lancet* 1985;i:400.

86 Mackenzie DW, Hay RJ. Capsule-deficient *Cryptococcus neoformans* in AIDS patients (letter). *Lancet* 1985;i:642.

87 Bottone EJ, Toma M, Johansson BE, Wormser GP. Poorly encapsulated *Cryptococcus neoformans* from patients with AIDS. I. Preliminary observations. *AIDS Research* 1986;2:211–218.

88 Bottone EJ, Wormser GP. Poorly encapsulated cryptococci from patients with AIDS. II. Correlation of capsule size observed directly in cerebrospinal fluid with that after animal passage. *AIDS Research* 1986;2:219–225.

89 Kaufman L, Reiss E. Serodiagnosis of fungal diseases. In: Lennette EH, ed. *Manual of Clinical Microbiology, 4th ed.* Washington, DC: American Society of Microbiology 1985:924–944.

90 Stockman L, Roberts GD. Corrected version. Specificity of the latex test for cryptococcal antigen; a rapid, simple method for eliminating interference factor. *J Clin Microbiol* 1983;17:945–947.

91 Bennett JE, Bailey JW. Control for rheumatoid factor in the latex test for cryptococcosis. *Am J Clin Path* 1971;56:360–365.

92 Mackinnon S, Kane JG, Parker RH. False positive cryptococcal antigen test and cervical prevertebral abscess. *JAMA* 1978;240:1982–1983.

93 McManus EJ, Jones JM. Detection of trichosporon beigelii antigen cross-reactive with *Cryptococcus neoformans* capsular polysaccharide in serum from a patient with disseminated trichosporon infection. *J Clin Microbiol* 1985;21:681–685.

94 Westerink MA, Amsterdam D, Petell RJ, Stramm MN, Apicella MA. Septicemia due to DF-2. Cause of a false-positive cryptococcal latex agglutination result. *Am J Med* 1987;83:155–158.

95 Baes H, VanCutsen J. Primary cutaneous cryptococcosis. *Dermatologica* 1985;171:357–361.

96 Gonyea EF. Cisternal puncture and cryptococcal meningitis. *Arch Neurol* 1973;28:200–202.

97 Stamm AM, Polt SS. False-negative cryptococcal antigen test. *JAMA* 1980;244:1359.

98 Gray LD, Roberts GD. Experience with the use of pronase to eliminate interference factors in the latex agglutination test for cryptococcal antigen. *J Clin Microbiol* 1988;26:2450–2451.

99 Hamilton JR, Noble A, Denning DW, Stevens DA. Performance of cryptococcus antigen latex agglutination kits on serum and cerebrospinal fluid specimens of AIDS patients before and after pronase treatment. *J Clin Microbiol* 1991;29:333–339.

100 Spickard A, Butler WT, Andriole V. The improved prognosis of cryptococcal meningitis with amphotericin B therapy. *Ann Intern Med* 1963;58:66–83.

101 Dismukes WE, Cloud G, Galis HA, et al. Treatment of cryptococcal meningitis with combination amphotericin B and flucytosine for four as compared with six weeks. *N Engl J Med* 1987;317:334–341.

102 Butler WT, Bennett JE, Alling DW, et al. Nephrotoxicity of amphitericin B. Early and late effects in 81 patients. *Ann Intern Med* 1964;61:175–181.

103 McCurdy DK, Frederic M, Elkinton JR. Renal acidosis due to amphotericin B. *N Engl J Med* 1968;278:124–128.

104 Johanet H, Saliou C, Marmuse JP, Benhamou G, Charleux H. Implantable devices for permanent venous access. A single-center prospective study comparing an AIDS population to a control population. *Ann Chir* 1991;45:497–501.

105 Raviglione MC, Battan R, Pablos-Mendez A, Aceves-Casillas P, Mullen MP, Tarata A. Infections associated with Hickman catheters in patients with acquired immunodeficiency syndrome. *Am J Med* 1989;86:780–786.

106 Bennett JE. Flucytosine. *Ann Intern Med* 1977;86:319–323.

107 Bennett JE, Dismukes WE, Duma RJ, et al. A comparison of amphotericin B alone and combined with flucytosine in the treatment of cryptococcal meningitis. *N Engl J Med* 1979;301:126–131.

108 Stamm AM, Diasio RB, Dismukes WE, et al. Toxicity of amphotericin B plus flucytosine in 194 patients with cryptococcal meningitis. *Am J Med* 1987;83:236–242.

109 Polsky B, Depman MR, Gold JWM, Balicich JH, Armstrong D. Intraventricular therapy of cryptococcal meningitis via a subcutaneous reservoir. *Amer J Med* 1968;24–28.

110 Holtom PD, Leal M, Riley K, Larsen R. Lack of survival benefit and frequent neurologic complications of intrathecal amphotericin B for cryptococcal meningitis. *Int Conf AIDS* (San Francisco). 1990;6:237 (abstract no. Th.B.461).

111 Hoprich R, Bozzette SA. Fluconazole. In: Dollery CT, ed. *Therapeutic Drugs* (suppl). London: Churchill-Livingston, 1992.

112 Grant SM, Clissold SP. Fluconazole—a review of the pharmacokinetic properties and therapeutic potential in superficial and systemic mycoses. *Drugs* 1990;39:877–916.

113 Adndt CAS, Walsh TJ, McCully CL, Balis FM, Pizzo PA, Poplack DG. Fluconazole penetration into cerebrospinal fluid: implications for treating fungal infections of the central nervous system. *J Infect Dis* 1988;157:178–180.

114 Dupont B, Drouhet E. Cryptococcal meningitis and fluconazole. *Ann Intern Med* 1987;106:778.

115 Stern JJ, Hartman BJ, Sharkey P, Rowland V, Squires KE, Murray HW, Graybill JR. Oral fluconazole therapy for patients with acquired immunodeficiency syndrome and cryptococcosis: experience with 22 patients. *Am J Med* 1988;85:477–480.

116 Larsen RA, Leal MA, Chan LS. Fluconazole compared with amphotericin B plus flucytosine for cryptococcal meningitis in AIDS. A randomized trial. *Ann Intern Med* 1990;113:183–187.

117 Berry AJ, Rinaldi MG, Graybill JR. Use of high-dose fluconazole as salvage therapy for cryptococcal meningitis in patients with AIDS. *Antimicrobial Agents and Chemotherapy* 1992;36:690–692.

118 Jones BE, Larsen RA, Bozzette SA, Haghighat D, Leedom JM, McCutchan JA. A phase II trial of fluconazole plus flucytoxine for cryptococcal meningitis. *Int Conf AIDS* (Florence) 1991;7:(abstract WB2337).

119 Perfect JR, Durack DT. Penetration of imidazoles and triazoles into cerebrospinal fluid of rabbits. *J Antimicrob Agents and Chemother* 1985;16:81–86.

120 Perfect JR, Savani DV, Durack DT. Comparison of itraconazole and fluconazole in the treatment of cryptococcal meningitis and candida pyelonephritis in rabbits. *Antimicrob Agents Chemother* 1986;29:579–583.

121 Denning DW, Tucker RM, Hanson LH, Hamilton JR, Stevens DA. Itraconazole therapy for cryptococcal meningitis and cryptococcosis. *Arch Intern Med* 1989;149:2301–2308.

122 de Gans J, Portegies P, Tiessens G, Schattenkerk JKME, van Boxtel CJ, van Ketel RJ, Stam J. Itraconazole compared with amphotericin B plus flucytosine in AIDS patients with cryptococcal meningitis. *AIDS* 1992;6:185–190.

123 De Matos B, Pohle HD, Hahn H, Ruf B. Liposomal amphotericin B: a new formulation in treating disseminated cryptococcosis. *Int Conf AIDS* 1991;7:258 (abstract no. W.B.2305).

124 Lazar JT, Ksionski GE. Efficacy and safety of amBisome (liposomal amphotericin B) in primary episodes of cryptococcosis in patients

with HIV infection. *Int Conf AIDS* 1991;7:226 (abstract no. W.B.2177).

125 Schurmann D, de Matos-Marques B, Grunewald T, Pohle HD, Hahn H, Ruf B. Safety and efficacy of liposomal amphotericin B in treating AIDS-associated disseminated cryptococcosis. *J Infect Dis* 1991;164:620–622.

126 Coker R, Tomlinson D, Harris J. Successful treatment of cryptococcal meningitis with liposomal amphotericin B after failure of treatment with fluconazole and conventional amphotericin B. *AIDS* 1991;5:231–232.

127 Powderly W, Medoff G. Amphotericin B. *Antimicrob Agents Chemo* 1986;29:579–583.

128 Bozzette SA, Larsen RA, Chiu J, et al. Fluconazole treatment of persistent Cryptococcus neoformans infection in AIDS. *Ann Intern Med* 1991;115:285–286.

129 Staib F, Seibold M, L'age M. Persistence of *Cryptococcus neoformans* in seminal fluid and urine under itraconazole treatment. The urogenital tract (prostate) as a niche for *Cryptococcus neoformans*. *Mycoses* 1990;33: 369–373.

130 Zuger A, Schuster M, Simberkoff MS, Rahal JJ, Holzman RS. Maintenance amphotericin B for cryptococcal meningitis in the acquired immunodeficiency syndrome (AIDS). *Ann Intern Med* 1988;109:592–593.

131 Rienes E, Gross PA. Cryptococcal meningitis: seven years of maintenance amphotericin therapy without progressive renal failure. *Am J Med* 1988;85:591–592.

132 Powderly WG, Saag MS, Cloud GA, et al. A controlled trial of fluconazole or amphotericin B to prevent relapse of cryptococcal meningitis in patients with acquired immunodeficiency syndrome. *N Engl J Med* 1992; 326:793–798.

133 De Gans J, Eeftinck-Schattenkerk JKM, van Ketel RJ. Intraconazole as maintenance therapy for cryptococcal meningitis in the acquired immunodeficiency syndrome. *Br Med J* 1988;296(6618):339.

134 Heel RC, Brogden RN, Carmine A, et al. Ketoconazole: a review of its therapeutic efficacy in superficial and systemic fungal infections. *Drugs* 1982;23:1–34.

135 Nightingale SD, Cal SX, Peterson DM, Loss SD, Gamble BA, Watson DA, Manzone CP, Baker JE, Jockusch JD. Primary prophylaxis with fluconazole against systemic fungal infections in HIV-positive patients. *AIDS* 1992;6:191–194.

136 Kronfeld M, Sprinz E, Zimmer P. Ketoconazole as a prophylactic agent against cryptococcal meningitis. *Int Conf AIDS* 1991;7:258 (abstract no. W.B.2307).

Magnetic resonance imaging update on brain abscess and central nervous system aspergillosis

DIETER R. ENZMANN

INTRODUCTION

Brain abscess continues to be an important central nervous system (CNS) infection, all the more so because it represents a curable disease. The discovery of antibiotics improved the outlook for patients with brain abscess, decreasing mortality from a high 70% rate to a range of 30% to 50% (1–4). It is ironic that a diagnostic imaging test, computed tomography (CT), has had as great an impact on the clinical outcome of brain abscess as has antibiotics (5–7). The availability of CT has been associated with a reduction of mortality from 41% to 4% (6,7). Magnetic resonance (MR) imaging carries on in the tradition of CT and currently represents the diagnostic modality of choice in the diagnosis and follow-up of brain abscess.

The reasons that these diagnostic tests have had such a positive impact on the prognosis of brain abscess are that the diagnosis is made earlier and more accurately, and the lesion is definitively localized. The combination of these factors has changed the neurosurgical approach to brain abscess from attempted surgical resection to simple aspiration and/or conservative medical management with antibiotics (6–8). The use of stereotactic CT or MR has further entrenched this simplified aspiration approach (9).

BRAIN ABSCESS STAGING

Brain abscess can be divided into two major stages: (a) the cerebritis stage and (b) the capsule stage. This staging of brain abscess was more important in the era of brain abscess resection since an abscess in the cerebritis stage could not be resected easily without significant damage to adjacent viable neural tissue, whereas, in the capsule stage, it could be more easily "shelled out." Surgical damage to adjacent neural tissue was less in the capsule stage. With the current, more conservative methods of treatment, this staging process is no longer important for neurosurgical planning, although it does yield information with regard to the rate at which an abscess is expected to resolve. Staging of brain abscess using pre- and postcontrast CT has been described in detail before and will not be repeated here (10).

The staging of a brain abscess using MR criteria is less well known and the MR findings, to some extent, can be extrapolated from the CT scan findings. It is important to reiterate that the presence of ring enhancement alone, be it on CT or on MR with gadolinium pentate (GdDTPA), does not differentiate these two stages. As with the CT criteria, delayed MR scans after injection of GdDTPA provide criteria for differentiating these stages. In the cerebritis stage, delayed scans will show thickening of the contrast-enhancing ring and filling in of the abscess center. In the capsule stage, for a period of up to 45 minutes, there is no significant change in the thickness of the contrast-enhancing ring of a cerebral abscess.

Because of the increased resolution of both CT and MR scanners, criteria exist for noncontrast scans. This means that the additional scanning time for delayed scans is not necessary. The key imaging sequence is the T2-weighted (T2W) sequence, which is very sensitive to the presence of abscess. In the cerebritis stage, one may see a large area of high signal, with scalloped borders representing the margins of edema in white matter. Within this large area may be a central, circular region of slightly lower signal intensity, representing the beginning of the necrotic center. No other features are noted within this area of high signal intensity. This is typical of the cerebritis stage.

In the capsule stage, one major, new finding appears, and that is a ring of low signal intensity around the necrotic center. This represents the collagen capsule. The necrotic center will increase in signal equal to that of surrounding edema. The MR appearance in the capsule stage, therefore, is a large area of high signal with scalloped outer borders representing vasogenic edema in white matter, a ring of relatively lower signal intensity near the center of this abnormality representing the capsule, and a high signal intensity center within the low signal ring representing purulent fluid. The low signal intensity represents formation of a collagen capsule which is proton poor and thus lacks MR signal and is depicted, therefore, as low signal intensity. In the capsule stage, the ring of enhancement on a GdDTPA-enhanced T1W image corresponds exactly to the ring of low signal intensity on the T2W sequence. These two features of the MR image are important since they form the basis for interpreting whether or not the abscess is responding favorably or unfavorably to antibiotic treatment.

The MR characteristics of an abscess usually do not allow a specific bacteriologic diagnosis. The appearance of the brain abscess and its progression through its stages depend more on the patient's immune status rather than on the type of offending organism. If the patient is immunocompromised, capsule formation is usually delayed or inhibited, and thus these typical findings may not be seen. For example, in acquired immunodeficiency syndrome (AIDS) patients with toxoplasmosis, the capsule stage of brain abscess is rarely seen (4,11,12). If the patients' immune system is intact, even unusual organisms such as fungi may produce typical encapsulated abscesses (13).

BRAIN ABSCESS TREATMENT AND IMAGING

Besides playing a key role in the diagnosis and localization of brain abscess, imaging tests are now becoming integral to treatment (6,9,14). This has occurred because of the important role of abscess aspiration in its treatment. CT and MR can both be used with a stereotactic frame in order to localize the abscess accurately and determine the best trajectory for its aspiration (14). Using this technique, previously inaccessible abscesses have now become accessible. In fact, virtually all intracranial abscesses can be aspirated, including those lying in deep structures (Figures 15.1,15.2). The aspiration serves two purposes: (a) It provides tissue for identification of the offending microorganism(s) and (b) it decompresses the necrotic center and thereby relieves the mass effect in the brain. A postaspiration scan, CT or MR, normally shows significant reduction in the size of the necrotic center, as evidenced by a decrease in the diameter of ring enhancement or size of the capsule depicted by CT or MR (Figures 15.1,15.2). The aspiration usually introduces a small amount of hemorrhage into the abscess center. This is usually not detected by CT but can be visualized by MR which is exquisitely more sensitive to the presence of blood in CNS tissue. At this point or just prior to the aspiration, an antibiotic regimen is begun; this is modified as culture results become available.

Since abscess size changes are not rapid, it is reasonable to repeat a CT or MR scan approximately a week after aspiration to determine the course of abscess evolution. After a week's interval, the abscess size should be smaller than the preaspiration size. The only reliable determinant for abscess size is the diameter of ring enhancement (CT or MR) or the low signal ring seen on T2W images (Figures 15.1,15.2). A decrease in the amount of surrounding vasogenic edema may be an ancillary sign of improvement.

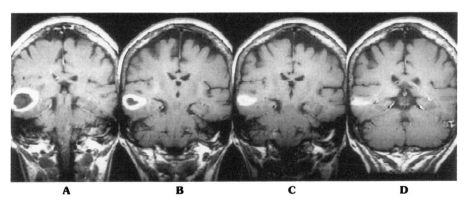

| A | B | C | D |

Figure 15.1 Serial coronal postcontrast (GdDTPA) T1-weighted (T1W) scans of a patient with a streptococcal brain abscess treated by a single aspiration and antibiotic treatment. **(a)** Pretreatment MR scan shows a large, right temporal lobe abscess, with the typical MR appearance of a thin rim of contrast enhancement around a low signal center. This abscess was aspirated once to identify the organism and to reduce its mass effect. **(b)** A scan performed 10 days later shows a marked decrease in the diameter of the ring enhancement. **(c,d)** Two subsequent postcontrast MR scans performed 19 days **(c)** and 35 days **(d)** after aspiration show continued decrease in diameter of the ring enhancement. This is the typical pattern of an abscess responding appropriately to treatment (in this case, after a single aspiration). Near-total resolution took place over a period of approximately one month.

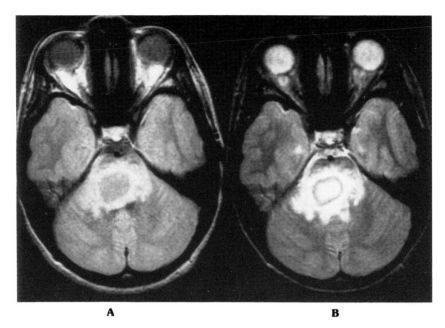

A   B

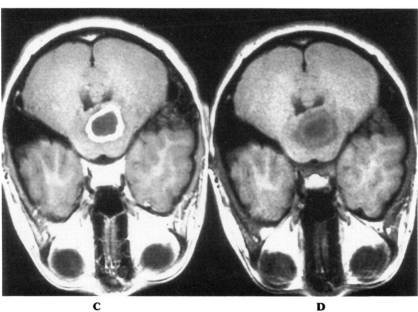

C   D

Figure 15.2 Serial MR and CT scans in a child with a brainstem abscess caused by *Hemophilus aphrophilous.* **(a,b)** First **(a)** and second **(b)** echo of a T2-weighted (T2W) sequence shows a large abscess in the mid-pons. The abscess has a moderate amount of surrounding high signal edema. A capsule has begun to form around the necrotic center, as evidenced by the low signal ring seen on the second echo **(b)**. **(c,d)** The pre- **(c)** and postcontrast (GdDTPA) **(d)** T1W images show the typical abscess findings of well-defined ring enhancement around a low signal center. The ring enhancement corresponds closely to the low signal ring seen on the T2W sequence indicative of capsule formation **(b)**.

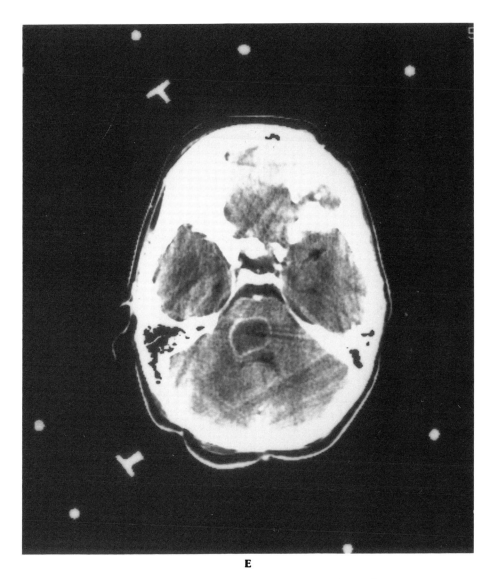

E

Figure 15.2 (continued) **(e)** Postcontrast CT scan performed in a stereotactic frame (note fiducial markers) shows abscess localization. The appearance of the contrast-enhancing abscess on the CT scan is quite similar to the postcontrast MR scan **(d)**.

If the response at this time is favorable, a follow-up CT or MR scan can be obtained 10 to 14 days later to insure that the abscess is continuing to resolve, i.e., the diameter of the capsule continues to decrease. If, at the first week's interval, the abscess diameter is the same or larger than the preaspiration diameter, reaspiration will be necessary

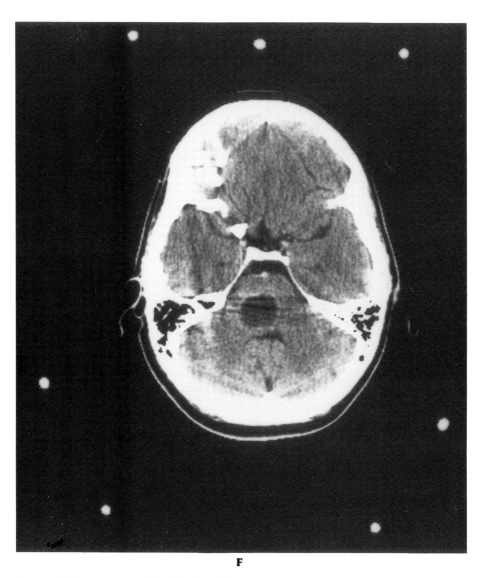

F

Figure 15.2 (continued) **(f)** After the first aspiration, a repeat scan was per-formed 11 days later, showing a similar-size, contrast-enhancing ring in the pons. The abscess being the same size or slightly larger on the imaging test is an indication for reaspiration. Another aspiration was therefore performed.

(Figures 15.2, 15.3). Multiple aspirations may be needed before the diameter of the capsule shows a definite favorable response by progressively decreasing in size. Each aspiration should be performed with the aid of a stereotactic device to insure accuracy in needle placement.

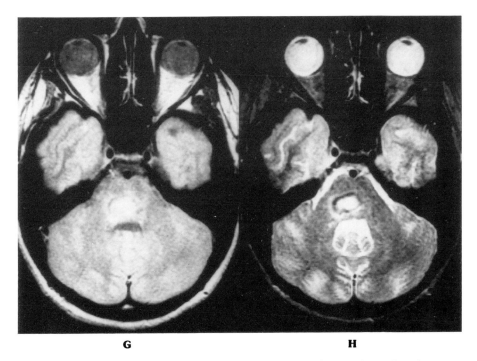

G   H

Figure 15.2 (continued) **(g,h,i)** MR scans performed nine days after the second aspiration show a decrease in size of the abscess on the T2W sequence ((**g**) first echo, **(h)** second echo) and on the postcontrast T1W scan **(i)**.

The process of aspiration causes small hemorrhages within the abscess which will be detectable on the MR scan. The appearance of hemorrhage should be expected and should not be taken as a sign of worsening. As the abscess heals, these hemorrhagic characteristics become more prominent. In fact, the final, residual scar in a totally healed abscess may in large part be residual hemosiderin deposition from hemorrhage in and around an abscess. The healing, as evidenced by decreasing size of the abscess capsule, continues to take place for a period of weeks to months after the cessation of antibiotic treatment. In immunocompetent hosts, complete resolution of the abscess may take on the order of three to four months. In immunosuppressed patients, monitoring of the abscess will require a longer period of time because healing may extend from several months to a year.

The aspiration technique is most applicable for solitary abscesses. In AIDS patients in whom multiple widespread abscesses may be present, this technique is usually not used. In these patients, if the CT or MR findings are suggestive, a presumptive diagnosis of toxoplasmosis is made, and appropriate therapy is instituted. As with the aspiration technique, the imaging tests are important in assessing the response to treatment. Since these abscesses are usually in the cerebritis stage, response can be quite rapid. The response can be gauged by a similar criterion, i.e., decreasing size of

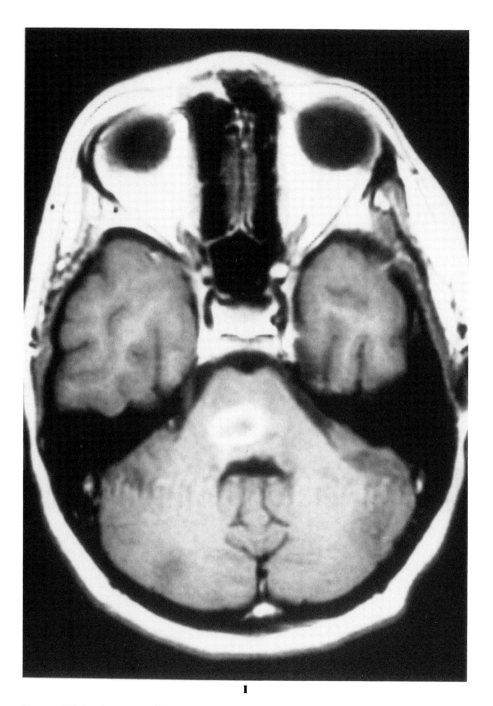

I

Figure 15.2 (continued)

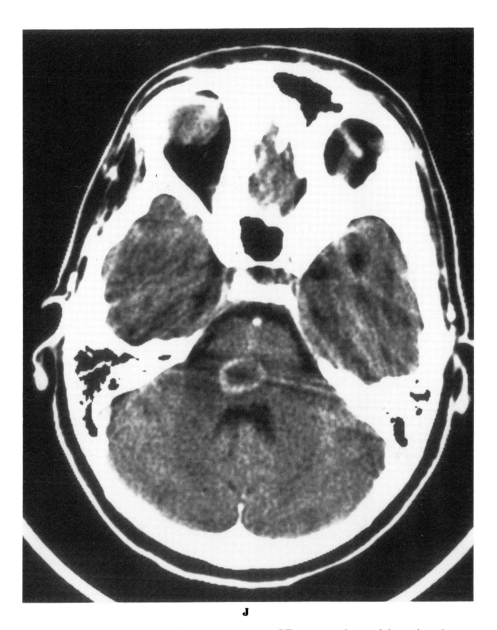

J

Figure 15.2 (continued) **(j)** A postcontrast CT scan performed four days later shows close correlation in abscess size between the CT scan and postcontrast MR scan.

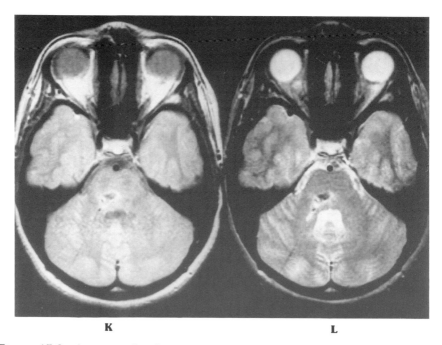

K   L

Figure 15.2 (continued) **(k,l,m,n)** This abscess required no further aspiration and showed continued improvement, as evidenced by an MR scan performed five weeks later. The T2W images (**(k)** first echo, **(l)** second echo) show a significantly smaller lesion, with only a nodular area of low signal intensity, surrounded by a small area of high signal intensity. Note that the needle track is evident on these images as a low signal straight line going through the right cerebellar hemisphere **(k,l)**.

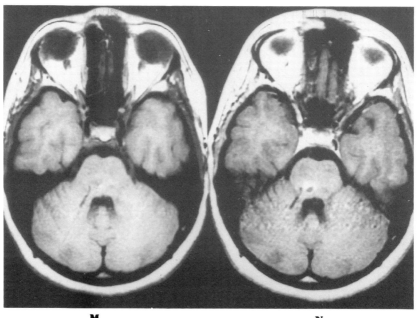

M   N

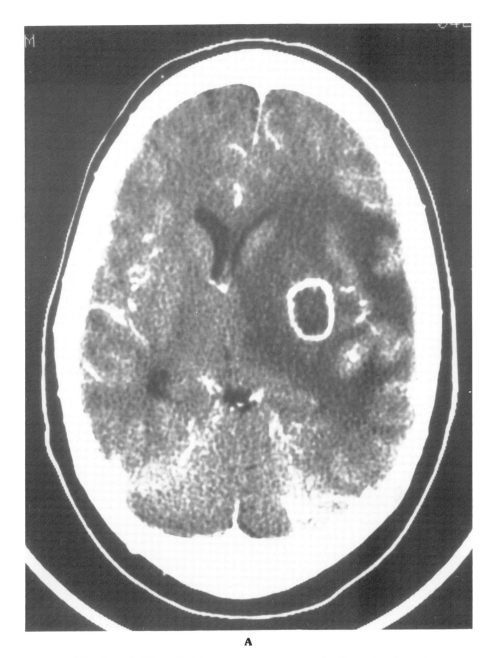

A

Figure 15.3 Serial CT and MR scans in a patient with idiopathic thrombocytopenic purpura with very low platelet counts, which limited the options of aspirat-
ing what turned out to be an *Aspergillus* abscess. **(a)** Postcontrast CT scan showing well-defined ring enhancement in the left basal ganglia region, with marked
amount of surrounding vasogenic edema typical of a brain abscess.

←————————————————————————————————————

Figure 15.2 (continued)   The pre- **(m)** and postcontrast **(n)** T1W images show
near-complete resolution of the abscess, which is now seen as a small area of
ring enhancement **(n).** The biopsy needle track is also visualized in these images
(m,n). This abscess required two aspirations before responding as defined by the
imaging criteria. Overall resolution of this abscess was on the order of 10 weeks.

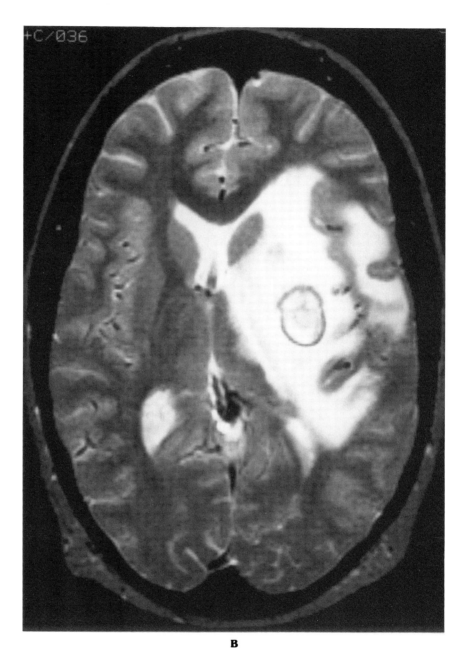

B

Figure 15.3 (continued) **(b,c,d)** The T2W MR scan performed two days later shows a well-defined ring of low signal intensity in the left basal ganglia region, indicative of an encapsulated abscess, with prominent surrounding high signal vasogenic edema.

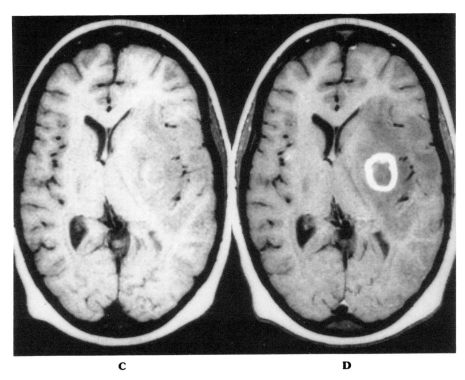

C   D

Figure 15.3 (continued) **(c)** the pre and postcontrast **(d)** T1W MR scans show well-defined ring enhancement comparable to the CT scan **(a)**. The subtle ring of increased signal intensity on the precontrast scan **(b)** turns out to be a clue to the diagnosis since this may represent petechial hemorrhage, which is a finding in CNS aspergillosis.

ring contrast enhancement. Many lesions, however, may not enhance with contrast, and, in such instances, the T2W scan becomes important. The criterion then rests with decreasing size of areas of abnormal high signal intensity on a T2W image. The response can be expected in a few days, and any lesions not responding within five to seven days become suspect for being something other than toxoplasmosis, either a different infection or possibly a tumor. In a *Toxoplasma* infection, the MR scan is the strongly preferred imaging technique, whereas, in the solitary brain abscess, the CT scan can be as effective as the MR scan when contrast enhancement of the capsule is present.

ASPERGILLOSIS

Aspergillus species have been significant causes of CNS fungal infection in immuno-suppressed hosts, with *Aspergillus fumigatus* being the most common species (15,16).

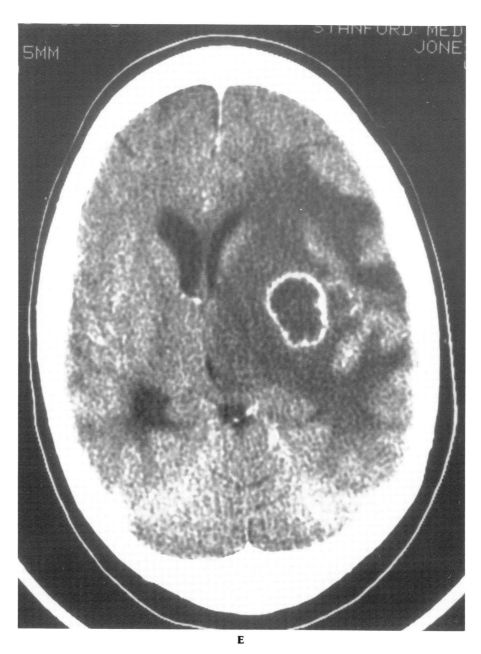

E

Figure 15.3 (continued) **(e)** Despite coverage with multiple antibiotics, the scan two weeks later shows an increase in the diameter of ring enhancement. This indicates a lack of response of the abscess to the treatment regimen.

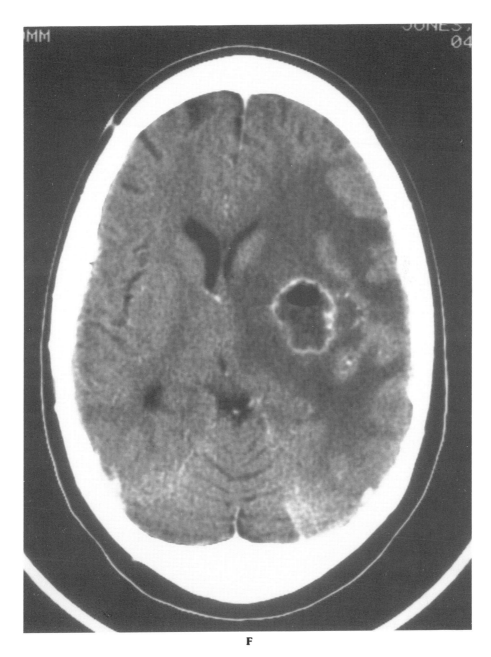

F

Figure 15.3 (continued)   **(f)** With great trepidation and planning, this abscess was aspirated once and *Aspergillus* was isolated. Note that, two weeks after aspiration, although the abscess had a "crenated" appearance, it has not substantially decreased in size.

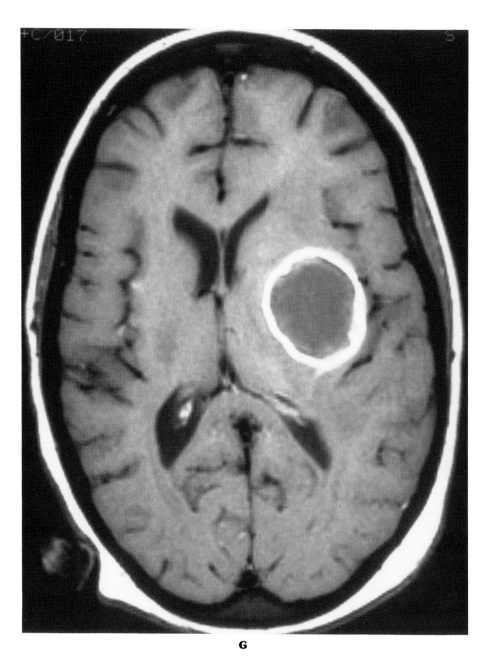

G

Figure 15.3 (continued) **(g)** Postcontrast (GdDTPA) T1W MR scan shows persistent increases in size of this *Aspergillus* abscess despite appropriate antifungal treatment for one month. The patient succumbed due to this abscess.

Aspergillus presented as a major CNS infection problem in early cardiac transplant patients. CNS involvement usually occurred in the clinical setting of a primary pulmonary infection, with secondary spread to the CNS. In the immunosuppressed host, CNS aspergillosis carries a very poor prognosis. With a change in the immuno-suppression regimen in cardiac transplant patients, i.e., primarily the institution of cyclosporin therapy, the incidence of CNS aspergillosis seems to have decreased (17). CNS aspergillosis, however, is making a comeback, but this time in the clinical setting of bone marrow transplant patients.

The CNS manifestation of aspergillosis infection is a function of the immune status of the patient rather than the specific characteristics of the organism itself. *Aspergillus* infections have been reported in seemingly immunocompetent hosts. In such instances, the *Aspergillus* infection may assume the character of a typical solitary brain abscess or granuloma (18). In the setting of the immunocompromised host, CNS aspergillosis usually presents with ill-defined, poorly marginated, rapidly enlarging lesions that seem to have the characteristics of both infarction and edema (Figure 15.4). This presentation has been seen in patients that were unable to mount a significant inflammatory response to this organism (15). These patients in particular had a poor prognosis, which was typical of cardiac transplant patients.

In bone marrow transplant patients, the CNS presentation of aspergillosis seems to have a greater variety of manifestations (Figures 15.5–15.7). Presumably, this reflects differences in the immunologic status of these patients, although the specific factors have not been identified. Aspergillosis can present in these patients just as in previous cardiac transplant patients, with the lesion being relatively diffuse, poorly marginated, and rapidly progressive. Contrast enhancement on either CT or MR may be minimal, reflecting a minimal inflammatory host response (15).

A less aggressive presentation is one where the infection is focal, somewhat better marginated, but still rapidly progressive (Figure 15.5). In these patients, contrast enhancement is evident and suggests the presence of a significant inflammatory response but one still unable to contain the organism. The imaging findings are of a focal infection that progresses rapidly enough so that a well-defined capsule is never fully formed (Figure 15.6). Contrast enhancement is irregular and spreads rapidly, indicating spread of the infection. The major difference between this presentation and the previously described form is the presence of contrast enhancement. Although the immune system is able to mount an inflammatory response, it seems to be insufficient. Treatment with amphotericin B and other antifungal agents appears to be ineffective in these two presentations. The rapid progression of the infection is an important diagnostic feature suggesting aspergillosis. Both of these presentations usually occur in the setting of primary pulmonary aspergillosis. When intraparenchymal hemorrhage can be identified, the diagnosis of aspergillosis is even more likely because of its propensity to invade vessel walls (15).

In bone marrow transplant patients, however, a third, more benign, form of CNS aspergillosis seems possible. In this presentation, multifocal disease is noted, but the individual lesions are circumscribed and exhibit ring contrast enhancement, indicating an appropriate inflammatory response (Figure 15.7). Despite immunosuppression, enough of a host response is mounted to limit the size of the lesions, despite their

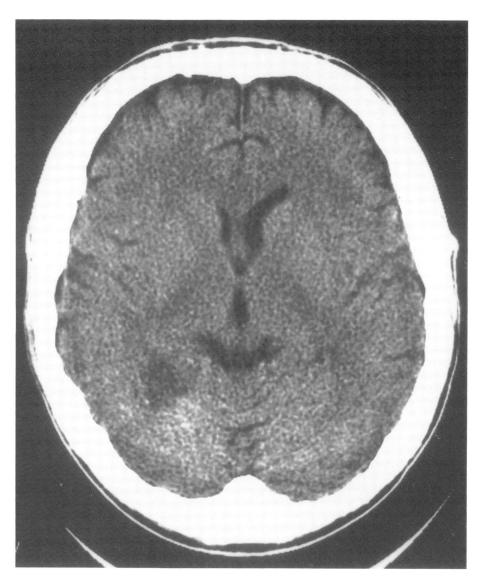

Figure 15.4 Noncontrast CT scan of a bone marrow transplant patient with pulmonary aspergillosis and sudden mental status change. Although no contrast was administered, the ill-defined region of low density in this patient given pulmonary aspergillosis is enough to suggest the diagnosis of CNS involvement by *Aspergillus*. Although the CT findings are nonspecific, in this patient population with the appropriate clinical history of pulmonary aspergillosis, this lesion should suggest CNS aspergillosis.

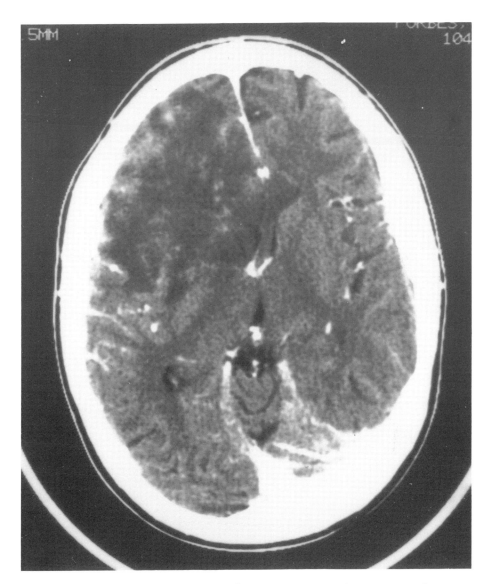

Figure 15.5   Postcontrast CT scan in a bone marrow transplant patient with aspergillosis in the right frontal lobe. In this patient, the presentation was that of a more diffuse process with multiple scattered foci of minimal contrast enhancement, but no well-defined single lesion. There was significant edema and mass effect.

widespread nature. In patients with this presentation, antifungal therapy may reverse the course of the disease and result in regression of the infection. The resolution of CNS infection, however, is markedly prolonged compared with abscesses in immuno-competent hosts. Regression of the infection is similar to that seen in other brain

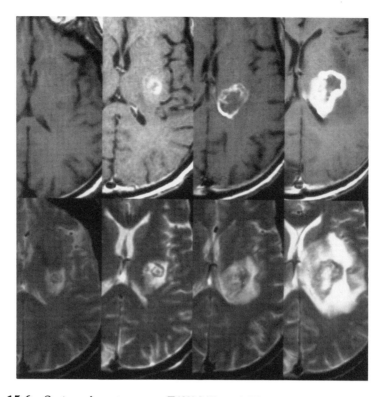

Figure 15.6   Series of postcontrast T1W MR and T2W MR (second echo only) scans of a cardiac transplant patient with aspergillosis. Typical of this brain infection is its rapid progression in immunocompromised hosts. **(a,b)** This first pair of scans shows no significant enhancement on the T1W MR scan **(a)**, but a mixed high and low signal lesion in the left basal ganglia region on the T2W MR scan **(b)**. **(c,d)** Two days later, the lesion has significantly progressed, now showing contrast enhancement **(c)** and an increased size of the ring center and the abnormal high signal edema region on the T2W MR scan **(d)**. **(e,f)** This rapid progression continued, with a marked increase in size of the contrast enhancing region **(e)**, with concomitant increase in lesion size on the T2W MR image **(f)**. This progression occurred over a period of nine days. Note the heterogeneity of the signal within the lesion. **(g,h)** Progression continued, as within seven days marked increase in contrast enhancement has occurred on the postcontrast T1W MR scan **(g)**, and edema greatly increased on the T2W MR scan **(h)**. This rapid progression of lesion size in an immunocompromised patient with known pulmonary aspergillosis is virtually diagnostic of CNS aspergillosis.

Figure 15.7   Bone marrow transplant patient with CNS aspergillosis. **(a,c)** T1W scans with GdDTPA contrast at two different levels in the brain show multiple lesions scattered throughout the cerebral white matter. These lesions have a clear ring-enhancing pattern despite their small size. **(b,d)** T2W scans show nonspecific, small, high signal lesions in the white matter where contrast enhancement is noted. Note that the use of contrast media makes the findings more apparent and provides additional diagnostic features.

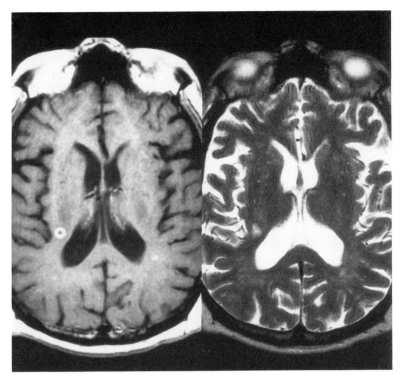

A   B

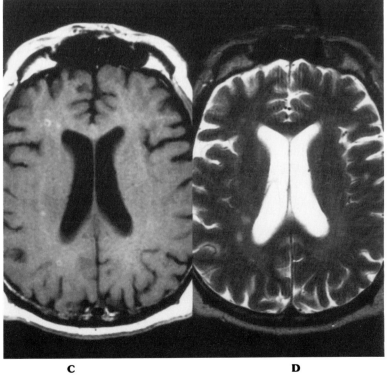

C   D

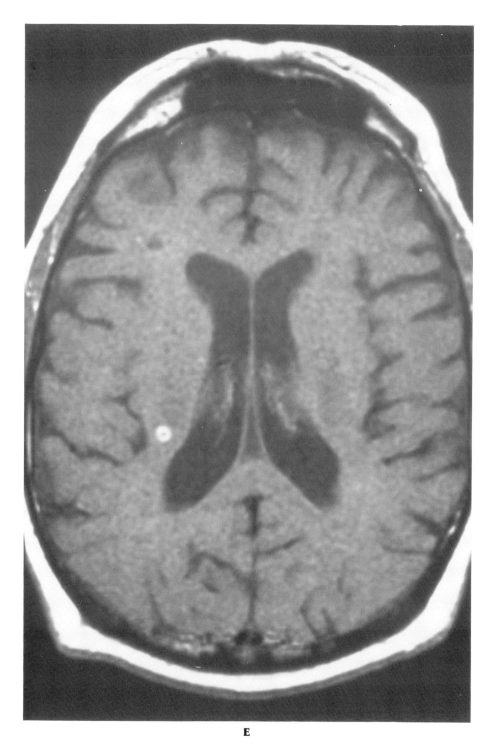

E

Figure 15.7 (continued) **(e,f)** T1W scans with GdDTPA performed one month later, after the institution of amphotericin B. The lesions, although still present, have shown a small, slow, but definite decrease in size, indicating a response to treatment.

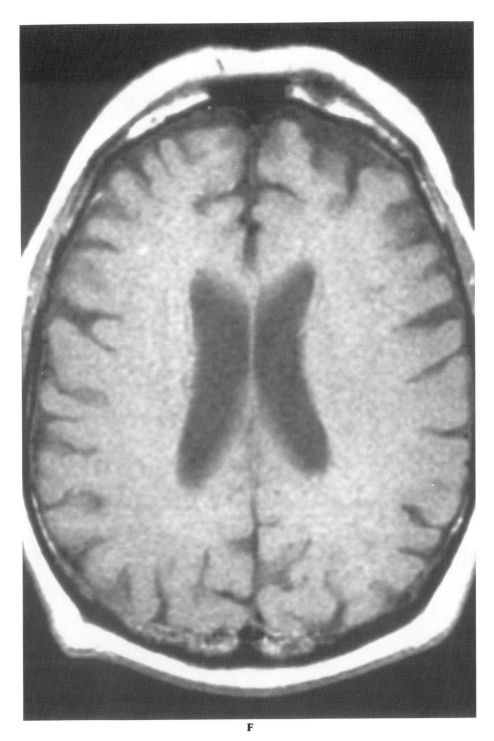

F

Figure 15.7 (continued)

abscesses, i.e., the diameter of ring contrast enhancement decreases over time (Figure 15.7). Imaging tests such as CT or MR with contrast enhancement play an important part in monitoring what turns out to be a relatively chronic CNS infection. While, in the past, CNS aspergillosis has usually heralded the demise of the patient, in the bone marrow transplant population, there appears to be a wide spectrum of responses to this infection, with some patients showing the ability to contain this infection and respond favorably to fungal treatment. The differences in the immunologic status of these bone marrow transplant patients and their different responses to CNS aspergillosis are not well defined and warrant further study.

REFERENCES

1 Ballantine HT, White J. Influence of the antibiotics on therapy and mortality. *New England J of Med* 1953;248(1):14–19.

2 Jooma OV, Pennybacker JB, Tutton GD. Brain abscesses: Aspiration, drainage or excision. *J Neurol Neurosurg Psychiatry* 1951;14:308–313.

3 Morgan H, Wood MW, Murphy F. Experience with 88 consecutive cases of brain abscess. *J Neurosurg* 1951;38:698–704.

4 Levy RM, Pons VG, Rosenblum ML. Central nervous system mass lesions in the acquired immunodeficiency syndrome (AIDS). *J Neurosurg* 1984;61:9–16.

5 Mampalam TJ, Rosenblum ML. Trends in the management of bacterial brain abscesses: A review of 102 cases over 17 years. *Neurosurg* 1988;23(4):451–458.

6 Rosenblum ML, Hoff JT, Norman D, Weinstein PR, Pitts L. Decreased mortality from brain abscesses since advent of computerized tomography. *J Neurosurg* 1978;49:658–668.

7 Ferriero DM, Derechin M, Berg BO. Outcome of brain-abscess treatment in children— reduced morbidity with neuroimaging. *Neurology* Apr 1986;36(4):149.

8 Le Beau J, Creissard P, Harispe L, Redondo A. Surgical treatment of brain abscesses and subdural empyema. *J Neurosurg* 1973;38:198–203.

9 Nauta HJW, Contreras FL, Weiner RL, Crofford MJ. Brain stem abscess managed with computed tomography-guided stereotactic aspiration. *Neurosurg* 1987;20(3):476–480.

10 Enzmann DR, Britt RH, Placone R. Staging of human brain abscess by computed tomography. *Radiology* 1983;146:703–708.

11 Handler M, Ho V, Whelan M, Budzilovich G. Intracerebral toxoplasmosis in patients with acquired immune deficiency syndrome. *J Neurosurg* 1983;59:994–1001.

12 Zee CS, Segall HD, Rogers C, Ahmadi J, Apuzzo M, Rhodes R. MR imaging of cerebral toxoplasmosis: Correlation of computed tomography and pathology. *J Comp Assist Tomo* 1985;9(4):797–799.

13 Steinberg GK, Britt RH, Enzmann DR, Finlay JL, Arvin AM. Fusairum brain abscess: Case report. *J Neurosurg* 1983;56:598–601.

14 Levy RM, Breit R, Russell E, Dal Canto MC. MRI-guided stereotaxic brain biopsy in neurologically symptomatic AIDS patients. *J Acquired Immune Deficiency Syndromes* 1991;4(3):254–260.

15 Enzmann DR, Brant-Zawadski M, Britt RH. CT of central nervous system infections in immunocompromised patients. *Amer J of Neurorad* May/June, 1980;1:239–243.

16 Grossman RI, Davis KR, Taveras JM, Flint Beal M, O'Carroll CP. Computed tomography of intracranial aspergillosis. *J Comp Assist Tomo* 1981;5(5):646–650.

17 Stinson EB, Oyer PE. Infectious complications in thoracic transplantation. In: Shumway SJ, Shumway NE, eds. *Thoracic Transplantation.* Boston: Blackwell Scientific Publications, in press.

18 Mukoyama M, Gimple K, Poser CM. Aspergillosis of the central nervous system. *Neurol* 1969;19:967–974.

Prophylaxis and treatment of infection in the bone marrow transplant recipient

DREW J. WINSTON

INTRODUCTION

The growth of bone marrow transplantation has been very rapid over the last 10 years. Whereas, prior to 1980, bone marrow transplantation was considered primarily a research tool for a limited number of diseases, the use of and indications for bone marrow transplantation have greatly expanded since 1980 (1,2). There are now more than 400 institutions worldwide performing transplants (2). Over 5,000 patients per year receive allogeneic marrow transplants from related or unrelated donors, while an even greater number of patients undergo autologous transplantation (2–4). Allotransplantation is now considered superior to alternative therapies for conditions such as the Wiskott-Aldrich syndrome, severe combined immunodeficiency disease, severe aplastic anemia, and chronic myelogenous leukemia. In addition, allotransplants are effective and widely used in the treatment of acute leukemias and lymphomas, although their value relative to other approaches is less clear (2). Similarly, autotransplants for solid tumors, lymphomas, and leukemias are commonly performed, with different degrees of success (3,4).

Accompanying this rapid progress of bone marrow transplantation has been a greater appreciation of the infectious complications that occur after transplantation. Many of the risk factors and common infections associated with bone marrow transplantation are now well defined as a result of clinical and laboratory studies performed over the last two decades (5,6). Effective strategies to prevent or treat these infections are now available. The purpose of this review is to provide an update of new approaches to the management of infections in bone marrow transplants and to emphasize recent developments and current controversies.

RISK FACTORS FOR INFECTION

The incidence and severity of infections observed in bone marrow transplants are determined by several factors related to the procedure itself. These include the type of transplant (allogeneic, syngeneic, or autologous), the degree of histocompatibility between the donor and recipient, the use of radiation as part of the pretransplant conditioning therapy, the types of immunosuppressive regimens given to prevent or treat graft-versus-host disease (GVHD), the presence and severity of GVHD, and graft failure (5,6). These risk factors also influence the timing of infections after transplantation. There are three time frames during which most posttransplant infections occur: (a) the first month after transplant, prior to marrow engraftment; (b) the second through third month after transplant, when engraftment has occurred; and (c) the late posttransplant period, three months or later after transplant.

During the first month after transplant, prior to marrow engraftment, granulocytopenia and damaged mucosal surfaces, as a consequence of pretransplant chemotherapy and radiation, are the predominant defects in host defenses. Similar to other granulocytopenic patients, patients are most susceptible to gram-negative and gram-positive aerobic bacterial infections and fungal infections. Reactivated herpes simplex viral infections of the oral cavity or genital area in patients seropositive for herpes simplex viral antibody are also common and occur in 70% to 80% of seropositive patients (7,8).

The bacterial infections during granulocytopenia are usually bacteremias or soft tissue infections. Bacterial pneumonias are uncommon (9). Most bone marrow transplant centers, including University of California at Los Angeles (UCLA), have witnessed an increasing incidence of gram-positive bacterial infections. As shown in Table 16.1, gram-positive bacteremias (especially staphylococci and streptococci) only accounted for approximately 25% of all documented bacteremias in granulocytopenic patients at UCLA in the late 1970s. Ten years later, in the late 1980s, these same gram-positive organisms accounted for about 60% of all bacteremias. In contrast, gram-negative bacteremias, especially cases due to *Pseudomonas aeruginosa*, decreased. The increased use of oral fluoroquinolones for prophylaxis and the liberal administration of intravenous antibiotics active against gram-negative organisms for empiric therapy have contributed to an even further decline in gram-negative infections (10,11). The high incidence of staphylococcal infections is partly related to the widespread utilization of indwelling central intravenous catheters (12), while the incidence of bacteremias due to viridans group streptococcus has risen with the use of the fluoroquinolones for gastrointestinal decontamination (13). Fortunately, the mortality from these gram-positive infections has been low (<5%), although septic shock and adult respiratory distress syndrome (ARDS) are potential complications of alpha streptococcal bacteremia (14). In one marrow transplant center, 123 of 832 patients (15%) developed viridans group streptococcal bacteremia sepsis. Ten patients experienced shock (1.2%), and six patients died (0.7%) (14).

Candida species, predominantly *Candida albicans* and *Candida tropicalis*, and *Aspergillus* species are the most common fungal pathogens in granulocytopenic marrow transplant patients (15–17). Occasionally, infections caused by *Trichosporon, Fusarium, Rhizopus*, or *Pityrosporum* are seen (18–20). Increased duration of granulocytopenia (especially in patients with graft failure), the presence of *Candida* in multiple surveillance cultures, and the use of total-body irradiation as part of the pretransplant conditioning regimen are risk factors for systemic *Candida* infection (15,16). *Aspergillus* infections are also associated with prolonged granulocytopenia, as well as local epidemiologic

Table 16.1 Bacteremic isolates during UCLA antibiotic trials in granulocytopenic patients

	Antibiotic Regimens					
	Amikacin carbenicillin vs. gentamicin/ carbenicillin	*Netilmicin/ carbenicillin vs. amikacin carbenicillin*	*Piperacillin/ amikacin vs. carbenicillin/ amikacin*	*Moxalactam/ piperacillin vs. moxalactam/ amikacin*	*Cefoperazone/ piperacillin vs. moxalactam/ piperacillin*	*Ceftazidime/ piperacillin vs. cefoperazone/ piperacillin vs. imipenem alone*
No. of Patients	295	193	272	297	187	403
Year	1977	1979	1982	1984	1986	1989
Organisms						
Gram-positive	14(25%)	15(27%)	32(47%)	24(44%)	29(52%)	69(61%)
Coagulase-negative staphylococci	1	0	7	3	10	21
Staphylococcus aureus	4	10	10	8	7	16
Streptococci	5	5	12	7	10	25
Other	4	0	3	6	2	7
Gram-negative	43(75%)	41(73%)	36(53%)	31(56%)	27(48%)	44(39%)
Pseudomonas aeruginosa	11	13	6	8	7	6
Escherichia coli	11	10	12	15	9	10
Klebsiella-Enterobacter-Serratia	15	15	6	5	5	13
Other	6	3	12	3	6	15
Total	57	56	68	55	56	113

factors such as heavy contamination of the hospital air during construction and inadequate filtration of outside air by the hospital air-treatment system (17,21,22).

During the second time frame for infection, the second through third month after transplant, when engraftment has occurred, patients continue to have profound impairment of both cellular and humoral immunity (23–25). Cellular immune deficiency is evident by cutaneous anergy to recall antigens and neoantigens, lower-than-normal numbers of T helper lymphocytes, and higher-than-normal numbers of T cytotoxic suppressor lymphocytes. Alveolar macrophage and neutrophil function may also be defective (26,27). Humoral deficiency is manifested by low numbers of lymphocytes bearing surface receptors for immunoglobulin and subnormal antibody responses to antigenic challenges, such as pneumococcal polysaccharides (28,29). Generally, these abnormalities are more severe and persist longer in patients with acute GVHD, which is the major risk factor for infection between day 30 and day 100 after transplant. Thus, autotransplants and syngeneic transplants not at risk for GVHD experience significantly fewer and less severe infections after engraftment than do allotransplants. Cytomegalovirus (CMV) interstitial pneumonia is the most severe infectious syndrome associated with GVHD (30–32). With more effective prevention of GVHD and CMV infection, the incidence of CMV pneumonia appears to be decreasing at many transplant centers. As shown in Figure 16.1, the overall incidence of interstitial pneumonia at UCLA was 32% before 1984 but only 12% from 1984 to 1989. The decline in pneumonia was due more to a decrease in CMV pneumonia (which now occurs in less than 5% of all patients) than to a change in the incidence of idiopathic interstitial pneumonia (which has been attributed to pulmonary toxicity of chemotherapy and radiation). Fever, wasting, pancytopenia, gastroenteritis, and hepatitis are other manifestations of CMV infection. CMV retinitis, however, is rarely seen (31,32). Cytotoxic T-cell and NK-cell activity against CMV-infected target cells is lower in marrow transplants who experience CMV infection (33), and the development of CMV-specific T-cell cytotoxicity may protect against development of symptomatic CMV disease (34).

Pulmonary aspergillosis is the other major infectious complication associated with acute GVHD, especially when higher doses of additional immunosuppressive therapy are given for treatment (16,17). Gram-positive infections related to indwelling intravenous catheters, gram-negative infections in patients with GVHD of the gastrointestinal tract, pulmonary infections due to adenovirus, respiratory syncytial virus, parainfluenza virus, influenza virus, or human herpes virus 6 (35–39), hemorrhagic cystitis due to BK virus or adenovirus (40,41), and enteric infections due to rotavirus or coxsackie virus (42, 43) are other significant, but usually less severe, infections in the early postengraftment period. Interstitial pneumonia due to *Pneumocystis carinii* is now rarely seen in marrow transplants since the routine use of prophylactic trimethoprim-sulfamethoxazole (44). Similarly, Epstein-Barr (EB)-virus-related clinical syndromes such as lymphoproliferative disease rarely occur, except in occasional patients who have received monoclonal anti-T-cell antibodies for severe GVHD (8,45,46). Reactivation of toxoplasmosis has been reported in some European marrow transplant centers (47) but is seen infrequently in the United States (48).

The third time frame for infection is after the third posttransplant month and is characterized by gradual recovery of both humoral and cellular immunity over many

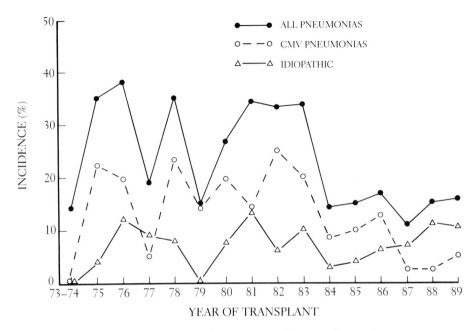

Figure 16.1   Incidence of interstitial pneumonia, by year of transplantation, among recipients of allogeneic marrow transplants at UCLA between 1973 and 1989.

months. This recovery, however, is seriously delayed by chronic GVHD which causes persistent and profound defects in both cellular and humoral immune responses (23–25,28). Fortunately, expect for varicella-zoster infections, autotransplants, syngeneic recipients, and allotransplants without GVHD experience relatively few late infections. In one review of late infections in 98 long-term survivors after bone marrow transplant (49), most allogeneic transplants without chronic GVHD or syngeneic transplants had either no or only one or two late infections. Fifty percent of the allogeneic patients with chronic GVHD had three or more late infections, for a total of 244 infections.

The single most frequent late infection is varicella-zoster infection, which occurs in 25% to 40% of allogeneic transplants and in as many as 28% of all autologous transplants (49–51). Most other late infections involve the respiratory tract (pneumonia, bronchitis, sinusitis) and are usually caused by encapsulated bacteria (*Streptococcus pneumoniae, Hemophilus influenzae*) or common respiratory viruses (49,52,53). Decreased secretory IgG production (54), impaired splenic function (55), inadequate opsonizing antibody (28,29), and the bronchopulmonary sicca syndrome characteristic of chronic GVHD (56) contribute to these frequent respiratory tract infections. The destructive effects of chronic GVHD on mucocutaneous surfaces also provide a route for infection by staphylococci and other skin bacteria. Late-onset interstitial pneumonia due to CMV or *Pneumocystis carinii* is uncommon but still must be an ongoing concern in patients with active GVHD. Most cases of late-onset interstitial pneumonia, however, are either idiopathic or caused by other organisms (30,57,58).

PREVENTION OF INFECTIONS DURING GRANULOCYTOPENIA

Various approaches have been used for prophylaxis of infection in marrow transplants during the period of granulocytopenia before marrow engraftment. The most elaborate approach is to isolate patients in laminar-air-flow rooms and administer concomitant sterile food and oral antimicrobial agents for gastrointestinal decontamination. Several studies have demonstrated the efficacy of laminar-air-flow isolation for prevention of infections and GVHD (59,60). Nonetheless, it does not improve survival, is not cost-effective, and is not recommended except in institutions where there is a persistent problem with endemic *Aspergillus* infections. Moreover, the benefits of laminar-air-flow units may well come from the simultaneously administered oral antimicrobial regimens that suppress the gastrointestinal flora. In most hospitals having adequate filtration of outside air, both allogeneic as well as autologous transplants can be performed safely in a standard single room without strict protective isolation (61).

Oral chemoprophylaxis in granulocytopenic patients has been greatly improved by the use of the new fluoroquinolones. In contrast to the oral nonabsorbable antibiotics which have frequent gastrointestinal side effects and trimethoprim-sulfamethoxazole which may cause myelosuppression and lacks antipseudomonal coverage, the fluoroquinolones are well-tolerated and very effective in the prevention of infections caused by *Pseudomonas aeruginosa*, β-lactam-resistant *Enterobacter* species, and other gram-negative bacilli (10). As shown in Table 16.2, the routine use of either prophylactic norfloxacin or ciprofloxacin in patients at three large oncology centers over one and a half to four years was associated with very infrequent colonization or infection by gram-negative bacillary organisms (62,63). An increase in quinolone-resistant, gram-negative bacilli was not encountered. On the other hand, gram-positive infections caused by coagulase-negative staphylococci and viridans group streptococci resistant to the quinolones were still common, but none were fatal. Nevertheless, since some transplant centers have occasionally witnessed rapidly fatal cases of viridans group streptococcal bacteremia complicated by shock and adult respiratory distress syndrome (ARDS), prophylactic intravenous vancomycin (500 mg every 12 hours) is sometimes given concomitantly with an oral fluoroquinolone (14,62,64).

Until recently, there had been no well-controlled, randomized trials in a large number of bone marrow transplant patients clearly establishing the efficacy of any oral antifungal agent for prophylaxis of serious fungal infections during periods of granulocytopenia. Prophylaxis with oral nystatin, clotrimazole, ketoconazole, and amphotericin B have all failed to produce consistently favorable results (65). Fluconazole, a new triazole antifungal agent active against many common fungal pathogens, was recently licensed. Results of a placebo-controlled, double-blind, multicenter trial of fluconazole prophylaxis (400 mg daily given orally or intravenously) in patients undergoing either allogeneic or autologous bone marrow transplantation are summarized in Table 16.3 (66). Both systemic and superficial fungal infections were significantly reduced by fluconazole. Fluconazole prevented infections by all *Candida* species except for *Candida krusei*, which is known to be resistant to fluconazole. Deaths from systemic fungal infection were also reduced by fluconazole (one fungal death in 179 fluconazole patients versus 10 fungal deaths in 177 placebo patients, $p < 0.001$) (66). The fluconazole was well

Table 16.2 Effects of routine oral fluoroquinolone prophylaxis on colonization and infection during chemotherapy-related granulocytopenia

Center	Fluoroquinolone	Duration of prophylaxis	Gram-negative colonization	Infection	Gram-negative fluoroquinolone resistance
Johns Hopkins (Karp, 62)	Norfloxacin (400 mg q. 12 h) + IV Vancomycin (500 mg q. 12 h)	15 months in 111 patients	Occasional non-*aeruginosa* pseudomonads (*Pseudomonas cepacia*, *Xanthomonas maltophilia*, *P. putida*)	Only 4 gram-negative infections (*P. aeruginosa*, *K. oxytoca*, *K. pneumoniae*, *Achromobacter*)	None
Utrecht (Dekker, 63)	Ciprofloxacin (500 mg q. 12 h)	4 years in 194 patients	Occasional non-*aeruginosa* pseudomonads	Only 1 gram-negative infection (*X. maltophilia*); 27 gram-positive bacteremias (*Staphylococcus epidermidis*, *Streptococcus viridans*) but none fatal	None
UCLA (Winston)	Norfloxacin (400 mg q. 12 h)	15 months in 205 patients	Rare non-*aeruginosa* pseudomonads	Only 3 gram-negative bacteremias (*X. maltophilia*, *Escherichia coli*, *Enterobacter*); 31 gram-positive bacteremias (*S. epidermidis*, *S. viridans*), but none fatal	None

Table 16.3 Fluconazole prophylaxis of proven fungal infections in bone marrow transplants

	Placebo	*Fluconazole*	*P* value*
No. of patients	177	179	
Systemic fungal infections	28(16%)[†]	5(3%)	<0.0001
Candida albicans	12	0	
Candida tropicalis	6	0	
Candida lusitaniae	2	0	
Candida parapsilosis	2	0	
Candida krusei	2	3	
Candida species	1	0	
Torulopsis glabrata	2	0	
Aspergillus species	2	1	
Mucorales	1	1	
Superficial fungal infections	59(33%)	15(8%)	<0.0001

*P value determined by Cochran-Mantel Haenzel test.
[†]One placebo patient had fungemia with both *C. albicans* and *C. tropicalis*, and another placebo patient had both disseminated aspergillosis and *C. parapsilosis* fungemia.
SOURCE Modified from Reference 66.

tolerated and not associated with any significant toxicity. One of the concerns about the prophylactic use of fluconazole, however, is an increase in the emergence of fungal pathogens persistent to fluconazole. An increase in *Candida krusei* colonization and infection was associated with prophylactic fluconazole at one marrow transplant center (67) but not in the multicenter trial (66). Surprisingly, only three systemic *Aspergillus* infections occurred in the 356 patients in the multicenter trial (Table 16.3). While fluconazole has been shown in animal studies to be active against *Aspergillus* at high doses (68), there is no clinical data from either the multicenter trial or any other study demonstrating its efficacy for prevention or treatment of *Aspergillus* infections. On the other hand, low-dose intravenous amphotericin B (0.25 mg/kg per day) has been employed as prophylaxis against invasive *Aspergillus* infection in allogeneic marrow transplants (69). It should be considered for the patient with a history of well-documented invasive aspergillosis prior to transplant and who is at risk for reactivation of disease.

Another approach for the reduction of early infections after marrow transplant is to accelerate recovery of the granulocyte count. In contrast to the demise of granulocyte transfusions due to untoward side effects and lack of clinically meaningful benefits (70,71), the recombinant hematopoietic growth factors (granulocyte-macrophage colony stimulating factor (GM-CSF) and granulocyte colony stimulating factor (G-CSF)) offer significant promise for shortening the duration of granulocytopenia and risk of infection (72). GM-CSF is currently approved for acceleration of myeloid recovery in patients undergoing autologous bone marrow transplantation for lymphoma or acute lymphocytic leukemia, while G-CSF is approved for use after chemotherapy in patients with nonmyeloid malignancies. The results of randomized, controlled trials of GM-CSF in autologous or allogeneic marrow transplants are summarized in Table 16.4

Table 16.4 Randomized, controlled trials of GM-CSF in autologous or allogeneic bone marrow transplants

Reference	Treatment	No. of Patients	Days to ANC* >500	Days to ANC >1000	Days in hospital	Days of fever	Days on antibiotics	Infections Bacteremia	Other	Total
Autotransplants										
Nemunaitis	Placebo vs. GM-CSF	63	26	33	33	8	27	6	13	19
(73)		65	19	26	27	8	24	9	2	11
Gulati	Placebo vs. GM-CSF	12		27	40			1	6	7
(74)		12		16	32			2	6	8
Advani	Placebo vs. GM-CSF	33	16	24	27			6	0	6
(75)		36	12	15	27			1	0	1
Gorin	Placebo vs. GM-CSF	47	21	30	28	2	22			22
(76)		41	14	17	23	4	19			16
Link	Placebo vs. GM-CSF	40	28		31		19			28
(77)		39	15		30		19			15
Allotransplants										
Powles	Placebo vs. GM-CSF	20	16		24		13			
(78)		20	13		24		16			

*ANC = Absolute Neutrophil Count

(73–78). The only consistent benefit of GM-CSF in all six trials was a shortening of the duration of granulocytopenia. Three trials found a reduction in the length of hospitalization, two demonstrated less antibiotic usage with GM-CSF, and three reported fewer infections in patients receiving GM-CSF. GM-CSF had no significant effect on the number of days of fever, and, in one trial, patients given GM-CSF actually experienced more fevers and received more antibiotics than the placebo patients (78). Thus, apart from shortening the length of granulocytopenia, the overall impact of GM-CSF on preventing infectious morbidity and mortality is not entirely clear. More selective use of GM-CSF or G-CSF in patients with graft failure or in patients with persistent granulocytopenia and life-threatening infection may be more beneficial and economical than routine use in all patients (79,80). Concerns about the long-term effects of these growth factors on GVHD and leukemia relapse also need to be addressed in additional controlled studies (78,81).

Acyclovir given intravenously (5 mg/kg every eight hours) or orally (400 mg five times daily) is highly effective prophylaxis against reactivation of herpes simplex virus infection during the early posttransplant period (82,83). The approximate cost to a patient for 28 days of acyclovir prophylaxis at UCLA is $10,000 for intravenous drug and $1,200 for oral drug. This high cost must be weighed against the fact that almost all herpes simplex infections in marrow transplants are localized infections that are easily treatable and rarely fatal. Thus, we do not recommend the use of acyclovir for prevention of herpes simplex viral infection unless a patient has a well-documented history of recurrent and severe infection during previous chemotherapy. Development of resistance or selection of naturally resistant strains of herpes simplex virus have also been concerns about the use of prophylactic acyclovir, although acyclovir resistance has been reported more frequently in patients given acyclovir for treatment of established infection than in patients on prophylaxis (84,85,86).

TREATMENT OF INFECTIONS DURING GRANULOCYTOPENIA

Successful treatment of the febrile granulocytopenic patient with suspected or documented infection requires prompt initiation of appropriate parenteral antimicrobial therapy. Previously, this therapy most often consisted of an aminoglycoside plus an antipseudomonal β-lactam drug (87,88). Several developments, however, have led to the utilization of alternative regimens in bone marrow transplant patients. Due to the use of other nephrotoxic drugs in marrow transplants (cyclosporine, amphotericin B), there is a frequent desire to avoid aminoglycosides. The incidence of *Pseudomonas aeruginosa* and other gram-negative infections has declined at many transplant centers, especially with the use of prophylactic oral fluoroquinolones (Table 16.2). On the other hand, the proportion of infections caused by gram-positive organisms has greatly increased (Table 16.1). The availability of new β-lactam drugs with broader and more potent antibacterial activity has also made it possible to design new approaches to empiric therapy.

Alternative empiric antimicrobial regimens now being used in febrile granulocytopenic patients include a double β-lactam combination (a third-generation cephalosporin such as ceftazidime or cefoperazone plus a ureidopenicillin such as piperacillin or mezlocillin), monotherapy with a third-generation cephalosporin (ceftazidime, cefoperazone) or imipenem, and vancomycin plus a third-generation cephalosporin (88). In choosing a particular regimen, the patient's own endogenous microflora, as well as the susceptibility pattern of organisms within the transplant center, must be considered. The cost of antibiotics and their administration may also be a factor. At UCLA, a double β-lactam combination (cefoperazone plus piperacillin or ceftazidime plus piperacillin) had been the regimen most frequently used in febrile, granulocytopenic marrow transplants, since several clinical studies had shown that these double β-lactam combinations are as effective as combinations of a β-lactam plus an aminoglycoside without the nephrotoxicity or ototoxicity associated with the aminoglycosides (89–91). However, we recently found, in a comparative, randomized trial, that imipenem alone (500 mg intravenously every six hours) was as effective as cefoperazone plus piperacillin or ceftazidime plus piperacillin and that the cost of imipenem therapy was approximately $2000 less per treatment course than combination therapy (92). Thus, we have switched to monotherapy with imipenem. Similar results have been achieved with ceftazidime monotherapy (93,94), although, in two studies, imipenem was more effective as monotherapy than ceftazidime (95,96). There has been concern over the emergence of resistant strains of *Pseudomonas aeruginosa* or *Enterobacter* species in patients receiving these β-lactam monotherapies (97,98), but the concomitant use of an oral fluoroquinolone to decontaminate the gastrointestinal tract may minimize this risk.

One of the more controversial issues in the management of febrile granulocytopenic patients is the use of intravenous vancomycin. Some investigators advocate vancomycin as part of the initial antimicrobial regimen in all patients in order to provide better coverage for the increasing number of gram-positive infections (99,100). Other investigators found the empiric use of vancomycin unnecessary and expensive (101). They recommend vancomycin only when clinical or microbiological data suggest a need (such as infection of a central intravenous catheter). It is argued that most gram-positive infections are indolent and allow the later modification of therapy, if necessary, without increased morbidity or mortality. Indeed, in our recent trial of β-lactam therapy in febrile granulocytopenic patients at UCLA (92), only two of 69 gram-positive infections (3%) initially treated with a double β-lactam combination or imipenem alone were fatal. Furthermore, there were only two fatal gram-positive superinfections during β-lactam therapy. Thus, we believe that routine inclusion of vancomycin in the initial empiric antibiotic regimen for febrile granulocytopenic patients is not always necessary. On the other hand, in transplant centers with frequent overwhelming infection caused by viridans group streptococcus uniformly susceptible to vancomycin, there may be a greater role for empiric usage of vancomycin (14,64).

Amphotericin B remains the "gold standard" for treatment of documented or suspected systemic fungal infection in the granulocytopenic patient and other immunocompromised patients. The most common situation in marrow transplants requiring amphotericin B is a patient who exhibits persistent or recurrent fever while receiving antibiotics and has no identifiable source of infection. Two common issues related to this empiric use of amphotericin B are the time at which therapy should be initiated and the duration of therapy. In randomized trials of empiric amphotericin B in granulocytopenic patients, the amphotericin B (0.5 to 0.6 mg/kg per day) was started after four to six days of antibacterial therapy and then continued until there was resolution of granulocytopenia (granulocyte count > 1,000/mm^3) (102,103). The amphotericin B was discontinued after recovery of the granulocyte count unless an invasive fungal infection had been documented. This is the approach that we follow at UCLA, although it is less than ideal. Amphotericin B itself is toxic and also enhances the risk of nephrotoxicity in patients on cyclosporine (104). Patients who develop renal failure on amphotericin B and cyclosporine frequently require reduction in their cyclosporine dose which may compromise its effects on GVHD. A new formulation of amphotericin (liposomal amphotericin B) appears less nephrotoxic and may improve the safety of empiric amphotericin B (105). Fluconazole is also currently being compared with empiric amphotericin B in randomized controlled trials, but its use for empiric therapy needs to be tempered by its lack of significant activity for *Aspergillus* which could be problematic in a patient with persistent fevers and undefined pulmonary infiltrates. Ketoconazole is less effective than amphotericin B for empiric therapy (106).

For documented *Candida* or *Aspergillus* infection, amphotericin B has been the most reliable agent despite its shortcomings. The published data on fluconazole therapy of candidemia or disseminated candidiasis are still very limited, especially in the granulocytopenic patient. Nevertheless, fluconazole has been used to treat invasive *Candida* infections in patients who either failed amphotericin B therapy or could not tolerate the toxicity of the drug. In one series of 16 patients with chronic disseminated (hepatosplenic) candidiasis treated with fluconazole, 14 responded (107). Several prospective, randomized trials comparing fluconazole with amphotericin B are in progress, and the results of these studies are needed for full assessment of the drug's efficacy. Similarly, despite promising reports of treatment of invasive aspergillosis with itraconazole, very few granulocytopenic patients were treated (108). More data are needed from controlled trials before itraconazole can be recommended as a replacement for amphotericin B in the therapy of *Aspergillus* infection.

PATHOGENESIS AND TREATMENT
OF INTERSTITIAL PNEUMONIA

Interstitial pneumonia occurs in 15% to 40% of allogeneic transplant patients and has a median onset of six to seven weeks after transplantation (30,31,57,109). CMV is associated with approximately one-half of the cases. Thus, the average incidence of CMV-related interstitial pneumonia among allotransplants is 15%. CMV interstitial pneumonia is uncommon after syngeneic transplantation (no cases reported in 100 identical twin transplants from Seattle) (110) and autologous transplantation (3.5% incidence) (32,111,112). Most other interstitial pneumonias are either idiopathic or, less commonly, caused by other viruses or *Pneumocystis carinii*. Idiopathic interstitial pneumonia has a similar incidence among allogeneic and syngeneic transplants and has been attributed to pulmonary toxicity of drugs and radiation (110,113). Attempts to identify an infectious etiology for these idiopathic pneumonias by special cultures, immunochemical stains, or molecular diagnostic techniques have generally been unsuccessful (113). Risk factors for the development of interstitial pneumonia are increasing age of the patient, presence of GVHD, conditioning with high dose rates of irradiation, the use of methotrexate as opposed to cyclosporine as prophylaxis against GVHD, and CMV infection either pretransplant (seropositive for CMV antibody) or posttransplant (culture positive for CMV) (30,31,57,109,113).

The pathogenesis of CMV interstitial pneumonia has been the subject of considerable speculation. Recent information suggests that CMV pneumonia may be mediated, not only by viral replication, but also by immunopathologic factors present in the host which are triggered either by GVHD or CMV (114). Previously, the high incidence of CMV pneumonia after allogeneic transplantation was attributed to the use of immunosuppressive agents and radiation before and after the transplant that impair the patient's ability to control replication and dissemination of the virus which destroys pulmonary tissues. However, despite a frequency of CMV infection similar to that in allogeneic transplants and the use of similar pretransplant immunosuppressive agents, CMV pneumonia is rare in both syngeneic twin transplants and in autologous transplants (32,110–112). On the other hand, GVHD, which is not an expected complication of syngeneic or autologous transplantation, is commonly associated with CMV interstitial pneumonia in allogeneic transplant recipients (30,31,57,109). At one transplant center, the incidence of CMV pneumonia in allotransplants with acute GVHD was 23%, which was significantly higher than the incidence of pneumonia in either allotransplants without GVHD (6%) or autotransplants (2%) (115). These observations suggest that immunologic reactions associated with GVHD may be involved in the development of CMV pneumonia. Indeed, the GVHD reaction in mice is associated with enhancement of CMV infection and development of CMV pneumonia (116,117). The use of an antiviral agent against CMV (ganciclovir) in mice challenged with CMV plus cells eliciting a GVHD reaction does not prevent the development of pneumonia despite the elimination of detectable virus in the lungs (118). Similarly, administration of ganciclovir to human allogeneic marrow transplants with CMV pneumonia reduces CMV titers in the lung but does not prevent death (119,120). In contrast, when CMV pneumonia in marrow transplants is treated with a combination of ganciclovir plus high doses of an immunomodulating agent like intravenous immune globulin, the survival rate is 30% to 75%, which is substantially better than that produced by treatment with either ganciclovir or intravenous immune globulin alone (121–128). The unifying hypothesis to explain these observations is that some component of the immune response to CMV is responsible for determining the occurrence and outcome of CMV pneumonia (129). CMV pneumonia in both patients and animals who receive marrow transplants is associated with an increase in the number of cytotoxic lymphocytes in the lungs (130,131). In athymic/nude mice, the absence of these T-cells prevents CMV pneumonia despite viral replication (132). Thus, the interstitial pneumonia associated with CMV infection may be an immunopathologic process mediated by a T-cell response to CMV antigens whose expression on the surface of infected lung cells is enhanced by GVHD. Blockage of this T-cell response by immunomodulating agents may explain the lower mortality of CMV pneumonia in human transplant recipients treated with intravenous immune globulin plus ganciclovir (121–128) and in mice treated with cyclophosphamide (133).

Open-lung biopsy was generally considered the procedure of choice for the diagnosis of CMV pneumonia (134). However, the centrifugation culture technique and direct immunochemical staining with CMV monoclonal antibodies have greatly enhanced the sensitivity of bronchoalveolar lavage for the diagnosis (135–137). Most cases of CMV pneumonia after marrow transplant can now be diagnosed by bronchoalveolar lavage without the need for an open-lung biopsy.

Previous attempts to treat CMV pneumonia either with antiviral agents (vidarabine, interferon, acyclovir, ganciclovir, foscarnet) or intravenous immune globulin alone failed (31,44). The overall survival using these approaches was only 20%. On the other hand, improved survival has been noted in uncontrolled trials that combined ganciclovir (7.5 to 10 mg/kg per day) with either a polyvalent intravenous immune globulin containing CMV antibody (500 mg/kg every other day) or a CMV hyperimmune globulin (400 mg/kg every other day). Overall survival reported from several transplant centers and the European Bone Marrow Transplant Group is 46% (Table 16.5) (121–128). Survival appears to be influenced by the severity of the pneumonia and the need for mechanical ventilation at the start of therapy. At the Wisconsin, Sloan-Kettering, Seattle, and City of Hope transplant centers, where patients requiring mechanical ventilation were excluded from therapy, survival was 50% to 85%. At the Innsbruck, Utrecht, and UCLA transplant centers, when patients requiring mechanical ventilation were not excluded, survival was only 0% to 38%. At UCLA, none of five patients on mechanical ventilation at the start of therapy survived. On the other hand, three of

Table 16.5   Treatment of CMV pneumonia in bone marrow transplants with intravenous immune globulin plus ganciclovir

Reference	Treatment	Response	Ventilator dependent at start of therapy
Wisconsin (Bratanow, 121)	Immune globulin (Gamimune) + ganciclovir	6/12 (50%)	No data
Sloan-Kettering (Emanuel, 122)	Immune globulin (Gammagard) + ganciclovir	7/10 (70%)	None
Seattle (Reed, 123)	CMV immune globulin (Cutter) + ganciclovir	13/24 (52%)	None (ventilator patients excluded)
City of Hope (Schmidt, 124)	Immune globulin (Gammagard) + ganciclovir	11/13 (85%)	None
Innsbruck (Aulitzky, 125)	Immune globulin (Sandoglobulin) + ganciclovir	1/4 (25%)	3 patients
Utrecht (Verdonk, 126)	CMV immune globulin (Cytotect) + ganciclovir	0/4 (0%)	2 patients
UCLA (Winston, 127)	Immune globulin (Gammagard) + ganciclovir	3/8 (38%)	5 patients
European Bone Marrow Transplant Group (Ljungman, 128)	Standard immune globulin or CMV immune globulin + ganciclovir	17/49 (35%)	2 patients
	Total	58/125 (46%)	

three patients with interstitial infiltrates on chest X-ray due to CMV but minimal respiratory symptoms survived. The European Bone Marrow Transplant Group also noted better survival rates among patients who were not hypoxic at time of diagnosis (54% versus 26%) and who had not received total body irradiation (75% versus 27%) (128). These data suggest that combination therapy with ganciclovir plus intravenous immune globulin is more likely to be effective when the diagnosis of CMV pneumonia is made early. The mechanism by which the combination of ganciclovir and intravenous immune globulin is effective is not clearly understood. As noted previously, CMV pneumonia may involve abnormal immune responses which are modified by the intravenous immune globulin (114,129). After a patient recovers on the ganciclovir plus intravenous immune globulin, maintenance therapy with ganciclovir (5 mg/kg per day, five to seven times each week) and intravenous immune globulin (500 mg/kg per day once weekly) should be continued for at least several more weeks to prevent relapses (122,123).

There is no treatment of proven value for idiopathic interstitial pneumonia. Corticosteroids have been used. Their efficacy is uncertain. Trimethoprim-sulfamethoxazole is the drug of choice for treatment of *Pneumocystis carinii* pneumonia. Parenteral pentamidine is given when the patient is allergic to sulfamethoxazole. Aerosolized ribavarin has been used in patients with parainfluenza virus pneumonia (37). Foscarnet may have a role in the treatment of patients with CMV infection resistant to ganciclovir (138), but it is not known whether foscarnet plus intravenous immune globulin is as effective as ganciclovir plus intravenous immune globulin.

TREATMENT OF OTHER CMV-RELATED DISEASES

There are no controlled studies supporting the efficacy of either ganciclovir or intravenous immune globulin for treatment of other CMV-related diseases after marrow transplantation. Ganciclovir alone has been used to treat CMV gastroenteritis, retinitis, and wasting syndrome (120,139). However, in a randomized, double-blind, placebo-controlled trial, treatment of CMV gastroenteritis with two weeks of ganciclovir was not associated with any clinical or endoscopic improvement when compared with a placebo and supportive care (140). Whether the addition of intravenous immune globulin to ganciclovir would improve efficacy is unknown and requires additional study.

PREVENTION OF CMV INFECTION AND DISEASE IN CMV-SERONEGATIVE PATIENTS

Blood products and bone marrow from CMV-seropositive donors are the most common sources of CMV infection in CMV-seronegative transplant recipients (31,32,141). CMV infection can be prevented in CMV-seronegative recipients with a CMV-seronegative bone marrow donor by using only CMV-seronegative blood products (Table 16.6) (142,143,144). If a CMV-seronegative patient has a CMV-seropositive bone

Table 16.6 Incidence of CMV infection in CMV-seronegative bone marrow transplants receiving CMV-seronegative blood or unscreened blood

Reference	Donor CMV serology	Blood products received	
		Unscreened	CMV-negative
Seattle (Bowden, 142)	CMV-negative	4/11 (36%)	1/17 (6%)
	CMV-positive	4/9 (44%)	2/7 (29%)
Minnesota (Miller, 143)	CMV-negative	14/44 (32%)	2/45 (4%)
	CMV-positive	7/17 (41%)	6/19 (32%)
UCLA (Winston, 144)	CMV-negative		1/29 (3%)
	CMV-positive		3/19 (16%)

marrow donor, CMV-seronegative blood products are less effective. Nonetheless, in a recent study at UCLA, we observed a low incidence of CMV infection (16%) even in CMV-seronegative patients with CMV-seropositive marrow donors when only CMV-seronegative blood products were used (144). These results suggest that blood products may be a greater source of CMV infection than the donor bone marrow. We currently recommend CMV-seronegative blood products for all CMV-seronegative patients, even if the bone marrow donor is CMV-seropositive. Because seronegative blood may not always be available, leukocyte-depleted blood transfusions may be an alternative to seronegative blood products (145).

Studies in animal models of CMV infection and in human bone marrow transplant recipients indicate that immune globulin or plasma containing CMV antibodies modifies the severity of CMV infection and reduces the incidence of CMV interstitial pneumonia in CMV-seronegative recipients (31,146). However, in view of the ability to prevent CMV infection by CMV-seronegative blood products alone, the need for immune globulin has been questioned. Although intravenous immune globulin is not necessary for prevention of CMV infection in CMV-seronegative patients when the patient has a CMV-seronegative donor and is receiving only CMV-seronegative blood products, other benefits may be associated with its use. In a recent randomized, controlled trial in CMV-seronegative marrow transplant patients with seropositive donors, an intravenous CMV immune globulin significantly reduced the incidence of CMV infection and viremia (147). In addition, as shown in Table 16.7, several trials have found a significantly lower incidence of acute GVHD in patients receiving prophylactic intravenous immune globulin (144,148,149). The mechanisms by which intravenous immune globulin reduces GVHD have not been clearly defined but may include inhibition of T-cell function, blockage of cytokines mediating GVHD, and antiidiotypic regulation of the expression of GVHD (150–153). A lower incidence of serious bacterial, fungal, and non-CMV viral infections has also been observed in marrow transplants receiving prophylactic intravenous immune globulin (148,154,155). Thus, intravenous immune globulin has the additional benefits of modifying GVHD and preventing other serious infections and is now commonly given with CMV-seronegative blood products in CMV-seronegative patients.

Table 16.7 Effect of intravenous immune globulin (IVIG) on acute graft-versus-host disease (GVHD)

Reference	IVIG regimen	Acute GVHD		P Value
		Controls	IVIG	
UCLA (Winston, 148)	1000 mg/kg Gamimune, once weekly, days −7 to +120	24/37 (65%)	13/38 (34%)	0.01
Seattle (Sullivan, 149)	500 mg/kg Gamimune, once weekly, days −7 to +90; once monthly, days +120 to +360 (adults only)	56/110 (51%)	37/108 (34%)	0.005
UCLA (Winston, 144)	1,000 mg/kg Sandoglobulin once weekly, days −7 to +120	11/23 (48%)	5/25 (20%)	0.04
	Total	91/170 (54%)	55/169 (33%)	

PREVENTION OF CMV INFECTION AND DISEASE IN CMV-SEROPOSITIVE PATIENTS

In CMV-seropositive transplant recipients, CMV disease usually develops as a consequence of reactivation of latent CMV infection (31, 32, 141). Studies of the molecular epidemiology of CMV infection after marrow transplantation show that CMV-seropositive patients can develop posttransplant pneumonia caused by a CMV strain genetically identical to a CMV isolate detected in the urine before transplant (156). Exogenous infection with a new and different CMV strain also occurs but is much less frequent.

Until recently, effective prophylaxis against CMV disease in CMV-seropositive patients had not been available. Trials of prophylactic vidarabine, interferon, and low-dose acyclovir showed no benefit (44). In a nonrandomized, controlled trial, high doses of prophylactic intravenous acyclovir (500 mg/m^2 every eight hours from five days before to 30 days after transplant) were associated with a decreased incidence of CMV infection and CMV disease (157). However, a 59% incidence of CMV infection and a 19% incidence of CMV-related pneumonia still occurred despite the high doses of acyclovir. In contrast, three recently completed randomized, controlled trials have shown that prophylactic ganciclovir significantly decreases both CMV infection and CMV disease in CMV-seropositive patients (Table 16.8) (158–160). At the City of Hope, the finding of CMV in cytology or shell-vial culture of routine bronchoalveolar lavage on day 35 after transplant in an asymptomatic patient is a significant risk factor for subsequent development of interstitial pneumonia (161). Forty patients with this finding were randomized to receive prophylactic ganciclovir or to observation. Five of 20 patients (25%) receiving ganciclovir developed CMV pneumonia compared with 14 of 20 controls (70%) ($p = 0.01$). In a second double-blind trial at Seattle, prophylactic ganciclovir or placebo was given only to asymptomatic patients excreting CMV after transplant (usually in the blood). One of the 37 ganciclovir patients (3%) and 15 of 35

Table 16.8 Randomized, controlled trials of ganciclovir for prevention of CMV infection or CMV disease in CMV-positive bone marrow transplants

Reference	Trial design	Results	Comments
City of Hope (Schmidt, 158)	Asymptomatic patients positive for CMV in bronchoalveolar lavage on day 35 after transplant randomized to ganciclovir or observation.	5/20 (25%) ganciclovir patients and 14/20 (70%) control patients developed CMV pneumonia.	12 patients developed CMV pneumonia without a previous lavage positive for CMV.
Seattle (Goodrich, 159)	Asymptomatic patients who excrete CMV after transplant randomized to ganciclovir or placebo; double-blinded.	1/37 (3%) ganciclovir patients and 15/35 (43%) placebo patients developed CMV disease (pneumonia, gastrointestinal).	35 patients developed CMV disease before detection of CMV excretion.
UCLA (Winston, 160)	CMV-seropositive patients randomized to receive ganciclovir or placebo for 1 week before transplant and then after transplant from time granulocyte count reaches 1000/mm^3 until day +120; double-blinded.	4/40 (10%) ganciclovir patients and 11/45 (24%) placebo patients developed CMV disease (pneumonia, gastrointestinal, wasting).	Ganciclovir-related neutropenia was frequent.

placebo patients (43%) subsequently developed CMV disease (pneumonia, gastroenteritis) ($p < 0.00001$). Finally, in a third double-blind trial at UCLA, prophylactic ganciclovir or placebo was given to all CMV-seropositive patients for one week pretransplant and then again after transplant from the time the granulocyte count was greater than 1,000 cells/mm^3 until day 120. Four of 40 ganciclovir patients (10%) and 11 of 45 placebo patients (24%) subsequently developed CMV disease (pneumonia, gastroenteritis, wasting syndrome) ($p = 0.09$).

Despite the impressive results, there are certain limitations to prophylactic ganciclovir in marrow transplants. Approximately 30% to 50% of patients require interruption of the ganciclovir prophylaxis due to reversible neutropenia (159,160). The ganciclovir must be given intravenously, usually through a central intravenous catheter, although an oral formulation of ganciclovir is under development (162). In the City of Hope and Seattle trials, a substantial number of patients at risk for CMV pneumonia escaped early detection despite routine cultures of bronchoalveolar lavage fluid, buffy coat, and other body fluids (158,159). These findings suggest that routine prophylaxis of all CMV-seropositive allotransplants, as was done in the UCLA study, may be the best approach for maximizing the efficacy of prophylactic ganciclovir.

Prophylactic CMV immune plasma and intravenous immune globulin have also been used in CMV-seropositive patients. Some studies showed a reduction in acute GVHD and interstitial pneumonia (148,149,163), while others found no benefit (164). In the largest study including 308 CMV-seropositive patients (149), 22% of control patients contracted interstitial pneumonia, compared with 13% of patients receiving intravenous immune globulin ($p = 0.02$). For patients ≥ 20 years old, there was a significant reduction in the incidence of acute GVHD (51% versus 34%, $p = 0.0051$) and in the risk of gram-negative septicemia and local infection among immune globulin recipients. Thus, the administration of prophylactic intravenous immune globulin to CMV-seropositive patients may reduce the risk for infection and interstitial pneumonia by modifying GVHD.

PREVENTION AND TREATMENT OF LATE INFECTIONS

Late bacterial infections and *Pneumocystis carinii* pneumonia associated with chronic GVHD can be prevented by continued prophylaxis with trimethoprim-sulfamethoxazole (165,166). An oral penicillin and aerosolized pentamidine are substituted in patients who cannot tolerate trimethoprim-sulfamethoxazole. Since patients with chronic GVHD have IgG deficiencies, monthly infusions of intravenous immune globulin may also be helpful (149). Unfortunately, the subnormal antibody response of these patients to pneumococcal and other antigenic stimuli limits the utility of the pneumococcal vaccine and other polysaccharide vaccines (28,29). Patients without GVHD, however, have improved humoral immunity six months or later after transplant and are suitable candidates for pneumococcal vaccination (29).

Intravenous acyclovir is the drug of choice for treatment of late varicella-zoster infections (167). A comparative study found high-dose oral acyclovir (800 mg five times daily) as efficacious as intravenous acyclovir in a small number of transplants with varicella-zoster infection (168). Due to the poor absorption of oral acyclovir, we still prefer intravenous acyclovir for initial therapy, especially if the patient is highly immunocompromised from GVHD. Therapy can be switched to oral acyclovir once the skin lesions begin to crust and heal. Oral acyclovir at a dose of 400 mg three times daily was also found in one study to be effective prophylaxis against varicella-zoster infection when it was given, but reactivation of infection frequently occurred after cessation of the drug (169). For seronegative patients exposed to a case of varicella-zoster, early administration of varicella-zoster immune globulin may reduce the risk of infection. Although a live attenuated varicella vaccine is available (170), its use in marrow transplants might be hazardous. Similarly, despite one study showing the apparent safety of a live attenuated trivalent vaccine directed against measles, mumps, and rubella in marrow transplants without GVHD or immunosuppressive treatment at two years after transplant, seroconversion occurred in a lower frequency than normal (171), and these live vaccines still need to be used with caution. Vaccination of marrow transplant recipients six months or more after transplantation with inactivated poliovirus reestablishes humoral immunity against poliovirus (172).

SUMMARY

Considerable progress has been made in the prophylaxis and treatment of infections in the bone marrow transplant recipient. Much of this progress is related to the availability of many new antimicrobial agents and biological products, as well as to an improved understanding of the pathogenesis of infections. Because of the expense associated with many of these agents and products, defensive strategies against infections must consider not only effectiveness but also cost (Table 16.9). It is now possible that a marrow transplant recipient could receive as many as five or six different prophylactic agents. While the use of an oral fluoroquinolone or oral fluconazole for prevention of serious bacterial and fungal infections is relatively inexpensive, the price of intravenous immune globulin and GM-CSF is considerably higher. Their routine use in all patients may not be economical. The results from ongoing trials comparing different dosing regimens of intravenous immune globulin and selectively using GM-CSF or G-CSF only in patients with suspected or documented infection will be important (80,173). On the other hand, the cost of providing CMV-seronegative blood products or prophylactic ganciclovir is justified by the high morbidity and mortality of CMV interstitial pneumonia in allotransplants. The low incidence of CMV disease in syngeneic transplants and autotransplants, however, makes CMV prophylaxis unnecessary. Similarly, in view of a recent controlled trial showing no benefit of intravenous immune globulin for prophylaxis of infections, intravenous immune globulin is also not needed in autotransplants (174). Trimethoprim-sulfamethoxazole is cheap prophylaxis for *Pneumocystis carinii* pneumonia, but the very low mortality from herpes simplex infection makes acyclovir a very expensive prophylaxis.

Treatment options for the infected bone marrow transplant recipient have also become broader. The decline of *Pseudomonas aeruginosa* and other gram-negative bacillary infections and the availability of newer, more potent β-lactam drugs makes monotherapy an appropriate and more cost-effective regimen for empiric therapy of many febrile patients. The introduction of fluconazole, itraconazole, and other newer antifungals offers promise for improving antifungal therapy, but these agents should not take the place of amphotericin B in a critically ill patient with suspected or documented fungal infection until results of ongoing controlled trials show equivalent efficacy. The role of biological response modifiers like macrophage colony-stimulating factor in the treatment of fungal infections also needs to be defined (175). Development of clinically applicable serologic tests for early detection of specific *Candida* or *Aspergillus* antigen is badly needed to help guide antifungal therapy. The combination of intravenous immune globulin plus ganciclovir has reduced mortality from CMV interstitial pneumonia, but prevention is still preferable to treatment. Although CMV infection and pneumonia are declining at many transplant centers, idiopathic interstitial pneumonias remain problematic. A better understanding of the pathogenesis of these idiopathic pneumonias as

Table 16.9   Cost of antimicrobial prophylaxis in bone marrow transplants

Agent	Regimen	Indication	Approximate cost to patient*
Norfloxacin	400 mg P.O. b.i.d. × 28 days	Prevent gram-negative bacillary infections during granulocytopenia	$232.00
Ciprofloxacin	500 mg P.O. b.i.d. × 28 days		284.00
Fluconazole	400 mg P.O. q.d. × 28 days	Prevent *Candida* fungal infections during granulocytopenia	1,160.00
GM-CSF[†]	250 μmg/m²/day IV × 21 days	Shorten posttransplant granulocytopenia	7,650.00
IVIG[‡]	500 mg IV q. weekly × 3 months 500 mg IV q. monthly × 9 months	Prevent or modify graft-versus-host disease and septicemia	35,000.00
CMV-negative blood products[§]		Prevent CMV infection in CMV-negative patient	3,000.00
Ganciclovir	6 mg/kg IV q.d. × 1 week before transplant 6 mg/kg IV q.d., Monday through Friday, between day 30 and 120 after transplant	Prevent CMV infection in CMV-seropositive patient	7,500.00
Trimethoprim-sulfamethoxazole	One double-strength tablet t.i.d. × 1 week before transplant; One double-strength tablet t.i.d. given twice weekly between day 30 and 150 after transplant	Prevent *Pneumocystis carinii* pneumonia	12.00
Acyclovir	5 mg/kg IV q. 8 h × 28 days	Prevent herpes simplex viral infection during granulocytopenia	7,200.00

*UCLA patient charge for antimicrobial agent. Does not include administration fees.
[†]GM-CSF = granulocyte-macrophage colony-stimulating factor.
[‡]IVIG = intravenous immune globulin.
[§]$57.00 additional charge for each unit of CMV-negative red blood cells or platelets. Based on average of 20 units of red blood cells and 50 units of single-donor or random-donor platelets per patient.

they relate to cytotoxic conditioning regimens and GVHD will likely lead to improved strategies for their prevention and treatment. An improved ability to predict, prevent, and modulate the GVHD reaction with newer molecular techniques and biological response modifiers will also likely contribute to a reduction in many of the early and late infections that occur after marrow engraftment (56).

REFERENCES

1 Bortin MM, Rimm AA. Increasing utilization of bone marrow transplantation. *Transplantation* 1986;42:229–234.

2 Bortin MM, Horowitz MM, Rimm AA. Increasing utilization of allogeneic bone marrow transplantation. Results of the 1988–1990 survey. *Ann Intern Med* 1992;115:505–512.

3 Advisory Committee of the International Autologous Bone Marrow Transplant Registry (ABMTR). Autologous bone marrow transplants: Different indications in Europe and North America. *Lancet* 1989;2:317–318.

4 Gale RP, Armitage JO, Dicke KA. Autotransplantation: Now and in the future. *Bone Marrow Transplant* 1991;7:153–157.

5 Meyers JD. Infections in marrow transplant recipients. In: Mandell GL, Douglas RG, Bennett JE, eds. *Principles and Practice of Infectious Diseases*. Third edition. New York: Churchill Livingstone, 1990:2291–2294.

6 Winston DJ, Ho WG, Champlin RE, Gale RP. Infectious complications of bone marrow transplantation. *Exp Hematol* 1984;12:205–215.

7 Meyers JD, Flournoy N, Thomas ED. Infection with herpes simplex virus and cell-mediated immunity after marrow transplant. *J Infect Dis* 1980;142:338–346.

8 Burns WH, Wingard JR. Viral infection following bone marrow transplantation. In: Baum SJ, Santos GW, Takaku F, eds. *Experimental Hematology Today—1987. Recent Advances and Future Directions in Bone Marrow Transplantation*. New York: Springer-Verlag, 1987:165–170.

9 Pannuti CS, Gingrich RD, Pfaller MA, Wenzel RP. Nosocomial pneumonia in adult patients undergoing bone marrow transplantation: a 9-year study. *J Clin Oncol* 1991;9:77–84.

10 Winston DJ. Use of quinolone antimicrobial agents in immunocompromised patients. In: Wolfson JS, Hooper DC, eds. *Use of Quinolone Antimicrobial Agents in Immunocompromised Patients*. Washington, DC: American Society for Microbiology, 1989:187–212.

11 Peterson FB, Buckner CD, Clift RA, et al. Laminar air flow isolation and decontamination: A prospective randomized study of the effects of prophylactic systemic antibiotics in bone marrow transplant patients. *Infection* 1986;14:115–121.

12 Winston DJ, Dudnick DV, Chapin M, Ho WG, Gale RP, Martin WJ. Coagulase-negative staphylococcal bacteremia in patients receiving immunosuppressive therapy. *Arch Intern Med* 1983;143:32–36.

13 Classen DC, Burke JP, Ford CD, et al. *Streptococcus mitis* sepsis in bone marrow transplant patients receiving oral antimicrobial prophylaxis. *Am J Med* 1990;89:441–446.

14 Villablanca JG, Steiner M, Kersey J, et al. The clinical spectrum of infections with Viridians Streptococci in bone marrow transplantation patients. *Bone Marrow Transplant* 1990;6:381–393.

15 Verfaille C, Weisdorf D, Haake R, Hostetter M, Ramsay NKC, McGlave P. Candida infections in bone marrow transplant recipients. *Bone Marrow Transplant* 1991;8:177–184.

16 Meyers JD. Fungal infections in bone marrow transplant patients. *Semin Oncol* 1990;17(suppl 6):10–13.

17 Wingard JR, Beals SU, Santos GW, Merz WG, Saral R. Aspergillus infections in bone marrow transplant recipients. *Bone Marrow Transplant* 1987;2:175–181.

18 Lowenthal RM, Atkinson K, Challis DR, Tucker RD, Biggs RC. Invasive *Trichosporon cutaneum* infection: an increasing problem in immunosuppressed patients. *Bone Marrow Transplant* 1987;2:321–327.

19 Blazer BR, Hurd D, Snover DC, Alexander JW, McGlave PB. Invasive *Fusarium* infection in bone marrow transplant recipients. *Am J Med* 1984;77:645–651.

20 Bufill JA, Lum LG, Caya JG, et al. *Pityrosporum* folliculitis after bone marrow transplantation. Clinical observations in five patients. *Ann Intern Med* 1988;108:560–563.

21 **Opal SM, Asp AA, Cannady PB, Morse PI, Burton LJ, Hammer PG.** Efficacy of infection control measures during a nosocomial outbreak of disseminated aspergillosis associated with hospital construction. *J Infect Dis* 1986; 153:634–637.

22 **Rotstein C, Cummings KM, Tidings J, et al.** An outbreak of invasive aspergillosis among allogeneic bone marrow transplants: a case-control study. *Infect Control* 1985;6:347–355.

23 **Witherspoon RP, Lum LG, Storb R.** Immunologic reconstitution after human marrow grafting. *Semin Hematol* 1984;21:2–10.

24 **Lum LG.** The kinetics of immune reconstitution after human marrow transplantation. *Blood* 1987;69:369–380.

25 **Witherspoon RP.** Suppression and recovery of immunologic function after bone marrow transplantation. *J Natl Cancer Inst* 1986;76: 1321–1324.

26 **Winston DJ, Territo MC, Ho WG, Miller MJ, Gale RP, Golde DW.** Alveolar macrophage dysfunction in human bone marrow transplant recipients. *Am J Med* 1982;73:859–866.

27 **Zimmerli W, Zarth A, Gratwohl A, Speck B.** Neutrophil function and pyogenic infections in bone marrow transplant recipients. *Blood* 1991; 77:393–399.

28 **Witherspoon RP, Storb R, Ochs HD, et al.** Recovery of antibody production in human allogenic marrow graft recipients: influence of time post-transplantation, the presence or absence of chronic graft versus host disease, and antithymocyte globulin treatment. *Blood* 1981;58:360–368.

29 **Winston DJ, Ho WG, Schiffman G, Champlin RE, Feig SA, Gale RP.** Pneumococcal vaccination of bone marrow transplant recipients. *Arch Intern Med* 1983;143:1735–1737.

30 **Meyers JD, Flournoy N, Thomas ED.** Nonbacterial pneumonia after allogeneic marrow transplantation: a review of ten years' experience. *Rev Infect Dis* 1982;4:1119–1132.

31 **Winston DJ, Ho WG, Champlin RE.** Cytomegalovirus infections after allogeneic bone marrow transplantation. *Rev Infect Dis* 1990; 12(suppl 7):S776–S792.

32 **Wingard JR, Piantadosi S, Burns WH, Zahurak ML, Santos GW, Saral R.** Cytomegalovirus infections in bone marrow transplant recipients given intensive cytoreductive therapy. *Rev Infect Dis* 1990;12(suppl 7):S793–S804.

33 **Bowden RA, Day LM, Amos DE, Meyers JD.** Natural cytotoxic activity against cytomegalovirus-infected target cells following marrow transplantation. *Transplantation* 1987;44:504–508.

34 **Reusser P, Riddell SR, Meyers JD, Greenberg PD.** Cytotoxic T-lymphocyte response to cytomegalovirus after human allogeneic bone marrow transplantation: pattern of recovery and correlation with cytomegalovirus infection and disease. *Blood* 1991;78:1373–1380.

35 **Shields AF, Hackman RC, Fife KH, Corey L, Meyers JD.** Adenovirus infections in patients undergoing bone-marrow transplantation. *N Engl J Med* 1985;312:529–533.

36 **Hertz MJ, Englund JA, Snover D, Bitterman PB, McGlave PB.** Respiratory syncytial virus-induced acute lung injury in adult patients with bone marrow transplants: a clinical approach and review of the literature. *Medicine* (Baltimore) 1989;68:269–281.

37 **Wendt CH, Weisdorf DJ, Jordan MC, Balfour HH, Hertz MI.** Parainfluenza virus respiratory infection after bone marrow transplantation. *N Engl J Med* 1992;326:921–926.

38 **Ljungman P, Gleaves CA, Meyers JD.** Respiratory virus infection in immunocompromised patients. *Bone Marrow Transplant* 1989;4:35–40.

39 **Carrigan DR, Drobyski WR, Russler SK, Tapper MA, Knox KK, Ash RC.** Interstitial pneumonitis associated with human herpesvirus-6 infection after marrow transplantation. *Lancet* 1991;338:147–149.

40 **Arthur RR, Shah KV, Baust SJ, et al.** Association of BK viruria with hemorrhagic cystitis in recipients of bone marrow transplants. *N Engl J Med* 1986;315:230–234.

41 **Ambinder RF, Burns W, Forman M, et al.** Hemorrhagic cystitis associated with adenovirus infection in bone marrow transplantation. *Arch Intern Med* 1986;146:1400–1401.

42 **Yolken RH, Bishop CA, Townsend TR, et al.** Infectious gastroenteritis in bone marrow transplant recipients. *N Engl J Med* 1982;306: 1009–1012.

43 **Townsend TR, Bolyand EA, Yolken RH.** Outbreak of Coxsackie A1 gastroenteritis: a complication of bone-marrow transplantation. *Lancet* 1982;1:820–823.

44 **Winston DJ, Ho WG, Gale RP, Champlin RE.** Treatment and prevention of interstitial pneumonia after bone marrow transplantation. In: Gale RP, Champlin RE, eds. *Progress in Bone Marrow Transplantation.* New York: Alan R. Liss, 1987:525–544.

45 **Lange B, Henle W, Meyers JD, et al.** Epstein-Barr virus-related serology in marrow transplant recipients. *Int J Cancer* 1980;26:151–157.

46 **Zutter MM, Martin PJ, Sale GE, et al.** Epstein-Barr virus lymphoproliferation after bone marrow transplantation. *Blood* 1988;72:520–529.

47 Deronin F, Gluckman E, Beauvais B, et al. Toxoplasma infection after human allogeneic bone marrow transplantation: clinical and serological study of 80 patients. *Bone Marrow Transplant* 1986;1:67–73.

48 Shepp DH, Hackman RC, Conley FK, Anderson JB, Meyers JD. *Toxoplasma gondii* reactivation identified by detection of parasitemia in tissue culture. *Ann Intern Med* 1985;103:218–221.

49 Atkinson K, Farewell V, Storb R, et al. Analysis of late infections after human bone marrow transplantation: role of genotypic nonidentity between marrow donor and recipient and of nonspecific suppressor cells in patients with chronic graft-versus-host disease. *Blood* 1982;60:714–720.

50 Locksley RM, Flournoy N, Sullivan K, et al. Infection with varicella-zoster virus after marrow transplant. *J Infect Dis* 1985;152:1172–1181.

51 Schuchter LM, Wingard JR, Piantadosi S, et al. Herpes zoster infection after autologous bone marrow transplantation. *Blood* 1989;74: 1424–1427.

52 Atkinson K, Storb R, Prentice RL, et al. Analysis of late infections in 89 long-term survivors of bone marrow transplantation. *Blood* 1979;53:720–731.

53 Winston DJ, Shiffman G, Wang D, et al. Pneumococcal infections after human bone marrow transplantation. *Ann Intern Med* 1979; 91:835–841.

54 Izutsu KT, Sullivan KM, Schubert MM, et al. Disordered salivary immunoglobulin secretion and sodium transport in human chronic graft-versus-host disease. *Transplantation* 1983;35: 441–446.

55 Dematrakopoulos GE, Tsokos GC, Levine AS. Recovery of splenic function after GVHD-associated functional asplenia. *Am J Hematol* 1982;12:77–80.

56 Ferrara JLM, Deeg HJ. Graft-versus-host disease. *N Engl J Med* 1991;324:667–674.

57 Wingard JR, Mellits ED, Sostrin MB, et al. Interstitial pneumonitis after allogeneic bone marrow transplantation. *Medicine* (Baltimore) 1988;67:175–186.

58 Wingard JR, Santos GW, Saral R. Late onset interstitial pneumonia following allogeneic bone marrow transplantation. *Transplantation* 1985; 39:21–23.

59 Buckner CD, Clift RA, Sanders JE, et al. Protective environment for marrow transplant recipients. A prospective study. *Ann Intern Med* 1978;89:893–901.

60 Storb R, Prentice RL, Buckner CD, et al. Graft versus host disease and survival in patients with aplastic anemia treated by marrow grafts from HLA-identical siblings. Beneficial effect of a protective environment. *N Engl J Med* 1983;308:302–307.

61 Russell JA, Poon MC, Jones AR, Woodman RC, Ruether BA. Allogeneic bone-marrow transplantation without protective isolation in adults with malignant disease. *Lancet* 1992; 339:38–40.

62 Karp JE, Dick JD, Merz WG. Systemic infection and colonization with and without prophylactic norfloxacin use over time in the granulocytopenic, acute leukemia patient. *Eur J Cancer Clin Oncol* 1988;24(suppl 1):S5–S13.

63 Dekker AW, Rozenberg-Arska M, Verdonk LF, Verhoef J. Longterm experience with ciprofloxacin for infection prevention in acute leukemia. *Program and Abstracts of the Sixth International Symposium on Infections in the Immunocompromised host.* Peebles, Scotland: 1990:100.

64 Akard L, Newton F, Black J, Hansen J. Prophylactic vancomycin prevents bacteremia by gram-positive organisms in neutropenic bone marrow transplant patients. *J Cell Biochem* 1992;16A:211.

65 Meunier F. Prevention of mycoses in immunocompromised patients. *Rev Infect Dis* 1987;9: 408–416.

66 Goodman JL, Winston DJ, Greenfield RA, et al. A controlled trial of fluconazole to prevent fungal infections in patients undergoing bone marrow transplantation. *N Engl J Med* 1992; 326:845–851.

67 Wingard JR, Merz WG, Rinaldi MG, Johnson TR, Karp JE, Saral R. Increase in *Candida krusei* infection among patients with bone marrow transplantation and neutropenia treated prophylactically with fluconazole. *N Engl J Med* 1991;325:1274–1277.

68 Patterson TF, Miniter P, Andriole VT. Efficacy of fluconazole in experimental invasive aspergillosis. *Rev Infect Dis* 1990;12(suppl 13):S281–S285.

69 Rousey SR, Russler S, Gottlieb M, Ach RC. Low-dose amphotericin B prophylaxis against invasive *Aspergillus* infections in allogeneic marrow transplantation. *Am J Med* 1991;91: 484–492.

70 Winston DJ, Ho WG, Young LS, Gale RP. Prophylactic granulocyte transfusions during human bone marrow transplantation. *Am J Med* 1980;68:893–897.

71 Winston DJ, Ho WG, Gale RP. Therapeutic granulocyte transfusions for documented infec-

tions: A controlled trial in ninety-five infectious granulocytopenic episodes. *Ann Intern Med* 1982;97:509–515.

72 **Metcalf D.** The colony stimulating factors: discovery, development and clinical applications. *Cancer* 1990;65:1286–1295.

73 **Nemunaitis J, Rabinowe SN, Singer JW, et al.** Recombinant granulocyte-macrophage colony-stimulating factor after autologous bone marrow transplantation for lymphoid cancer. *N Engl J Med* 1991;324:1773–1778.

74 **Gulati SC, Bennett CL.** Granulocyte-macrophage colony-stimulating factor (GM-CSF) as adjunct therapy in relapsed Hodgkin disease. *Ann Intern Med* 1992;116:177–182.

75 **Advani R, Chao NJ, Horning SJ, et al.** Granulocyte-macrophage colony-stimulating factor (GM-CSF) as an adjunct to autologous hematopoietic stem cell transplantation for lymphoma. *Ann Intern Med* 1992;116:183–189.

76 **Gorin NC, Coiffier B, Pico J, et al.** Granulocyte-macrophage colony-stimulating factor (GM-CSF) shortens aplasia duration after autologous bone marrow transplantation (ABMT) in non-Hodgkin's lymphoma. A randomized placebo-controlled double-blind study. *Blood* 1990; 76(Suppl 1):S42a.

77 **Link H, Bougaerts M, Carella A, et al.** Recombinant human granulocyte-macrophage colony stimulating factor (RH-GM-CSF) after autologous bone marrow transplantation for acute lymphoblastic leukemia and non-Hodgkin's lymphoma: a randomized double-blind multicenter trial in Europe. *Blood* 1990;76(suppl 1):152a.

78 **Powles R, Smith C, Milan S, et al.** Human recombinant GM-CSF in allogeneic bone marrow transplantation for leukemia: double-blind, placebo-controlled trial. *Lancet* 1990;2: 1417–1420.

79 **Nemunaitis J, Singer JW, Buckner CD, et al.** Use of recombinant human granulocyte-macrophage colony-stimulating factor in graft failure after bone marrow transplantation. *Blood* 1990;76:245–253.

80 **Anaissie E, Legrand C, Elting L, Gutterman J, Vadhan-Raaj S, Bodey GP.** Randomized trial of antibiotics (Ab) plus granulocyte-macrophage colony-stimulating factor (GM-CSF) for febrile episodes in neutropenic cancer (Ca) patients. In: *Program and Abstracts of the 30th Interscience Conference on Antimicrobial Agents and Chemotherapy.* Washington DC: American Society for Microbiology, 1990:129.

81 **Nemunaitis J, Singer JW, Buckner CD, et al.** Long-term follow-up of patients who received recombinant human granulocyte-macrophage colony stimulating factor after autologous bone marrow transplantation for lymphoid malignancy. *Bone Marrow Transplant* 1991;7:49–52.

82 **Saral R, Burns WH, Laskin OL, Santos GW, Leitman PS.** Acyclovir prophylaxis of herpes simplex virus infections. *N Engl J Med* 1981; 301:63–67.

83 **Wade JC, Newton B, Flournoy N, Meyers JD.** Oral acyclovir for prevention of herpes simplex virus reactivation after marrow transplantation. *Ann Intern Med* 1984;100:823–828.

84 **McLaren C, Chen MS, Ghazzouli I, Saral R, Burns WH.** Drug resistance patterns of herpes simplex virus isolates from patients treated with acyclovir. *Antimicrob Agents Chemother* 1985;28:740–744.

85 **Wade JC, McLaren C, Meyers JD.** Frequency and significance of acyclovir-resistant herpes simplex virus isolated from marrow transplant patients receiving multiple courses of treatment with acyclovir. *J Infect Dis* 1983;148: 1077–1082.

86 **Ambinder RF, Burns WH, Leitman PS, Saral R.** Prophylaxis: a strategy to minimize antiviral resistance. *Lancet* 1984;1:1154–1155.

87 **Klastersky J, Zinner SH, Calandra T, et al.** Empiric antimicrobial therapy for febrile granulocytopenic cancer patients: lessons from four EORTC trials. *Eur J Cancer Clin Oncol* 1988;24(suppl 1):S35–S45.

88 **Hughes WT, Armstrong D, Bodey GP, et al.** Guidelines for the use of antimicrobial agents in neutropenic patients with unexplained fever. *J Infect Dis* 1990;161:381–396.

89 **Winston DJ, Ho WG, Bruckner DA, Gale RP, Champlin RE.** Controlled trials of double beta-lactam therapy with cefoperazone plus piperacillin in febrile granulocytopenic patients. *Am J Med* 1988;85(suppl 1A):21–30.

90 **Anaissie EJ, Fainstein V, Bodey GP, et al.** Randomized trial of beta-lactam regimens in febrile neutropenic patients. *Am J Med* 1988; 84:581–589.

91 **DeJace P, Klastersky J.** Comparative review of combination therapy: two beta-lactams versus beta-lactam plus aminoglycoside. *Am J Med* 1986;80(suppl 6B):29–38.

92 **Winston DJ, Ho WG, Bruckner DA, Champlin RE.** Beta-lactam antibiotic therapy in febrile granulocytopenic patients. A randomized trial comparing cefoperazone plus piperacillin, ceftazidime plus piperacillin, and imipenem alone. *Ann Intern Med* 1991;115: 849–859.

93 **Pizzo PA, Hathorn JW, Hiemenz J, et al.** A randomized trial comparing ceftazidime alone with combination antibiotic therapy in cancer

patients with fever and neutropenia. *N Engl J Med* 1986;315:552–558.

94   **Schuchter L, Kaelin W, Petty B, et al.** Ceftazidime (C) vs. ticarcillin and gentamicin (TG) in febrile neutropenic bone marrow transplant (BMT) patients (pts): a prospective, randomized, double-blind trial. *Blood* 1988;72(suppl 1):406a.

95   **Liang R, Yung R, Chiu E, et al.** Ceftazidime versus imipenem-cilastatin as initial monotherapy for febrile neutropenic patients. *Antimicrob Agents Chemother* 1990; 34:1336–1341.

96   **Rolston KVI, Berkey P, Bodey GP, et al.** A comparison of imipenem to ceftazidime with or without amikacin as empiric therapy in febrile neutropenic patients. *Arch Intern Med* 1992;152:283–291.

97   **Winston DJ, McGrattan MA, Busuttil RW.** Imipenem therapy of *Pseudomonas aeruginosa* and other serious bacterial infections. *Antimicrob Agents Chemother* 1984;26:673–677.

98   **Johnson MP, Ramphal R.** Beta-lactam resistant *Enterobacter* bacteremia in febrile neutropenic patients receiving monotherapy. *J Infect Dis* 1990;162:981–983.

99   **Karp JE, Dick JD, Angelopulas C, et al.** Empiric use of vancomycin during prolonged treatment-induced granulocytopenia. Randomized, double-blind, placebo-controlled clinical trial in patients with acute leukemia. *Am J Med* 1986;81:237–242.

100   **Shenep JL, Hughes WT, Roberson PK, et al.** Vancomycin, ticarcillin and amikacin compared with ticarcillin-clavulanate and amikacin in the empirical treatment of febrile, neutropenic children with cancer. *N Engl J Med* 1988;319:1053–1058.

101   **Rubin M, Hathorn JW, Marshall D, Gress J, Steinberg SM, Pizzo PA.** Gram-positive infections and the use of vancomycin in 550 episodes of fever and neutropenia. *Ann Intern Med* 1988;108:30–35.

102   **Pizzo PA, Robichaud KJ, Gill FA, Witebsky FG.** Empiric antibiotic and antifungal therapy for cancer patients with prolonged fever and granulocytopenia. *Am J Med* 1982;72: 101–111.

103   **EORTC International Antimicrobial Therapy Cooperative Group.** Empiric antifungal therapy in febrile granulocytopenic patients. *Am J Med* 1989;86:668–672.

104   **Kennedy MS, Deeg HJ, Siegel M, Crowley JJ, Storb R, Thomas ED.** Acute renal toxicity with combined use of amphotericin B and cyclosporine after marrow transplantation. *Transplantation* 1983;35:211–215.

105   **Lopez-Berestein G.** Liposomal amphotericin B in the treatment of systemic mycoses in patients with cancer. In: Holmberg K, Meyer RD, eds. *Diagnosis and Therapy of Systemic Fungal Infections.* New York: Raven Press 1989;159–166.

106   **Fainstein V, Bodey GP, Elting L, et al.** Amphotericin B or ketoconazole therapy for fungal infections in neutropenic cancer patients. *Antimicrob Agents Chemother* 1987; 31:11–15.

107   **Anaissie E, Bodey G, Kantarjan H, et al.** Fluconazole therapy for chronic disseminated candidiasis in patients with leukemia and prior amphotericin B therapy. *Am J Med* 1991;91:142–150.

108   **Denning DW, Tucker RM, Hanson LH, Stevens DA.** Treatment of invasive aspergillosis with itraconazole. *Am J Med* 1989;86: 791–800.

109   **Weiner RS, Bortin MM, Gale RP, et al.** Interstitial pneumonitis after bone marrow transplantation. Assessments of risk factors. *Ann Intern Med* 1986;104:168–175.

110   **Appelbaum FR, Meyers JD, Fefer A, et al.** Nonbacterial nonfungal pneumonia following marrow transplantation in 100 identical twins. *Transplantation* 1982;33:265–268.

111   **Pelego R, Hill R, Appelbaum FR, et al.** Interstitial pneumonitis following autologous bone marrow transplantation. *Transplantation* 1986;42:515–517.

112   **Winston DJ, Ho WG, Champlin RE.** Cytomegalovirus infection and interstitial pneumonia after bone marrow transplantation. In: Champlin RE, ed. *Bone Marrow Transplantation.* Boston: Kluwer Academic Publishers, 1990:113–128.

113   **Meyers JD, Flournoy N, Wade JC, et al.** Biology of interstitial pneumonia after marrow transplantation. In: Gale RP, Champlin RE, eds. *Progress in Bone Marrow Transplantation.* New York: Alan R. Liss, 1983:405–423.

114   **Zia JA.** Understanding human cytomegalovirus infection. In: Champlin RE, Gale RP, eds. *New Strategies in Bone Marrow Transplantation.* New York: Wiley-Liss, 1991:319–334.

115   **Wingard JR, Chen DY-H, Burns WH, et al.** Cytomegalovirus infection after autologous bone marrow transplantation with comparison to infection after allogeneic bone marrow transplantation. *Blood* 1988;71:1432–1437.

116   **Dowling JN, Wu BC, Armstrong JA, Hu M.** Enhancement of murine cytomegalovirus infection during graft-vs-host reaction. *J Infect Dis* 1977;135:990–994.

117 Grundy JE, Shanley JD, Shearer GM. Augmentation of graft-versus-host reaction by cytomegalovirus infection resulting in interstitial pneumonitis. *Transplantation* 1985;39: 548–553.

118 Shanley JD, Pomeroy C, Via CS, Shearer GM. Interstitial pneumonitis during murine cytomegalovirus infection and graft-versus-host reaction: effect of ganciclovir therapy. *J Infect Dis* 1988;158:1391–1394.

119 Shepp DH, Dandliker PS, de Miranda P, et al. Activity of 9-[2-hydroxy-1-(hydroxlmethyl)-ethoxymethyl] guanine in the treatment of cytomegalovirus pneumonia. *Ann Intern Med* 1985;103:368–373.

120 Winston DJ, Ho WG, Bartoni K, et al. Ganciclovir therapy for cytomegalovirus infections in recipients of bone marrow transplants and other immunosuppressed patients. *Rev Infect Dis* 1988;10(suppl 3):S547–S553.

121 Bratanow NC, Ash RC, Turner PA, et al. Successful treatment of serious cytomegalovirus (CMV) disease with 9(1,3-dihydroxy-2-propoxymethyl) guanine (ganciclovir, DHPG) and intravenous immunoglobulin (IVIG) in bone marrow transplant (BMT) patients. *Exp Hematol* 1987;15:41.

122 Emanuel D, Cunningham I, Jules-Elysee K, et al. Cytomegalovirus pneumonia after bone marrow transplantation successfully treated with the combination of ganciclovir and high-dose intravenous immune globulin. *Ann Intern Med* 1988;109:777–782.

123 Reed EC, Bowden RA, Dandliker PS, Lilleby KE, Meyers JD. Treatment of cytomegalovirus pneumonia with ganciclovir and intravenous cytomegalovirus immunoglobulin in patients with bone marrow transplants. *Ann Intern Med* 1988;109:783–789.

124 Schmidt GM, Kovacs A, Zaia JA, et al. Ganciclovir/immunoglobulin combination therapy for the treatment of human cytomegalovirus-associated interstitial pneumonia in bone marrow allograft patients. *Transplantation* 1988; 46:905–907.

125 Aulitzky WE, Tilg H, Niederwieser G, Hack M, Meister B, Huber C. Ganciclovir and hyperimmunoglobulin for treating cytomegalovirus infection in bone marrow transplant recipients. *J Infect Dis* 1988;158:488–489.

126 Verdonk LF, De Gast GC, Dekker AW, De Weger RA, Schuurman HJ, Rozenberg-Arska M. Treatment of cytomegalovirus pneumonia after bone marrow transplantation with cytomegalovirus immunoglobulin combined with ganciclovir. *Bone Marrow Transplant* 1989;4:187–189.

127 Winston DJ, Ho WG, Champlin RE. Ganciclovir and intravenous immunoglobulin in bone marrow transplants. In: Champlin RE, Gale RP, eds. *New Strategies in Bone Marrow Transplantation*. New York: Wiley-Liss, 1991:337–348.

128 Ljungman P, Engelhard D, Link H, et al. Treatment of interstitial pneumonitis due to cytomegalovirus with ganciclovir and intravenous immune globulin: experience of European Bone Marrow Transplant Group. *Clinical Inf Dis* 1992;14:831–835.

129 Grundy JE, Shanley JD, Griffiths PD. Is cytomegalovirus interstitial pneumonia in transplant recipients an immunopathological condition? *Lancet* 1987;2:996–999.

130 Bowden RA, Dobbs S, Kopecky KJ, Crawford S, Meyers JD. Increased cytotoxicity against cytomegalovirus-infected target cells by bronchoalveolar lavage cells from bone marrow transplant recipients with cytomegalovirus pneumonia. *J Infect Dis* 1988;158:773–779.

131 Shanley JD, Via CS, Sharrow SO, Shearer GM. Interstitial pneumonitis during murine cytomegalovirus infection and graft-versus-host reaction. Characterization of bronchoalveolar lavage cells. *Transplantation* 1987; 44:658–662.

132 Shanley JD. Murine cytomegalovirus pneumonitis in T-cell deficient nude mice. In: *Abstracts of the 12th Herpesvirus Workshop*, Philadelphia, 1987.

133 Shanley JD, Pesanti EL, Nugent KM. The pathogenesis of pneumonitis due to murine cytomegalovirus. *J Infect Dis* 1982;146:388–396.

134 Springmeyer SC, Silvestri RC, Sale GE, et al. The role of transbronchial biopsy for the diagnosis of diffuse pneumonitis in immunocompromised marrow transplant recipients. *Am Rev Respir Dis* 1982;126:763–765.

135 Emanuel D, Peppard J, Stover D, Gold J, Armstrong D, Hammerling V. Rapid immunodiagnosis of cytomegalovirus by bronchoalveolar lavage using human and murine monoclonal antibodies. *Ann Intern Med* 1986;104:476–481.

136 Cordonnier C, Escudier E, Nicolas JC, et al. Evaluation of three assays on alveolar lavage fluid in the diagnosis of cytomegalovirus pneumonitis after bone marrow transplantation. *J Infect Dis* 1987;155:495–500.

137 Crawford SW, Bowden RA, Hackman RC, Gleaves CA, Meyers JD, Clark JG. Rapid detection of cytomegalovirus pulmonary infection by bronchoalveolar lavage and centrifugation culture. *Ann Intern Med* 1988;108; 180–185.

138 Drobyski WR, Knox KK, Carrigan DR, Ash RC. Foscarnet therapy of ganciclovir-resistant cytomegalovirus in marrow transplantation. *Transplantation* 1991;52:155–157.

139 Erice A, Jordan MA, Chace BA, Fletcher C, Chinnock BJ, Balfour HH. Ganciclovir treatment of cytomegalovirus disease in transplant recipients and other immunocompromised hosts. *J Am Med Assoc* 1987;257:3082–3087.

140 Reed EC, Wolford JL, Kopecky KJ, et al. Ganciclovir for the treatment of cytomegalovirus gastroenteritis in bone marrow transplant patients: a randomized, placebo-controlled trial. *Ann Intern Med* 1990;112:505–510.

141 Meyers JD, Flournoy N, Thomas ED. Risk factors for cytomegalovirus infection after human marrow transplantation. *J Infect Dis* 1986;153:478–488.

142 Bowden RA, Sayers M, Flournoy N, et al. Cytomegalovirus immune globulin and seronegative blood products to prevent primary cytomegalovirus infection after marrow transplantation. *N Engl J Med* 1986; 314:1006–1010.

143 Miller WJ, McCullough J, Balfour HH, et al. Prevention of cytomegalovirus infection following bone marrow transplantation: a randomized trial of blood product screening. *Bone Marrow Transplant* 1991;7:227–234.

144 Winston DJ, Ho WG, Bartoni K, Champlin RE. Intravenous immunoglobulin and cytomegalovirus (CMV)-seronegative blood products for prevention of CMV infection and disease in bone marrow transplants. In: Program and Abstracts of 31st Interscience Conference on Antimicrobial Agents and Chemotherapy. Washington, DC: American Society for Microbiology, 1991:221.

145 Bowden RA, Slichter SJ, Sayers MH, Mori M, Cays MJ, Meyers JD. Use of leukocyte-depleted platelets and cytomegalovirus-seronegative red blood cells for prevention of primary cytomegalovirus infection after marrow transplant. *Blood* 1991;78:246–250.

146 Winston DJ, Ho WG, Champlin RE. Use of DHPG (ganciclovir) and intravenous immune globulin in bone marrow transplants. In: Gale RP, Champlin RE, eds. *Bone Marrow Transplantation: Current Controversies.* New York: Alan R. Liss, 1989:533–551.

147 Bowden RA, Fisher LD, Rogers K, Cays M, Meyers JD. Cytomegalovirus (CMV)-specific intravenous immunoglobulin for the prevention of primary CMV infection and disease after marrow transplant. *J Infect Dis* 1991; 164:483–487.

148 Winston DJ, Ho WG, Lin CH, et al. Intravenous immune globulin for prevention of cytomegalovirus infection and interstitial pneumonia after bone marrow transplantation. *Ann Intern Med* 1987;106:12–18.

149 Sullivan KM, Kopecky KJ, Jacom J, et al. Immunomodulatory and antimicrobial efficacy of intravenous immunoglobulin in bone marrow transplantation. *N Engl J Med* 1990; 323:705–712.

150 Kawada K, Terasaki PI. Evidence for immunosuppression by high-dose gammaglobulin. *Exp Hematol* 1987;15:133–136.

151 Leung DY, Bruns JC, Newburger JW, Geha RS. Reversal of lymphocyte activation in vivo in the Kawasaki syndrome of intravenous gammaglobulin. *J Clin Invest* 1987;79:468–472.

152 Cohen J. Cytokines as mediators of graft-versus-host disease. *Bone Marrow Transplant* 1988;3:193–197.

153 Dietrich G, Kazatchkine MD. Normal immunoglobulin G (IgG) for therapeutic use (intravenous Ig) contains antiidiotypic specificities against an immunodominant, disease-associated, cross-reactive idiotype of human antithyroglobulin autoantibodies. *J Clin Invest* 1990;85:620–625.

154 Petersen FB, Bowden RA, Thornquist M, et al. The effect of prophylactic intravenous immune globulin on the incidence of septicemia in marrow transplant recipients. *Bone Marrow Transplant* 1987;2:141–147.

155 Graham-Pole J, Camitta B, Casper J, et al. Intravenous immunoglobulin may lessen all forms of infection in patients receiving allogeneic bone marrow transplantation for acute lymphoblastic leukemia: a Pediatric Oncology Group study. *Bone Marrow Transplant* 1988;3:559–566.

156 Winston DJ, Huang ES, Miller MJ, et al. Molecular epidemiology of cytomegalovirus infections associated with bone marrow transplantation. *Ann Intern Med* 1985;102:16–20.

157 Meyers JD, Reed EC, Shepp DH, et al. Acyclovir for prevention of cytomegalovirus infection and disease after allogeneic marrow transplantation. *N Engl J Med* 1988; 318:70–75.

158 Schmidt GM, Horak DA, Niland JC, et al. A randomized controlled trial of prophylactic ganciclovir for cytomegalovirus pulmonary infection in recipients of allogeneic bone marrow transplants. *N Engl J Med* 1991;324:1005–1011.

159 Goodrich JM, Mori M, Gleaves CA, et al. Early treatment with ganciclovir to prevent cytomegalovirus disease after allogeneic bone

marrow transplantation. *N Engl J Med* 1991; 325:1601–1607.

160   Winston DJ, Ho WG, Bartoni K, et al. Ganciclovir prophylaxis of cytomegalovirus infection and disease in allogeneic bone marrow transplants: results of a placebo-controlled, double-blind trial. *Ann Intern Med* 1993;118:179–184.

161   Schimdt GM, Zaia J, Horak D, et al. Human cytomegalovirus (HCMV) detection in routine bronchoalveolar lavage (BAL) specimens as a prediction for interstitial pneumonia (IP) in allogeneic bone marrow transplant (BMT). *Blood* 1988;72(suppl 1):405.

162   Drew WL, Lalezari J, Busch D, et al. In vivo antiviral efficacy of oral ganciclovir. *Antiviral Res* 1991;15(suppl 1):127.

163   Winston DJ, Pollard RB, Ho WG, et al. Cytomegalovirus immune plasma in bone marrow transplant recipients. *Ann Intern Med* 1982;97:11–18.

164   Ringdén O, Pihlstedt P, Volin L, et al. Failure to prevent cytomegalovirus infection by cytomegalovirus hyperimmune plasma: a randomized trial by the Nordic Bone Marrow Transplantation Group. *Bone Marrow Transplant* 1987;2:299–305.

165   Sullivan KM, Dahlberg S, Storb R, et al. Infection acquisition and prophylaxis in chronic graft-versus-host disease (GVHD). *Blood* 1983; 62:230A.

166   Sullivan KM, Meyers JD, Flournoy N, Storb R, Thomas ED. Early and later interstitial pneumonia following human bone marrow transplantation. *Int J Cell Cloning* 1986; 4(suppl 1):107–121.

167   Shepp DH, Dandliker PS, Meyers JD. Treatment of varicella-zoster virus infection in severely immunocompromised patients. A randomized comparison of acyclovir and vidarabine. *N Engl J Med* 1986;314:208–212.

168   Ljungman P, Lonnqvist B, Rindén O, Shinhoj P, Gharton G. Oral acyclovir for treatment of herpes zoster in marrow transplant recipients. In: *Program and Abstracts of the Fifth International Symposium on Infections in the Immunocompromised Host.* Noordwijkerhout, Netherlands, 1988:103.

169   Ljungman P, Lonnqvist B, Gharton G, Rindén O, Sundqvist CA, Wahren B. Clinical and subclinical reactivation of varicella zoster virus in immunocompromised patients. *J Infect Dis* 1986;153:840–847.

170   Gehrson AA, Steinberg S, The National Institute of Allergy and Infectious Diseases Varicella Vaccine Collaborative Study Group. Persistence of immunity to varicella in leukemic children immunized with live attenuated varicella zoster. *N Engl J Med* 1989;320: 892–897.

171   Ljungman P, Fridell E, Lonnqvist B, et al. Efficacy and safety of vaccination of marrow transplant recipients with a live attenuated measles, mumps, and rubella vaccine. *J Infect Dis* 1989;159:610–615.

172   Engelhard D, Handsher R, Naparstek E, et al. Immune response to polio vaccination in bone marrow transplant recipients. *Bone Marrow Transplant* 1991;8:295–300.

173   Graham-Pole J, Amylon M, Elfenbein G, et al. Prophylactic intravenous immunoglobulin (IVIG) after allogeneic marrow transplant (BMT): Preliminary analysis of a dose-randomizing study. *J Cell Biochem* 1992;Suppl 16A:213.

174   Wolff SN, Fay JW, Greer JP, Brown RA, Herzig GP, Herzig RH. High-dose weekly intravenous immunoglobulins (IVIG) for the prevention of infection in patients (PTS) undergoing autologous bone marrow transplantation (ABMT) and intense therapy for acute leukemia: a study of the North American Bone Marrow Transplant Group. *J Cell Biochem* 1992;Supple 16A:217.

175   Nemunaitis J, Meyers JD, Buckner CD, et al. Phase I trial of recombinant human macrophage colony-stimulating factor in patients with invasive fungal infections. *Blood* 1991;78:907–913.

Toxoplasmosis in the non-AIDS immunocompromised host

D. M. ISRAELSKI
J. S. REMINGTON

INTRODUCTION

Toxoplasma gondii is among the most common causes of latent infection of humans throughout the world. This chronic latent infection is associated with cysts in multiple organs and appears to be an active process of cyst disruption and reformation, ordinarily unaccompanied by clinical evidence of disease or tissue destruction (1). Immunologically normal individuals with acute acquired *Toxoplasma* infection usually have a self-limited clinical course and do not require specific treatment directed at the parasite. Limitation of the spread and containment of the latent form of the infection is compromised when there is a severe defect in the immune system and especially in cell-mediated immunity. This is most clearly evidenced in the tragic and frequent occurrence of toxoplasmosis in individuals with the acquired immunodeficiency syndrome (AIDS). Although this has received widespread attention in the literature, the subject of toxoplasmosis in patients who are immunocompromised by other conditions has been relatively neglected in the literature since Ruskin and Remington published their review nearly 16 years ago (2).

The non-AIDS immunocompromised individual is at risk for development of a wide variety of infectious complications, depending on the nature and degree of immunosuppression. Apart from its high incidence in individuals with AIDS, toxoplasmosis has only occasionally been reported to cause disease in the immunocompromised patient. Reviews of the occurrence of infections in patients with lymphoproliferative or myelopoietic malignancies infrequently list *Toxoplasma* as a cause of opportunistic infectious disease (3,4). The administration of antineoplastic drugs to patients with malignancy and unrecognized active *Toxoplasma* infection may lead to dissemination of *Toxoplasma* and death (2,5–7). Similarly, *Toxoplasma* infection may disseminate in transplant recipients who are receiving immunosuppressive agents and in patients with collagen vascular disease on high-dose corticosteroids (2,8–16). The unusual occurrence, protean clinical manifestations, and devastating consequences of toxoplasmosis in the non-AIDS immunocompromised host emphasize the need for clinical acumen in the diagnosis and management of this disorder.

Toxoplasma gondii has three infectious forms. Oocysts result from the enteroepithelial cycle in cats, the definitive host for *Toxoplasma*, and are a major cause of infection in humans in contact with cat feces, objects, or food contaminated with cat feces. Thus, the mechanisms of the spread of *Toxoplasma* are presumptively by the oral route; others include congenital transmission and blood transfusion (17). Tissue cysts, which contain a few or several thousand bradyzoites, are found in multiple tissues and organs throughout the body and cause a latent infection, probably for the entire life span of the host; cysts in raw or undercooked meat are a source of the infections in humans. Cysts in tissues are only rarely associated with an inflammatory response. "Rupture" of cysts, when it occurs in the immunocompromised host, leads to release of bradyzoites, which invade contiguous cells (and thereby become tachyzoites), and recrudescence of active infection. The crescent-shaped tachyzoite form is found mainly during acute infection and can invade all types of mammalian cell.

The mechanisms by which infection with *Toxoplasma* is maintained in a quiescent state are incompletely understood. The advent of AIDS and its associated immunologic abnormalities have revealed how important a severe disturbance of T lymphocyte function is as an important factor predisposing to development of toxoplasmosis in the immunocompromised host. This is, at least in part, due to an abnormality in production of cytokines critical to resistance against this organism (18–22).

CLINICOPATHOLOGICAL FEATURES

Toxoplasmosis has been found to be associated with a wide variety of conditions that result in immunosuppression (Table 17.1) and has been reported to involve nearly every organ system in non-AIDS immunocompromised patients (Tables 17.2,17.3,17.4). Clinical syndromes associated with toxoplasmosis in non-AIDS immunocompromised patients are most frequently encephalitis (2,6,16), myocarditis (13,24), and pneumonitis (26,144,149). In addition, cases of widely disseminated *Toxoplasma* infection have been described (5,12,27–31). The majority of cases in non-AIDS immunocompromised patients have occurred in individuals with malignancies (2,5,7,16,31), most frequently Hodgkin's lymphoma, and in recipients of heart (14,15,30,32–39), bone marrow (8,9,11–13,40–45), and renal (27,46–60) transplants (Table 17.1).

Clearly, toxoplasmosis can be present in the immunosuppressed patient without malignancies, including those on corticosteroids (10,28,59,61–64) or with systemic lupus erythematosus (SLE) (27,28,65–67). Thus, patients on immunosuppressive regimens may be seriously predisposed to development of toxoplasmosis.

In this review, we found 161 cases of toxoplasmosis that have been identified in the literature since 1953. We chose only those patients for whom there were sufficient clinical details and in whom the diagnosis was made by histopathology, or, in a setting of a suggestive clinical syndrome, concomitant significant changes in antibody titers and/or response to specific anti-*Toxoplasma* treatment. Of these 161 cases, 60% had fever, 14% presented with pneumonitis, 13% had evidence of myocarditis, 9% had hepatosplenomegaly, 15% had lymph node enlargement, and 7% had rash (Table 17.5). Given the vagaries associated with analysis of cumulative case reports and the complexity of the

Table 17.1   Predisposing conditions in 212* reported
cases of toxoplasmosis in the immunocompromised host

Underlying condition	Cases
Malignancy	
Hodgkin's lymphoma	59
Non-Hodgkin's lymphoma	12
Acute lymphocytic leukemia	11
Chronic lymphocytic leukemia	6
Acute myelogenous leukemia	7
Chronic myelogenous leukemia	9
Hairy cell leukemia	3
Angioimmunoblastic lymphadenopathy	4
Myeloma	2
Breast	3
Ovarian	2
Thymoma	2
Lung	1
Seminoma	1
Melanoma	1
Myelodysplastic syndrome	1
Chromophobe adenoma	1
Neuroblastoma	1
Waldenstrom's macroglobulinemia	1
Polycythemia vera	1
Organ transplantation	
Heart/heart-lung	24
Renal	22
Bone marrow	21
Liver	2
Collagen-vascular disease	
Systemic lupus erythematosus	8
Scleroderma	2
Corticosteroids	5

*See text for references.

individual underlying conditions in published reports, it cannot be concluded that these symptoms and signs were necessarily caused by toxoplasmosis (Table 17.5). Furthermore, the nature and degree of immunosuppression associated with the underlying conditions varied and may have influenced the clinicopathologic features of toxoplasmosis in the non-AIDS immunocompromised patient.

Central nervous system

Toxoplasmosis is an unusual cause of central nervous system (CNS) infections in non-AIDS immunocompromised patients (52,68). Nonetheless, our review confirms that

Table 17.2 Organ system infection with *Toxoplasma* in 52 transplant patients

Organ system	Bone marrow	Heart/heart-lung	Renal	Total
Number of case reports	20	15	17	52
Brain	16	9	12	37
Eye	1			1
Lung	7	2	7	16
Heart	11	10	9	30
Esophagus	1			1
Peritoneum				0
Liver	2	1	3	6
Spleen				0
Pancreas			2	2
Adrenal	1		2	3
Kidney	2		3	5
Testes			2	2
Muscle	1	1	5	7
Bone marrow	1	1		2
Lymph nodes	2		1	3
Skin	1			1
Salivary glands			1	1
Thyroid			1	1
Parathyroid			1	1

SOURCE See text for references.

encephalitis is the most common manifestation of toxoplasmosis in the non-AIDS immunocompromised host. Findings referable to the CNS in such cases include coma, seizures, alteration in mental status, motor weakness, cranial nerve disturbances, sensory disturbances, cerebellar signs, retinochoroiditis, meningeal signs, and movement disorders (6,16,49).

Of the 161 cases of toxoplasmosis in the immunocompromised host for which adequate information was available, 103 (64%) had encephalitis (Table 17.6). Altered mental status, manifested as lethargy, confusion, and disorientation, occurred in 67% of the cases. Other common features of toxoplasmic encephalitis were seizures in 28% and motor weakness in 25% of patients (6,16). Headache was stated to occur in only 17% of the reported cases: this low frequency likely reflects underreporting of headache rather than an actual low occurrence of this symptom.

Signs and symptoms associated with toxoplasmic encephalitis can be grouped into focal and nonfocal findings. Focal neurologic abnormalities included focal seizures, cranial nerve abnormalities, motor weakness, cerebellar signs, and meningeal signs. Nonfocal findings consisted of headache, altered mental status, lethargy, stupor, and coma. In the cases of toxoplasmic encephalitis in the non-AIDS immunocompromised patients identified in this literature review, 26% had focal presentations (6,8–10,12, 17,26,32,38,39,43,59,69–88), 40% had nonfocal presentations (5,11,12,14,17,27,

Table 17.3 Organ system infection with *Toxoplasma* in 49 patients with lymphoproliferative disease

Organ system	Hodgkin's lymphoma	Non-Hodgkin's lymphoma	Total
Number of case reports	41	8	49
Brain	34	6	40
Eye	4	2	6
Lung	5	3	8
Heart	6	3	9
Peritoneum		1	1
Liver		2	2
Spleen		3	3
Adrenal	1		1
Kidney	1		1
Muscle	1		1
Bone marrow	1	1	2
Lymph nodes		2	2

SOURCE See text for references.

Table 17.4 Organ system infection with *Toxoplasma* in 20 patients with leukemia

Organ system	Acute lymphocytic leukemia	Acute myelogenous leukemia	Chronic lymphocytic leukemia	Chronic myelogenous leukemia	Total
Number of case reports	11	3	1	5	20
Brain	7	2	1	5	15
Eye	1				1
Lung	3	1			4
Heart	5	1		1	7
Liver	2	1			3
Spleen	1				1
Pancreas	3				3
Kidney	2				2
Bone marrow	1				1
Lymph nodes	2				2

SOURCE See text for reference.

28,30–32,34,36,38,42,44,46,49,51,52,58,61,63,80,89–108), and 34% had both fo-cal and nonfocal presentations (5,10,13,26,28,31,34,37,40,41,47,48,53,54,56,57,59, 60,63,64,78,89,93,105,109–118). Miscellaneous neurologic disorders such as papill-edema, ataxia, aphasia, movement disorders, abnormal reflexes, and psychosis oc-curred in 1% to 5% of the cases (6,16) (Table 17.6).

In general, there were few abnormalities in the cerebrospinal fluids (CSF) of the

Table 17.5 Symptoms and signs reported concomitant with toxoplasmosis in immunocompromised patients

Condition	No. of cases	Fever	Dyspnea	Pneumonitis	Myocarditis	Hepato-splenomegaly	Lymph node enlargement	Rash
Malignancy								
Hodgkin's lymphoma	45	29	1	4	1	7	14	1
Lymphoma	8	6		3	1	2	1	1
Angioimmunoblastic lymphadenopathy	4	3	1		1	1	3	1
Acute lymphocytic leukemia	11	7		2	3	2	1	4
Acute myelogenous leukemia	4	4			1			2
Chronic lymphocytic leukemia	3	1		1			2	
Chronic myelogenous leukemia	4	4	1	1		1	2	
Hairy cell leukemia	2	1			1			
Breast cancer	2	2	2	1				
Melanoma	1	1						
Myeloma	2	2						
Transplant								
Heart	22	12		2	3			
Bone marrow	20	5	1	4	5		1	1
Renal	19	13	3	3	4	2		1
Liver	2	2	3					
SLE	7	3			1			
Corticosteroids	5	2		1				1
Total	161	97(60)	12(7)	22(14)	21(13)	15(9)	24(15)	12(7)

SOURCE: See text for references.

Table 17.6 Signs and symptoms reported in non-AIDS immunocompromised patients with toxoplasmic encephalitis

Condition	Cases of encephalitis	Head-ache	Altered mental status	Seizures	Coma	Cranial nerve abnor-mality	Motor weak-ness	Sensory changes	Cerebellar abnor-malities	Meningeal signs	Chorio-retinitis
Malignancy											
Hodgkin's lymphoma	38	4	16	5	10	8	12	3	3	4	5
Lymphoma	6		5		3					1	2
Angioimmunoblastic lymphadenopathy	1		2					1			
Acute lymphocytic leukemia	6	2	5	6	1	1	2				
Acute myelogenous leukemia	2	1	2	1							
Chronic lymphocytic leukemia	1										
Chronic myelogenous leukemia	4		2				3			1	
Hairy cell leukemia	1		2								
Breast cancer	1		1								
Myeloma	2	1	2		1	1					
Transplants											
Heart	8		6	3	1		1				3
Bone marrow	15	3	8	6	2	3	5				2
Renal	10	5	12	6	1		1	2	1		1
Liver	1									3	
Systemic lupus erythematosus	6	1	4	1	1		1		1		
Steroids	2	1	1	1			1				1
Total†	103(64)	18(17)	69(67)	29(28)	20(19)	14(14)	25(25)	8(8)	5(5)	9(9)	15(15)

Miscellaneous conditions reported were
*Movement disorder 5(5), papilledema 2(1), dysphasia 3(2), abnormal reflexes 7(4), ataxia 3(3), aphasia 4(3), psychosis 2(1).
†Number (percent).
SOURCE See text for references.

patients with toxoplasmic encephalitis. In most cases, results of the analysis were normal. The most common abnormalities reported included slight mononuclear pleocytosis and slightly elevated protein levels (5,31). Hypoglycorrhachia was reported to occur in 5% of individuals with toxoplasmic encephalitis (59). In our review of 53 cases of toxoplasmic encephalitis for which results of CSF analyses were fully reported (5–7,10,12,13,27,28,31,36,40,41,43,46,48,49,59,61,64,69–72,75,79,80,83,84,86,99, 101,110–112,114,116–124), the mean white blood cell count was 20/mm^3 (range 0 to 154), mean glucose value was 63 mg/dL (range 23 to 250), and mean protein value was 100 mg/dL (range 35 to 350).

Giemsa stains of CSF may be diagnostic since visualization of *Toxoplasma* in the CSF constitutes a definitive diagnosis (41,125). The frequency with which parasites are identified in the CSF of patients with toxoplasmic encephalitis has not been determined.

Involvement of the brain with *Toxoplasma* may be focal, multicentric, or diffuse. The classical anatomic feature of toxoplasmic encephalitis consists of small foci of perivascular inflammation and collection of microglial cells and astrocytes (31). *Toxoplasma* infection induces microglial cells to proliferate and form nodules. In the non-AIDS immunocompromised host, these microglial nodules are highly variable in stage of development and size and may be associated with necrosis. The degree of CNS pathology reflects the severity of immunosuppression and may vary from localized microglial nodule formation with surrounding gliosis to a fulminant necrotizing process (31). The larger, more severe lesions may result from acute vasculitis that often surrounds zones of coagulation necrosis (31).

The immune response of the brain to *Toxoplasma* infection is characterized by a mixed cellular infiltrate. Small lesions may be characterized by focal aggregates of lymphocytes and microglial cells. Larger, granulomatous lesions that contain macrophages, lymphocytes, plasma cells, and, less commonly, neutrophils may coalesce to form the inflammatory and necrotizing response to *Toxoplasma* infection (49). Both necrotizing and nonnecrotizing granulomatous lesions have been observed. Focal parenchymal lesions may have central zones of necrosis surrounded by mixed cellular infiltrates. Perivascular round cell infiltrates with necrosis of vessel walls may be a prominent feature of focal granulomatous lesions or may be present independently (16,49).

Focal lesions exhibit varying degrees of reactive astrocytosis at their periphery. Tachyzoites have been found within the parenchymal and perivascular infiltrates (31,49,60), as well as at the center of coagulative necrosis, and more abundantly at the periphery of necrotic foci in the brain (31,49).

Anatomical areas of frequent involvement include basal ganglia, corticomedullary junction, thalamus, and diffusely across the gray and white matter of the cerebrum and cerebellum (13,28,31,37,45,49,60). Diffuse cerebral involvement is frequently accompanied by necrosis of the pituitary gland (28). The leptomeninges are ordinarily spared. Nonspecific changes (e.g., vacuolation) within neurons and Purkinje cells and loss of Nissl substance may occur (16,49,126).

Clearly, encephalitis is related to unimpeded parasitization and destruction of brain parenchyma, but additional mechanisms may be responsible for the hemorrhagic or thrombotic infarction which results from toxoplasmic cerebral vasculitis (31). Henry et al. (127) described a thickening, with intense reticulum fiber deposition without evidence of parenchymal damage by *Toxoplasma*, in patients with cerebral lymphoma and toxoplasmic encephalitis. These findings suggested the possibility that, in these patients, normal lymphoid cells specifically induced the vasculitis. This obliterative vasculitis, unassociated with direct parasite infestation, may be part of the spectrum of histopathologic changes in toxoplasmic encephalitis. The contribution of inflammatory cells and chemically mediated destruction to the pathogenesis of an obliterative, occlusive, hypertrophic arteritis which leads to discrete coagulative necrosis in toxoplasmic encephalitis deserves further elucidation (127,128). Theoretically, occlusive hypertrophic arteritis results when *Toxoplasma* invades the vessel wall and induces segmental necrosis, followed by fibroreticular hyperplasia and vascular occlusion (128,129).

Since cerebral lesions may be devoid of inflammatory cellular response and since isolated tachyzoites have been identified in neutrophils (123), macrophages (123), neurons (49,91,92), glia (49,91,92), vascular endothelium (49,91,92), and pericytes (49,91,92), granulomatous lesions, and perivascular infiltrates (49,91,92), it appears unlikely that hypersensitivity plays a major role in the pathogenesis of toxoplasmic encephalitis in non-AIDS immunosuppressed patients (129).

A precise rapid diagnosis of toxoplasmic encephalitis can be made by electron microscopy (45), as well as by the highly specific and sensitive immunoperoxidase histologic staining method (130).

Eye

Ocular toxoplasmosis, most often a result of reactivation of latent infection, may be the first manifestation of a life-threatening infectious disease in the immunocompromised patient. Cyst rupture and release of parasites which disseminate to or contiguously infect retinal tissue may result in sight-threatening disease, when mechanisms of normal host immunity (which maintain encysted forms in a quiescent state) are abrogated by immunosuppressive treatments or rendered incompetent by underlying disease. Early diagnosis allows for prompt administration of treatment, often sparing sight (131).

The underlying conditions reported in association with toxoplasmic retinochoroiditis are heterogeneous and include angioimmunoblastic lymphadenopathy (99), common mixed variable immunodeficiency syndrome (132), and thymoma (133); more frequently, toxoplasmic retinochoroiditis has been reported in cases of Hodgkin's and non-Hodgkin's lymphoma (34,65,88,96,101,118,134). In this review, we identified 17 reported cases of toxoplasmic retinochoroiditis in non-AIDS immunocompromised patients (8,14,34,36,43,46,65,88,96,99,101,110,118,132–134); of these, 12 (71%) had an accompanying toxoplasmic encephalitis (8,14,34,36,43,46,88,96,99,101,110,118). Fever was recorded in five (29%) (43,88,101,110,118). It is noteworthy that, of the 16 cases where sufficient histopathologic details were provided (8,34,36,43,46,65,88,96, 99,101,110,118,132–134), 11 (69%) had toxoplasmic encephalitis (8,34,36,43,46,88, 96,99,101,110,118), three had evidence of toxoplasmic myocarditis (14,36,43), and, in one, *Toxoplasma* was isolated from the blood (132).

Toxoplasmic retinochoroiditis should be suspected in immunocompromised patients (especially those seropositive for toxoplasma antibodies) who complain of decreased visual acuity (134) and who, on ophthalmoscopic examination, have exudative retinal lesions and vitreal haziness with mild anterior chamber reaction (118,134). In contrast to the immunocompetent patient, the absence of anterior chamber reaction on ophthalmoscopic examination of immunocompromised patients does not preclude the diagnosis of toxoplasmic chorioretinitis (88). Lesions may involve one (65,88,134) or both (118) eyes.

The consistent absence of retinal scarring at the time of diagnosis in well-described reports (65,88,118,134) suggests the possibility that dissemination of *Toxoplasma* to the eye, rather than intraocular reactivation of latent infection, is the pathogenic mechanism for the development of toxoplasmic retinochoroiditis. Moreover, gross pathology of retinal lesions reveals a primarily perivascular pattern (65,131), which has been interpreted by others as being reflective of hematogenous dissemination to the retina (65,88). The occurrence of toxoplasmic retinochoroiditis in seronegative recipients of hearts transplanted from seropositive donors (14,36) is further strong, presumptive evidence for the likelihood that this entity follows hematogenous dissemination to the eye.

Toxoplasmosis in the immunocompromised patient should be considered in the differential diagnosis of any inflammatory or necrotizing retinitis distributed along the course of retinal vessels (65). Toxoplasmic retinochoroiditis may be severe and result in destruction of retinal tissues in the macular area and optic disk (65,118). Microscopic examination has demonstrated tachyzoites and *Toxoplasma* cysts with little surrounding retinal inflammation (65,88). Subsequent proliferation of glial cells and lymphoplasmacytic infiltration of residual tissue may provide the pathologic basis for diminished visual acuity (88,118). In toxoplasmic retinochoroiditis, the optic nerve may be atrophic, with both tachyzoites and *Toxoplasma* cysts present in all laminar regions (65,88). In contrast, despite extensive infestation of the retina, parasites may only rarely, if at all, infect the choroid. Choroiditis, therefore, is likely a secondary inflammatory response to the infection and necrosis in the retina (88).

In a patient with non-Hodgkin's lymphoma and with a postmortem diagnosis of toxoplasmic retinochoroiditis, who had been treated with a prolonged course of high doses of corticosteroids, histopathologic sections of the retina revealed extensive necrosis but only scant associated inflammation (65). The absence of retinal inflammation in the presence of extensive necrosis by *Toxoplasma* is consistent with experimental results in immunosuppressed animals (135). Thus, retinal destruction in immunocompromised patients with toxoplasmosis may be a result of suppression of cell-mediated immunity to replication of *Toxoplasma* in contrast to a secondary hypersensitivity reaction. Thus, while corticosteroids are indicated for prevention and treatment of iridocyclitis, vitritis, or papillitis in the immunocompetent patient with toxoplasmic retinochoroiditis (136), their use in the immunocompromised patient, who may have a different pathological basis for retinochoroiditis, is controversial.

Heart

Toxoplasma infection of the heart may or may not lead to clinically significant disease. This form of myocarditis has been recognized in patients with Hodgkin's and non-Hodgkin's lymphoma who were receiving chemotherapy (5,27,31). Toxoplasmic myocarditis has been reported more frequently in patients with acute lymphocytic leukemia than in those with other types of hematologic malignancies and is well described in recipients of allogeneic bone marrow and orthotopic cardiac transplants (8,13–15,44,137,138) (Tables 17.2,17.4).

Immunocompromised patients with toxoplasmic myocarditis may present with congestive heart failure (8,17,89), pericarditis (139), and arrhythmias (8,43,53), including bundle branch block due to lesions in the conducting system (139,140). In patients who are severely immunosuppressed, untreated toxoplasmic myocarditis is almost always fatal in days to weeks (12,17,28,31,53,139).

Despite the well-described occurrence of toxoplasmic myocarditis, descriptions of the pathology associated with this disorder are sparse. At autopsy, the heart may appear grossly normal, hypertrophic, or dilated, and show petecchial hemorrhages and grayish-yellow mottling due to focal necrosis (8,12,31,139). Microscopically, there is focal necrosis with edema and a cellular infiltrate composed of lymphocytes, plasma cells, histiocytes, and occasionally eosinophils (8,31,76,139). Myocardial cell fibers packed with tachyzoites have been described (13). These "pseudocysts" (accumulations of large numbers of intracellular organisms but not a true cyst) seldom generate an inflammatory response such as is seen following cell rupture and release of tachyzoites. Rupture of the pseudocyst leads to release of extracellular tachyzoites which are then free to parasitize surrounding normal cells and evoke mononuclear cell invasion and cell death (8). The focal fibrosis that follows healing of the necrotic foci is suggestive of the diagnosis of toxoplasmic myocarditis (15). The suppression of chemotaxic responses in patients receiving immunosuppressive agents may result in unimpeded parasitization and absence of an inflammatory response. Thus, the presence of myocyte necrosis, unaccompanied by an inflammatory response or fibrotic replacement of individual myocytes, in the appropriate setting should suggest the possibility of toxoplasmic myocarditis (15,76). In such cases, immunohistochemical staining techniques may be valuable in identification of *Toxoplasma* organisms (130).

Lung

Although it is not usually clinically apparent, toxoplasmic pneumonitis has been recognized as a cause of respiratory insufficiency in non-AIDS immunocompromised patients (Table 17.5). In our review of 39 cases with autopsy evidence of *Toxoplasma* infection of the lung (11,12,17,27,28,31,32,36–38,42,44,47,53,54,55,57–60,63,66, 82,84,89,95,102,108,113,141–143), only 15 (38%) had clinical evidence of pneumonitis before death (12,28,44,54,55,58,60,66,82,102,108,113,142). A recent review of the literature, which used strict diagnostic criteria, identified 12 cases of toxoplasmic pneumonitis in non-AIDS immunocompromised patients (144). Associated underlying illnesses included lymphoma (82,145), renal transplantation (26,108), multiple myeloma (146), bone marrow transplantation (147), hepatorenal transplantation (26), and oat cell carcinoma (148).

The clinical and radiologic features of toxoplasmic pneumonitis are not specific. Patients are usually febrile and complain of fever, dyspnea, and nonproductive cough.

Rales may be appreciated over the involved lung (144,149). Toxoplasmic encephalitis may be associated with, preceded by, or follow onset or development of pneumonia (21,31,82). The limited number of carefully described cases does not allow for determination of whether there are radiologic criteria that might be helpful to distinguish toxoplasmic pneumonitis from other infectious and noninfectious diseases that affect the lungs of these patients. In the appropriate clinical setting, however, the presence of a milliary pattern or patchy interstitial infiltrates on chest radiography should suggest the possibility of toxoplasmosis. Abnormal chest radiographs have been reported with interstitial and alveolar (28), bilateral interstitial (26,57,108), lobar (26,55), and diffuse nodular (142,150) infiltrates. Whether these radiographic abnormalities were related to toxoplasmosis was not always clear. Furthermore, often the diagnosis of toxoplasmic pneumonitis is confounded by the coexistence of other pathogens in the lungs of these patients (151). Consequently, the diagnosis of toxoplasmic pneumonitis has often been putative and based on identification of the parasite at extrapulmonary sites or by serologic criteria (12,44,146).

Definitive diagnosis can be established rapidly by fiberoptic bronchoscopy with Giemsa or eosin-methylene blue-stained preparations of bronchoalveolar lavage (BAL) or fluid or transbronchial biopsy material (26,108,147,152), or by open lung biopsy (145).

In this context, however, it is instructive to note a case of a patient with Hodgkin's lymphoma who had a negative BAL smear and who went on to die of toxoplasmic pneumonitis (82). BAL specimens can be cultured by traditional methods of mouse inoculation, but this may be impractical due to the necessity for animal facilities and time required for processing. Recently described methods for the successful culture of *T. gondii* in cell cultures two days after inoculation, using an immunofluorescence assay, have been employed successfully in patients with toxoplasmic pneumonitis and AIDS (152).

Microscopically, focal fibrosis has been observed surrounding areas of interstitial pneumonia. Alveolar capillaries may be markedly congested with abundant hemosiderin-laden macrophages (82). Tachyzoites may be present in multiple foci of necrosis, with complete ablation of the normal pulmonary architecture (28,31). Extensive interstitial pneumonitis with thickened hyaline membrane, alveoli-containing, sparse round cell infiltrates, and large prominent alveolar lining cells have been described (28). Groups of encysted parasites have been found within alveolar lining cells and in intraalveolar macrophages (28).

Other organs

There is great variability in cutaneous *Toxoplasma* lesions in the immunocompetent patient with acute acquired toxoplasmosis (Tables 17.2–17.4)(153). Nodular, purpuric, papulopustular, lichenoid, vegetating, and erythema multiformelike lesions have all been observed grossly (139,154–156); necrosis, vasculitis, perivasculitis, periadenexal inflammation, and granulomas have been described microscopically (115). The diagnosis in most cases of toxoplasmic dermatitis was presumptive and was based on serologic test results alone. Thus, the diagnosis of toxoplasmosis as a cause of dermatologic lesions in such cases must be accepted with caution. There is a report of a definitively diagnosed case of *Toxoplasma* infection of the skin in a 16-year-old who had received a bone marrow transplant and presented with purpuric nodules (115). Skin biopsy in this case revealed the presence of *Toxoplasma* cysts and extracellular tachyzoites, without an accompanying inflammatory response in the epidermis or dermis (115).

Acute acquired *Toxoplasma* infection is a cause of lymphadenopathy in immunocompetent individuals. In the setting of normal host immunity, the characteristic triad of florid reactive follicular hyperplasia, irregular clusters of epithelioid histiocytes and focal subcapsular distention (often encroaching on and blurring the margins of the germinal centers), and focal distention of the subcapsular and trabecular sinuses by reactive monocytoid B-cells (157–161) is highly suggestive of toxoplasmic lymphadenitis. In a recent study, polymerase chain reaction (PCR) (using four oligonucleotides corresponding to the genome of *T. gondii*) contributed little diagnostic utility over application of the classic pathologic triad to the evaluation of cases of suspected toxoplasmic lymphadenitis in immunocompetent individuals (161); however, *Toxoplasma* has only rarely been identified in lymph nodes of immunocompetent individuals with toxoplasmic lymphadenitis (157–160,162). An alternative explanation, therefore, for the lack of predictive value of the current *Toxoplasma* PCR is that the pathology of toxoplasmic lymphadenitis in the immunocompetent individual is a result of the humoral response to *Toxoplasma*. In contrast, the frequent observation of numerous *Toxoplasma* cysts in lymph node sections obtained from immunocompromised patients who died with disseminated toxoplasmosis (5,17,28,31,44,59,89,163) suggests a different pathogenic mechanism for toxoplasmic lymphadenitis in the cases that occur in patients with normal immunity. Thus, if toxoplasmic lymphadenitis in immunocompromised patients results from decreased immunity to replication of *Toxoplasma* and not an inflammatory response to the parasite, we would suspect histopathologic features in this setting to be different from the classic triad observed in immunocompetent individuals. In addition, if the mechanism of toxoplasmic lymphadenitis in immunocompromised patients primarily reflects parasite burden and not inflammatory response, a sensitive PCR should reveal the presence of *T. gondii*, in contrast to lymph nodes obtained from immunocompetent individuals with acute acquired toxoplasmosis. Unfortunately, there are insufficient data to definitively address these issues.

In our review, 10 patients were identified with toxoplasmic lymphadenitis by histopathology, and four (40%) of these, in fact, had lymphadenopathy at presentation of toxoplasmosis. Six of the cases of histopathologically proven toxoplasmic lymphadenitis were associated with disseminated toxoplasmosis, including involvement of brain, heart, pancreas, bone marrow, peripheral nerve, gastrointestinal, and genitourinary tracts (17,28,31,44,59,89).

Importantly, of these patients with lymphadenopathy and histopathologically proven toxoplasmic lymphadenitis, three had Hodgkin's disease. Furthermore, of 27 cases of non-AIDS immunocompromised patients presenting with lymphadenopathy at the time of diagnosis of toxoplasmosis (5,11,80,81,84,96,103,107,132,163–167), 21 occurred in patients with lymphoproliferative disorders (5,80,84,89,96,103,107,163, 164,166,167). Thus, the possibility of coincidence of *Toxoplasma* and lymphoproliferative disorders may make the evaluation and management of lymphadenopathy in non-AIDS immunocompromised patients fraught with therapeutic and diagnostic challenges (5,89,163,164,167).

Histopathologically demonstrated toxoplasmic myositis has been reported in a renal transplantation recipient (50) and in a patient with hairy cell leukemia (97). Other cases reported must be regarded as presumptive, since they were diagnosed based on serologic changes in *Toxoplasma* antibody titers (119,168,169). Skeletal muscles are commonly found to be involved on postmortem evaluation of non-AIDS immunocompromised patients with disseminated toxoplasmosis (15,44,47,48,57,58,61,82,113,166).

Disseminated toxoplasmosis in the non-AIDS immunocompromised host has involved the gastrointestinal tract, including pancreas (17,28,31,58,108,139), liver (7,12, 55,57–59,95,108,166,170), spleen (7,12,59,89,170), and colon (59), as well as the peritoneum (89), kidneys (17,31,44,47,53,57,101,139), and testicles (28,57). Adrenal, pituitary, thyroid, and parathyroid glands have all been found to be involved on postmortem examination of patients with disseminated toxoplasmosis (12,28,54,57,58,82,95).

UNDERLYING CONDITIONS PREDISPOSING TO TOXOPLASMOSIS IN THE NON-AIDS IMMUNOCOMPROMISED PATIENT

Malignancies

Toxoplasmosis is a relatively uncommon opportunistic infectious disease in the cancer patient (5–7,17,28,29,31,49,59,63,71–74,77–84,87–90,92–94,96,97,99–104, 107,109,110,112–114,117,119,122,133,134,139,145,148,150,163,164,166,170–174). A review of patients seen at Memorial Sloan Kettering Cancer Center in New York between 1967 and 1978 identified 39 cases of toxoplasmosis in patients with malignancies (5,7). In the majority, toxoplasmosis was diagnosed at the time of progression of their cancer (7). Thirty-three of the 39 patients were receiving corticosteroids, alkylating agents, antimetabolites, or radiation therapy, and 10% were in remission when toxoplasmosis was diagnosed (5,7). The frequency of occurrence of toxoplasmosis in the variety of neoplastic disorders reported by Hakes et al. ranged from two per 10,000 patients with breast cancer to 366 per 10,000 patients with chronic lymphocytic leukemia (7). These estimates reflect the prevalence of *Toxoplasma* infection in patients seen at Memorial Sloan Kettering Cancer Center during the years of study and not an absolute rate of development of toxoplasmosis, since toxoplasmosis in cancer patients most often results from reactivation of latent infection.

Toxoplasmosis in cancer patients has most frequently been described in association with Hodgkin's disease (2,5,16,31,163). It has also been associated with lymphosarcoma and reticulum cell sarcoma (159), acute and chronic leukemias (2,5,31,105,139,175), multiple myeloma (124), myeloid metaplasia (94), and, less frequently, with other hematologic or lymphoproliferative disorders, e.g., hairy cell leukemia (97,174) and angioimmunoblastic lymphadenopathy (31,80,99,166). Toxoplasmosis has also been recognized in patients with solid tumors, usually associated with antineoplastic treatment (e.g., breast (7,28,92), ovarian (7,173), thymus (114), and lung carcinoma (148)).

It has also been reported to complicate chromophobe adenoma (114), neuroblastoma (5), seminoma (92), and melanoma (31).

Although the most common malignancy associated with toxoplasmosis is Hodgkin's disease, toxoplasmosis is unusual in patients with this disease (4). In one report, it was estimated to occur in 3% of individuals with Hodgkin's disease (7). In a review of 81 non-AIDS immunocompromised patients with toxoplasmosis, 32 (40%) had Hodgkin's disease (2). In our review of 217 cases of toxoplasmosis in non-AIDS immuno-compromised individuals, 59 (27%) had Hodgkin's disease (Table 17.1). Those patients without clinical evidence of encephalitis were most often symptomatic with fever (Table 17.7). Autopsy studies reveal that, in patients with lymphoproliferative disease and toxoplasmosis, the most common organs involved were brain, eye, lung, and heart. Approximately 80% had toxoplasmic encephalitis. It is noteworthy that there was wide dissemination of *Toxoplasma* to other organ systems, including the gastrointestinal tract, musculoskeletal system, and endocrine glands (Table 17.3).

The mechanisms by which Hodgkin's disease predisposes to development of toxoplasmosis have not been well characterized. Whether Hodgkin's disease or the immunosuppressive agents used for its treatment are of greater importance in suppressing immunity against *Toxoplasma* is unclear. Hodgkin's disease is associated with both quantitative and qualitative defects in cell-mediated immunity (115,176–182). Lymphocyte proliferation to *Toxoplasma* antigen has been found to be impaired in patients with *Toxoplasma* infection and Hodgkin's disease (183,184). Clearly T-cell dysfunction associated with Hodgkin's disease, augmented by the use of immunosuppressive therapies, predisposes to development of toxoplasmosis. While most reported cases of toxoplasmosis in patients with Hodgkin's disease occurred in the setting of treatment with cytotoxic agents at the time of the diagnosis, several cases have been reported in which toxoplasmosis was temporally remote from the last cycle of chemotherapy (7,112) and occurred even prior to initiation of chemotherapy (113). This has been dramatically described in a patient who presented with stage IIIB Hodgkin's disease for which treatment was delayed because of severe toxoplasmic encephalitis (113).

Distinguishing Hodgkin's disease from acute acquired *Toxoplasma* infection may be difficult, especially since both of these disorders can produce lymphadenopathy, the most common manifestation of acute acquired toxoplasmosis in the immunologically normal patient. Toxoplasmic lymphadenitis, not uncommon in immunocompetent patients with acute acquired toxoplasmosis, has been reported only infrequently in patients with toxoplasmosis and underlying lymphoproliferative disorders. Moreover, since these disorders may coexist, multiple biopsies may be necessary for a definitive diagnosis and appropriate subsequent management (5,112,113).

Identification of toxoplasmosis in patients with active lymphoproliferative disease is crucial since treatment of these two conditions is different. In addition, treatment of neoplasia may lead to reactivation of latent, or worsening of an already active, *Toxoplasma* infection, with resulting morbidity. Patients with leukemia and toxoplasmosis generally present with fever (5,16,17,31,53,71,79,86,97,119,170). Definitive demonstration of transfusion-related acute acquired infection has been reported in two patients with leukemia (17). Fortunately, the occurrence of transfusion-related toxoplasmosis is uncommon and unlikely to be a significant cause of toxoplasmosis in patients with

Table 17.7 Symptoms reported in 45 patients with Hodgkin's disease and toxoplasmic encephalitis

Symptoms	Number (percent)
Fever	28 (62)
Lymph node enlargement	15 (33)
Neurologic symptoms	38 (84)
Coma	9 (20)
Seizures	5 (11)
Altered mental status	16 (36)
Hemiparesis	12 (27)
Cranial nerve changes	11 (24)
Sensory changes	3 (7)
Cerebellar signs	3 (7)
Chorioretinitis	5 (11)
Headache	4 (9)
Dysphagia	3 (7)
Meningeal signs	4 (9)
Movement disorder	1 (2)

SOURCE References 5,6,28,31,49,59,69,72,74,77,78,82–84,89,90, 102–104,110,113,117,118,122,134,163,164.

leukemia (185). Wide dissemination of *Toxoplasma* infection in patients with leukemia has been reported to involve liver (31), spleen (31,170), pancreas (17,31,139), kidney (17,31,139), bone marrow (17,29), and lymph nodes (17).

Infections are the primary cause of morbidity and mortality in hairy cell leukemia (174). Hairy cell leukemia may increase the susceptibility to *Toxoplasma* infection because of dysfunction in the monocyte/macrophage cells which serve as important effector cells in host defense against this pathogen (186–188).

Toxoplasmic myositis and encephalitis have been observed in patients undergoing chemotherapy for this disease (97,174). In one study, two of 22 patients with hairy cell leukemia had a febrile illness accompanied by significant changes in IgG antibody titer and were judged clinically to have toxoplasmosis (189). In a more recent study, three of 15 patients with hairy cell leukemia had significant changes in their *Toxoplasma* serologic test titers; this was considered by the investigators to suggest reactivation of chronic *Toxoplasma* infection (190).

Organ transplantation

Toxoplasmosis is a well-recognized, though uncommon, opportunistic infection in patients with transplants. The brain is the most common organ site involved; however, pneumonitis and myocarditis were reported more frequently in patients with heart/ heart-lung and bone marrow transplants than in patients with lymphoproliferative disease (Tables 17.2,17.5).

Heart/heart-lung In heart transplant recipients (14,15,30,32–38,76,88,138,143, 150,191–193), central nervous system infections occur primarily in the first 90 days after surgery (126,194) and are a major cause of morbidity (32). Infections, in general, account for as many as 54% of cardiac transplant recipient deaths (34). In a recently reported series, 13 (3%) of 417 heart/heart-lung transplant recipients developed CNS infection, and two (15%) of the 13 were due to *Toxoplasma* (34). Similarly, the series reported from Stanford revealed intracranial infection from nonviral agents to occur in 25 (14%) of 182 recipients of heart/heart-lung transplants, and four of the 25 were due to cerebral toxoplasmosis (32). Between 7% and 20% of all cardiac transplantations in the United States, England, and the Netherlands are between seronegative recipients and seropositive donors (35,38,193,195,196). In addition, heart/heart-lung transplant recipients with toxoplasmosis are at risk for development of disseminated infection involving multiple organs (15,26,30,32,37,138,143,151) (Table 17.2).

Toxoplasmosis in heart/heart-lung transplant recipients occurs following transplantation of a (mismatched) heart from a *Toxoplasma* seropositive donor to a seronegative recipient (Table 17.8). Infection in the donor heart is reactivated in the recipient in the presence of immunosuppressive therapy. In this setting, dissemination and death have occurred in as brief a period as three weeks (32).

Twenty-four cases of toxoplasmosis were identified in our review of toxoplasmosis in heart transplant recipients (Table 17.1). Eighteen of these were definitely proven by demonstration of *Toxoplasma* organisms on endomyocardial biopsy or at necropsy (13,15,32,38,43,45,59,191). The remainder were diagnosed presumptively in an appropriate clinical setting of a seronegative recipient of a heart from a seropositive donor with fever, constitutional symptoms, and fourfold or greater rise in serologic test titers for *Toxoplasma* antibodies. Fever was a common finding (15,30,36,38,138,191). Signs and symptoms of disease began as early as the twelfth postoperative day to as late as 301 days after transplantation (14,32). Pneumonitis (138), myocarditis (15,138), and encephalitis were the major clinical syndromes associated with toxoplasmosis in heart transplant recipients (14,16,32,34,36–38,138) (Tables 17.5,17.6). The presence of tachyzoites and/or cysts on endomyocardial biopsy performed routinely in evaluation of heart transplant rejection may be an early finding in subclinical *Toxoplasma* infection and lead to the institution of life-saving therapy. Moreover, *Toxoplasma* infection, rather than graft-versus-host disease, may lead to rejection in heart transplant recipients (15,33,76). *Toxoplasma* infection observed on routine endomyocardial biopsy has allowed prompt diagnosis of cardiac rejection caused by *Toxoplasma* (33). However, the interstitial mononuclear cell infiltrates that follow release of parasites from infected myofibers are similar to those observed in acute rejection (76,191). Therefore, it is frequently unclear whether acute rejection is related to graft-versus-host response or reactivation of transplanted *Toxoplasma* infection. This differential diagnosis is critical, since immune-mediated heart rejection is usually treated with increased immunosuppressive drugs, an intervention that may exacerbate *Toxoplasma* infection (37). Tragic cases of disseminated toxoplasmosis have been precipitated by erroneous findings of heart transplant rejection in mismatched patients, who subsequently underwent treatment with high doses of corticosteroids (33,34,37). The finding of eosinophils on endo-

Table 17.8   *Toxoplasma* infection transmitted through organ transplantation

Organ system	No	Probable	Definite	Unknown
Bone marrow	X*			
Heart/heart-lung			X	
Renal			X	
Liver				X

*A case of toxoplasmosis in a seronegative recipient of bone marrow from a donor with acute acquired *Toxoplasma* infection has been reported (165).
SOURCE see text for references.

myocardial biopsy may alert the pathologist to suspect toxoplasmosis versus acute transplant rejection (38,76). A high index of suspicion of toxoplasmosis in serologically mismatched patients is warranted and should prompt careful review of all endomyocardial biopsies, since early medical intervention may prevent significant morbidity and mortality. Eight of the heart transplant recipients diagnosed antemortem with toxoplasmosis were treated. Six of the eight improved, whereas each of the seven who did not receive treatment died of complications of disseminated *Toxoplasma* infection (15,34,37,136).

Bone marrow   Although bone marrow transplant recipients are at high risk for opportunistic infections, the rate of occurrence of toxoplasmosis in these patients is low (8,9,11–13,40–45,115,165). In 2,000 bone marrow transplant patients at the Fred Hutchinson Cancer Research Center, 10 cases of toxoplasmosis were reported (44). Toxoplasmosis should be suspected in *Toxoplasma* antibody-positive recipients of allogeneic bone marrow who present with fever, shortness of breath, cough, tachyarrhythmias, congestive heart failure, or signs and symptoms referable to the CNS 30 to 100 days following bone marrow transplantation. The 21 cases included in our analysis had sufficient data reported to make a definitive diagnosis of toxoplasmosis either by histopathologic criteria (8,9,11–13,41,43,45,115) or isolation of parasites from the blood of patients with a clinical course suggestive of toxoplasmosis and who responded to specific treatment (11,44). The conditions for which patients underwent allogeneic bone marrow transplantation were varied, although most cases reported were acute myelogenous leukemia (8,11,13,43); other associated underlying conditions have included chronic myelogenous leukemia (8,45,115), acute lymphocytic leukemia (11,12), aplastic anemia (11,12,115), and Burkitt's lymphoma (41).

Although unusual, acute acquired toxoplasmosis in the post-bone-marrow-transplantation state has been observed in a seronegative recipient of a seronegative donor (11). Recipients of allogeneic bone marrow transplantation are at increased risk for complications of acute acquired *Toxoplasma* infection, since cellular and humoral immune defense mechanisms are severely impaired during the post-bone-marrow-transplant period. This possibility of acquiring the infection is limited, however, because the patient is hospitalized during this period. In a recent report, a 12-year-old seronegative recipient of a bone marrow from a donor with serologic evidence of acute *Toxoplasma* infection developed prolonged fevers without clear etiology. Although animal inoculation and cell line culture of whole blood and bone marrow failed to isolate the parasite, a polymerase chain reaction detected *Toxoplasma* in both blood and bone marrow biopsy from the patient (165). The authors who reported this unusual case speculated that donor immune T-cells were removed by the use of Campath-IG and treatment with cyclosporin A (165).

Clinical disease in these patients generally reflects encephalitis, myocarditis, and pneumonitis. These are sufficiently well-recognized entities in the post-bone-marrow-transplant period that their appearance in the appropriate context should suggest the diagnosis of toxoplasmosis. The dominant clinical picture is that of a diffuse encephalitis or myocarditis complicated by congestive heart failure or arrhythmias (8,11). Similar to the other types of non-AIDS immunocompromised patients, encephalitis has been reported in the majority of cases of toxoplasmosis in bone marrow transplantation recipients (8,11,12,44). Involvement of the heart by *Toxoplasma* has been increasingly recognized as a cause of death after bone marrow transplantation (43). The association of myocarditis and interstitial pneumonitis has been commonly observed (8,11,12,44). In fact, of the reported cases we reviewed, the rate of myocardial and lung involvement was higher in bone marrow transplant recipients than in any other group of non-AIDS immunocompromised patients. Whether the idiopathic interstitial pneumonitis described in several cases was caused by disseminated *Toxoplasma* infection versus other conditions associated with lung disease in these patients is unclear (8,11).

Graft-versus-host disease treated with high doses of corticosteroids was temporally related to development of toxoplasmosis in six of eight cases reported by Beelen et al. and Derouin (8,11). Of 21 cases of toxoplasmosis in bone marrow transplant recipients, 13 had received additional immunosuppression with corticosteroids within weeks of the development of signs and symptoms of toxoplasmosis (8,9,11–13,43,44).

Unusual manifestations of toxoplasmosis have been described in bone marrow transplant recipients. A patient with acute lymphoblastic leukemia developed biopsy-proven toxoplasmic encephalitis and hemolytic uremic syndrome, presumed to be on the basis of toxoplasmosis (9). Tachyzoites were seen in the CSF of a patient with Burkitt's lymphoma who presented with multiple brain lesions on computed tomography (CT) scan but with a negative brain biopsy (41). Leyva described the first histopathologically documented case of toxoplasmosis presenting with cutaneous nodules (115). Hirsch described a case of biopsy-proven toxoplasmic hepatitis (12). In addition to the usual sites of organ involvement, *Toxoplasma* has been shown on autopsy studies to involve the adrenals, kidney, muscle, bone marrow itself, and lymph nodes (Table 17.2).

The protean manifestations and their relatively uncommon occurrence contribute to difficulties in diagnosis of toxoplasmosis in the bone marrow transplant recipient. Moreover, serology is of no value in the diagnosis of active infection in bone marrow recipients (11).

The existence of pretransplant antibodies to *Toxoplasma* is the major discriminatory test for evaluating those bone marrow recipients at greatest risk for development of toxoplasmosis. Unfortunately, serial changes in *Toxoplasma* antibody titers cannot be relied upon to diagnose toxoplasmosis in the post-bone-marrow state. In a recent systematic, clinical, and serologic follow-up of 241 bone marrow transplant recipients,

154 had a positive pretransplant *Toxoplasma* serology (11,137). Of these, 11 had severe toxoplasmosis, and, in 10 of them, the serology of the donor was negative at the time of transplantation. These observations suggest the possibility of protection of bone marrow transplant recipients against development of toxoplasmosis by the (seropositive donor) marrow (11,137). Furthermore, in the 87 seronegative recipients, clinical toxoplasmosis was not observed, suggesting that the risk of transmission from either transplantation or the environment is extremely low. Of the 11 cases of toxoplasmosis reported in that study, six had chronic myelogenous leukemia as their pretransplant diagnosis (Derouin F, personal communication). Details of other cases of toxoplasmosis in bone marrow transplant recipients substantiate the observation of seropositivity as a risk factor for development of disseminated toxoplasmosis (13,43). Thus, while there may be a rationale for prophylaxis of certain groups of bone marrow transplant recipients in the posttransplant stage (Derouin), this is, at present, controversial (197). Nevertheless, the lack of predictive value of serology and high risk of reactivation of chronic infection in the posttransplant state underscore the importance of determining *Toxoplasma* antibody titers in all patients prior to allogeneic bone marrow transplantation.

Renal Clinical and serological data reveal that the potential risk of developing *Toxoplasma* infection after renal transplantation is very low. Of 73 consecutive kidney transplant recipients, nine had serologic evidence of either acute acquired (198) or reactivation *Toxoplasma* infection (199). None of the patients with serologic evidence of active *Toxoplasma* infection developed clinical disease (199). Antibody titers to toxoplasma in renal transplant recipients indicate that the immunosuppressive regimens used may favor reactivation of the infection (133).

Recently, it has been clearly demonstrated that disseminated toxoplasmosis may occur in *Toxoplasma* seronegative recipients who receive renal allografts from seropositive donors (26,53,54,108). It is likely that, in these cases, *Toxoplasma* was transmitted to the recipient through the transplanted organ and rapidly disseminated in the setting of immunosuppressive treatments. Moreover, renal transplantation from a donor with acute acquired *Toxoplasma* infection has led to disastrous consequences (53). Whether clinically significant toxoplasmosis ever occurs in renal allograft recipients with pretransplant immunity to *Toxoplasma* is uncertain. Toxoplasmosis in patients who are recipients of renal transplants may present as an encephalitis (26–28,46–48,51–54,57–60,75,92,108), myocarditis (54,60), and pneumonitis (26,28,58,108). In these cases, postmortem evaluation generally has revealed disseminated infection with involvement of liver (47,55,57,58,108), pancreas (28,58,108), recipient kidney (47,53,57), muscle (48,57), lymph nodes (28), salivary (28), thyroid (28), pituitary (28), adrenal (28), and parathyroid (27) glands (Table 17.2).

Liver *Toxoplasma* in liver transplant recipients is rare (98,121). In a recent series, only one case of toxoplasmosis occurred in 101 consecutive liver transplantations (121). The patient was not treated and had a self-limited infection which was diagnosed by buffy coat inoculation into tissue culture (98). In the one case reported in the literature of fatal *Toxoplasma* infection in a liver transplant recipient, the likely cause was the increasing immunosuppressive regimens (200).

Miscellaneous conditions

Systemic lupus erythematosus Infection is a major cause of death in patients with systemic lupus erythematosus (SLE). A recent retrospective study noted that 33% of 1,103 patients with SLE died from infection (201). A more recent analysis of 50 patients with SLE found 44 fatal infections, two of which were due to *Toxoplasma* (62). The predisposing factor determined by logistic regression analysis of the major individual variables for development of opportunistic infection was prednisone administration (62).

Each of the cases of histologically proven toxoplasmosis in patients with SLE occurred while the affected individuals were receiving immunosuppressive agents. Toxoplasmic encephalitis, frequently misdiagnosed as lupus cerebritis and treated with increasing doses of corticosteroids, has resulted in disastrous consequences (10,28,44,59,61,117). Recent evidence suggests that high titers to *Toxoplasma* antibodies are significantly more common in patients with SLE than in normal controls (202).

Corticosteroid treatment Experiments performed in animal models provide convincing evidence of the effect of corticosteroids in predisposing to dissemination of latent *Toxoplasma* infection (203). For instance, animals pretreated with cortisone have increased susceptibility to infection with *Toxoplasma* (204). The administration of corticosteroids to rats, which are ordinarily highly resistant, increased their susceptibility to toxoplasmosis and most likely led to their death (203,205).

The immunosuppressive effects of large doses of corticosteroids have been associated with worsening of ocular toxoplasmosis and destruction of the eye in some cases (206,207). Nicholson and Wolcheck reported a woman with a lymphoproliferative disorder of unknown type who developed widespread bilateral retinal necrosis while receiving prolonged systemic steroid therapy.

The case described by Nicholson and others is intriguing because it raises the question of whether corticosteroids should ever be used in immunocompromised individuals for treatment of toxoplasmic retinochoroiditis. Whereas the antiinflammatory response of corticosteroids may prove beneficial in immunocompetent patients, the impaired ability to limit replication of *Toxoplasma* in immunocompromised individuals is exaggerated by corticosteroid administration.

Development of toxoplasmosis in the setting of corticosteroid administration is well reported. Since corticosteroids are frequently used in combination with cytotoxic agents for prevention of transplant rejection and for treatment of malignancies, it is often difficult to accurately assess the degree to which corticosteroids alone predispose to reactivation of latent *Toxoplasma* infection. Nevertheless, dissemination of *Toxoplasma* infection has been known to occur in patients whose only treatment was with corticosteroids (59,66). Disastrous consequences of corticosteroid-containing treatment regimens for lymphoproliferative and myelopoietic disorders have developed when the clinical diagnosis of toxoplasmosis was missed (27,28,59,65,66,114). Treatment with high doses of corticosteroids in bone marrow transplant recipients with graft-versus-host disease (8,11,12,43,44,208), heart transplant recipients with rejection (14,33,36,76), or patients with suspected complications of SLE (59,61–64) has been followed by fatal dissemination of infection. These case reports are highly suggestive of the role of cortico-steroids alone as a risk factor in the development of toxoplasmosis.

COINFECTION WITH *TOXOPLASMA* AND OTHER ORGANISMS

In our review, 76 (37%) of 206 cases for whom sufficient information was available had coinfections (Table 17.9). Viruses, most notably cytomegalovirus (CMV), were the most frequent cause of the coexisting infection. CMV occurred in 24 (32%) (11,12,28,31,38,41,42,44,45,79,87–89,94,102,105,111,121,151,166,172,184) of 76 cases where coinfections were described; these represented 28% of all infections reported in association with toxoplasmosis in the non-AIDS immunocompromised patient (Table 17.10).

Whether the frequent concurrence of CMV and toxoplasmosis represents a marker for the severity of immunosuppression of the patient or a process whereby CMV and *Toxoplasma* favor replication and ongoing activity of the other infection is uncertain. Acute CMV infection in mice has been shown to predispose to reactivation of latent *Toxoplasma* infection (209). Furthermore, experiments in vitro suggest a permissive effect of CMV on the replication of *Toxoplasma* (210). In addition, cases have been described in which focal areas of necrosis were infected with both *Toxoplasma* and CMV (166). Other significant viral pathogens in the setting of toxoplasmosis in the non-AIDS immunocompromised patient have included herpes simplex virus (7,28,31, 38,53,79,105,173,174), varicella-zoster virus (7,27,45,92,118,134,174), and progressive multifocal leukoencephalopathy (7,87) (Table 17.10). Coexistent infectious diseases also were caused by bacteria (7,17,27,28,37,44,53,59,79,99,102,124,134,139,

Table 17.9   Coinfections in case reports of toxoplasmosis in immunocompromised patients

Condition	Number of coinfection reported (total case reports reviewed)
Malignancy*	
Hodgkin's lymphoma	13(59)
Non-Hodgkin's lymphoma	3(12)
Acute lymphocytic leukemia	5(11)
Acute myelogenous leukemia	0 (7)
Chronic lymphocytic leukemia	0 (6)
Chronic myelogenous leukemia	1 (9)
Transplants†	
Renal	8(22)
Heart (heart/lung)	6(24)
Bone marrow	10(21)
Liver	2 (2)

*SOURCE References 7,17,28,31,59,79,84,88,89,94,102,104,112,124,134,172–174,232.
†SOURCE References 8,11,12,27,28,32–34,36,38,41,44,52–54,58,60,114,115,121,143,151,200.

Table 17.10 Types of coinfection in 76* non-AIDS immunocompromised patients with toxoplasmosis

Type		Number
Bacterial		26
Fungal		16
Aspergillus	4	
Candida	8	
Torulopsis	2	
Histoplasma	1	
Cryptococcus	1	
Viral		45
CMV	24	
HSV	11	
VZV	7	
PML	2	
Adenovirus	1	
Other		7
P. carinii	3	
M. tuberculosis	3	
M. avium- intracellularae	1	

*76 of 206 cases had coinfections. Infections do not add up to 76 since several individuals had multiple coinfections at time of diagnosis of toxoplasmosis.
SOURCE See text for references.

151), fungi (8,11,28,37,52,54,88,89,104,143,192), *Pneumocystis carinii* (28,33,166), *Mycobacterium tuberculosis* (60,114,118), and *Mycobacterium avium-intracellularae* (7) (Table 17.10).

DIAGNOSIS

The severity and outcome of *Toxoplasma* infection in the immunocompromised patient depends on the nature and extent of the immunosuppression. Immunocompromised patients with toxoplasmosis are a heterogeneous group. It is important to gauge suspicion and diagnostic evaluation upon the specific underlying immunosuppression and clinical presentation. Thus, whereas toxoplasmosis most often occurs as a reactivation of chronic latent infection in patients whose normal host immunity has been compromised by endogenous or iatrogenic conditions, other groups of immunocompromised patients (e.g., heart and renal transplant recipients) develop toxoplasmosis by transmission of the infection via the transplanted organ, with exacerbation caused by adjuvant immunosuppressive drug regimens (Table 17.8). For this reason, it is important to evaluate patients with malignancies who will undergo cytotoxic chemotherapy or patients in need of organ transplantation at the earliest available time. In patients with Hodgkin's disease and other lymphoproliferative disorders, it is advisable to obtain *Toxoplasma* serologies at their earliest presentation. Individuals who are seropositive should be considered at risk for development of toxoplasmosis. Moreover, the frequency of toxoplasmosis in patients with lymphoproliferative disease is so low that a systematic study in this group has not been possible.

It is especially important to obtain a baseline *Toxoplasma* serology as part of the pre-bone-marrow-transplant evaluation, since serologies are most often without predictive value in the diagnosis of toxoplasmosis in the recipient of a bone marrow transplant. In contrast, patients undergoing heart/heart-lung and renal transplantation, should be considered at risk for the development of toxoplasmosis if they are a seronegative recipient of an organ from a seropositive donor (Table 17.8). Thus, it is important to test pre-organ-donor serum for *Toxoplasma* antibodies whenever feasible. Serologic diagnosis of active *Toxoplasma* infection may be complicated by immunosuppressive therapy and/or the patient's underlying condition. Thus, in the bone marrow transplant recipient, *Toxoplasma* titers are as likely to be increased, decreased, or unchanged after transplantation in patients with or without active infection (11). Serial measurements of antibody titers in the bone marrow posttransplant period are not useful for diagnosis of active *Toxoplasma* infection since more than 50% of patients' titers will have a significant decrease or seroreversion of their titers (11).

Heart transplant recipients who are seropositive prior to transplantation will frequently have significant rises in antibody titers without evidence of active disease (14). When serologic evidence of reactivation (a fourfold or greater rise in serial IgG antibody titers) has been observed in seropositive heart transplant recipients, none have convincingly been demonstrated to have clinical disease (14,38,138). Therefore, elevation of titers cannot, at present, be used to discriminate active from quiescent infection.

In addition to their frequent lack of predictive value in diagnosis of toxoplasmosis in the bone marrow recipients, false-positive *Toxoplasma* fluorescent antibody tests may occur in patients with antinuclear antibodies (211), thereby confounding the ability to make a specific serological detection of infection in patients with SLE. Passive transfer of *Toxoplasma* antibodies in patients receiving blood products may further complicate the diagnosis. Furthermore, clinically important false-positive IgM enzyme-linked immunosorbent assay (ELISA) results have been reported in individuals who have received rabbit anti-thymocyte globulin (ATG). This may reflect a cross-reactivity between human antibody to rabbit ATG and the conjugated rabbit antibody used as a reagent in the ELISA (212). If toxoplasmosis is to be diagnosed confidently in non-AIDS immunocompromised patients in the absence of histopathology, results of serology must be viewed as ancillary, to be used in combination with careful clinical evaluation.

Serology may be used in lieu of a definitive diagnosis to presumptively identify *Toxoplasma* as the cause of chorioretinitis. Measurement of local antibody production in aqueous humor may establish the diagnosis (213,214). In a retrospective study of 22 patients with toxoplasmic retinochoroiditis where *Toxoplasma* antibodies and total IgG were determined, 16 (73%) had a positive coefficient, indicating local antibody production (214).

The tissue culture method for isolation of *Toxoplasma* is at least as sensitive as inoculation (215) and has the advantage that it may be performed in routine clinical virology laboratories without need for animal facilities. *Toxoplasma* may be isolated within a few days to a week after tissue culture inoculation (152,215).

Experimental methods currently under development for detection of active *Toxoplasma* infection include IgA (216,217) or IgE (218) antibody, methods for detection of *Toxoplasma* antigen in blood (219) or urine (23), and PCR (143,165,220). These methods are not standardized as yet and cannot be recommended for routine evaluation of the non-AIDS immunocompromised patient with suspected toxoplasmosis.

TREATMENT

Our review substantiates the observations of Ruskin and Remington that, in immunocompromised individuals with toxoplasmosis, the infection is often lethal if untreated (Table 17.11). Among 48 patients in whom the diagnosis of toxoplasmosis was made early enough to begin specific treatment, 32 (67%) improved. This is in marked contrast to the severe morbidity or mortality in 89 (99%) of the 90 individuals who never received treatment (Table 17.11). The high mortality in the untreated group of immunocompromised patients reflects the fact that these were generally debilitated and severely immunocompromised individuals who often had multiple opportunistic infections. Therefore, although toxoplasmosis contributed to a poor prognosis, it was not necessarily the proximate cause of death.

At present, the exact dosing schedule for treatment of toxoplasmosis in non-AIDS immunocompromised patients has not been defined. However, much has been learned from the research into treatment of toxoplasmic encephalitis in patients with AIDS. The combination of the dihydrofolate reductase inhibitor, pyrimethamine, and the dihydropteroate synthetase inhibitor, sulfadiazine, remains the treatment of choice. In patients with encephalitis, we and others prefer higher dosages than have been previously recommended. Since pharmacokinetics of pyrimethamine vary widely between individuals and even within the same individual on different days (221,222), and given the life-threatening nature of this disorder, it would be optimal to achieve uniformly high blood levels of pyrimethamine in order to assure maximal therapeutic benefit. At present, we recommend that pyrimethamine be given as a loading dose of 100 to 200 mg and then 50 to 75 mg per day thereafter until acute signs and symptoms of toxoplasmosis have resolved. The sulfonamide component is essential to the effective treatment inasmuch as erratic absorption of pyrimethamine may not allow for complete toxoplasmacidal activity. The remarkable synergism achieved when sulfonamide is added to pyrimethamine makes this component crucial for maximal benefit. We recommend four to six grams, per day, of sulfadiazine for acute management.

After treatment of the acute stage of toxoplasmosis, the necessity for maintenance therapy is not clear. Whenever possible, concomitant immunosuppressive regimens should be minimized. This may allow for restitution of normal host immune mechanisms and result in containment of active *Toxoplasma* infection. Thus, in patients on corticosteroids who can be tapered to relatively less immunosuppressive dosages, the

Table 17.11   Effect of treatment on outcome of toxoplasmosis in the non-AIDS immunocompromised host

Condition	Number of cases	Treatment	Improved	No Treatment	Dead/ Deteriorated
Malignancy					
Hodgkin's lymphoma	35	12	8	23	23
Lymphoma	8	1		7	7
Angioimmunoblastic lymphadenopathy	3	1	1	2	2
Acute lymphocytic leukemia	11	6	5	5	4
Acute myelogenous leukemia	4	3		1	1
Chronic lymphocytic leukemia	2	1	1	1	1
Chronic myelogenous leukemia	7	2	2	5	5
Hairy cell leukemia	2	2	2		
Breast cancer	2			2	2
Transplant					
Heart	15	8	6	7	7
Bone marrow	20	7	4	13	13
Renal	16	3	2	13	13
SLE	8	1		7	7
Steroids	5	1	1	4	4
Totals	138	48(35)*	32(67)†	90(65)*	89(99)‡

*Number (percent total).
†Number (percent treated).
‡Number (percent not treated).
SOURCE See text for references.

patient with toxoplasmosis may be effectively managed with only an acute treatment regimen.

While the combination of pyrimethamine and sulfonamides are effective (Table 17.11), they frequently lead to adverse reactions that require discontinuation of one or both drugs. Folinic acid, 5 to 10 mg/day, may be used to forestall emergence of bone marrow toxicity associated with pyrimethamine. Folic acid should not be used since it may antagonize the anti-*Toxoplasma* activity of pyrimethamine.

Alternative regimens have been studied. Clindamycin may be considered to be an effective alternative to sulfadiazine when used in combination with pyrimethamine in patients with histories of severe allergy to sulfonamides. Spiramycin has proved ineffective in the prevention and treatment of toxoplasmosis in patients with AIDS, although it has not been investigated in non-AIDS immunocompromised patients. Sluitters et al. described two cases of seroconversion in seronegative heart transplant recipients despite prophylaxis with spiramycin (38). The macrolide/azalide drugs (clarithromycin, azithromycin, and roxithromycin) and the hydroxynapthoquinone, 566C80, have in vivo activity in mouse models against *Toxoplasma* (223–226), but sufficient data on their effectiveness in humans are not yet available. Clinical trials with these drugs are presently in progress.

Interferon gamma has been shown to be effective in the treatment of *Toxoplasma* infection in animal models (227). Also, in animal models, the combination of gamma interferon with antibiotics has been shown to enhance the activity of the antibiotic in curing *Toxoplasma* infection (223,228). Whether other biologics with activity in animal models (e.g., IL1 (229), IL2 (230), IFN-β (231) or TNF (229)) will have therapeutic usefulness in the management of toxoplasmosis in the non-AIDS immunocompromised patient remains to be determined.

For primary prophylaxis in patients who are at risk for development of toxoplasmosis, it has been suggested that seronegative recipients of a heart transplant from a sero-positive donor be given pyrimethamine. Hakim and others have shown this interven-tion to be effective (35). Analysis of published series reveal 19 seronegative recipients of hearts from seropositive donors who did not receive pyrimethamine prophylaxis. Thir-teen (68%) developed clinical evidence of toxoplasmosis associated with a definitive diagnosis either by endomyocardial biopsy or presumptively by a fourfold rise in IgG antibodies (14,38,138). In contrast (44,138,192), of 24 serologically mismatched recipi-ents who received six weeks' pyrimethamine prophylaxis, only two developed evidence of *Toxoplasma* infection proven by either endomyocardial biopsy or rise in *Toxoplasma* antibody titers. These two were treated with pyrimethamine and sulfadiazine and had a mild clinical course (138). Whether routine primary prophylaxis with pyrimethamine or trimethoprim-sulfamethoxazole should be administered to heart and bone marrow transplant recipients at high risk for development of toxoplasmosis will require a multicentered, prospective, comparative clinical trial to decide.

REFERENCES

1 Remington JS, Desmonts G. Toxoplasmosis. In: Remington JS, Klein JO, eds. *Infectious Diseases of the Fetus and Newborn Infant, Third Edition.* Philadelphia: The W.B. Saun-ders Company, 1990:89–195.

2 Ruskin J, Remington JS. Toxoplasmosis in the compromised host. *Ann Intern Med* 1976;84: 193–199.

3 Bodey GP, Rodriguez V, Chang H-Y, Nar-bvoni G. Fever and infection in leukemic patients. *Cancer* 1987;41:1610–1622.

4 Notter DT, Grossman PL, Rosenberg SA, Remington JS. Infections in patients with Hodgkin's disease: A clinical study of 300 consecutive adult patients. *Rev Infect Dis* 1980;2:761–800.

5 Carey RM, Kimball AC, Armstrong D, Lieber-man PH. Toxoplasmosis, clinical experiences in a cancer hospital. *Am J Med* 1973;54:30–38.

6 Graveleau PH, Henin D, Masson M, Daumas-Duport C, Graveleau J, Cambier J. Acquired cerebral toxoplasmosis: three anatomoclinical cases (English translation). *Rev Neurol* 1984; 140(5):330–342.

7 Hakes TB, Armstrong D. Toxoplasmosis—problems in diagnosis and treatment. *Cancer* 1983;52(8):1535–1540.

8 Beelen DW, Mahmoud HK, Mlynek ML, Schmidt U, Richter HJ, Schaefer UW. Toxo-plasmosis after bone marrow transplantation. *Immun Infect* 1986;14:183–187.

9 Bergin M, Menser MA, Procopis R, et al. Central nervous system toxoplasmosis and he-molytic uremic syndrome (Letter to the Editor). *N Engl J Med* 1987;317(24):1540–1541.

10 Dubin HW, Courter MH, Harrell ER. Toxo-plasmosis: a complication of corticosteroid and

cyclophosphamide treated lupus erythematosus. *Arch Dermatol* 1971;104:547–550.

11 Derouin F, Gluckman E, Beauvais B, et al. Toxoplasma infection after human allogeneic bone marrow transplantation: clinical and serological study of 80 patients. *Bone Marrow Transplant* 1986;1(1):67–73.

12 Hirsch R, Burke BA, Kersey JH. Toxoplasmosis in bone marrow transplant recipients. *J Pediatr* 1984;105(3):426–428.

13 Lowenberg B, Van Gijn J, Prins E, Polderman AM. Fatal cerebral toxoplasmosis in a bone marrow transplant recipient with leukemia. *Transplantation* 1983;35(1):30–34.

14 Luft BJ, et al. Primary and reactivated toxoplasma infection in patients with cardiac transplants: clinical spectrum and problems in diagnosis in a defined population. *Ann Intern Med* 1983;99:27–31.

15 McGregor CG, Fleck DG, Nagington J, Stovin PG, Cory-Pearce R, English TA. Disseminated toxoplasmosis in cardiac transplantation. *J Clin Pathol* 1984;37(1):74–77.

16 Luft BJ, Remington JS. Toxoplasmosis of the central nervous system. In: Remington JS, Swartz MN, eds. *Current Clinical Topics in Infectious Diseases, 6*. New York: McGraw-Hill Book Company, 1985:315–358.

17 Siegel SE, Lunde MN, Gelderman AH, et al. Transmission of toxoplasmosis by leukocyte transfusion. *Blood* 1971;37(4):388–394.

18 McCabe RE, Luft BJ, Remington JS. Effect of murine interferon gamma on murine toxoplasmosis. *J Infect Dis* 1984;150:961–962.

19 Suzuki Y, Conley FK, Remington JS. Importance of endogenous IFN-γ for prevention of toxoplasmic encephalitis in mice. *J Immunol* 1989;143(6):2045–2050.

20 Suzuki Y, Remington JS. The effect of anti-IFN-γ antibody on the protective effect of LYT-2⁺ immune T cells against toxoplasmosis in mice. *J Immunol* 1990;144(5):1954–1956.

21 Subauste CS, Remington JS. Role of gamma interferon in *Toxoplasma gondii* infection. *Eur J Clin Microbiol Infect Dis* 1991;10(2):58–67.

22 Suzuki Y, Orellana MA, Schreiber RD, Remington JS. Interferon-γ: The major mediator of resistance against *Toxoplasma gondii*. *Science* 1988;240:516–518.

23 Huskinson J, Stepick-Biek P, Remington JS. Detection of antigens in urine during acute toxoplasmosis. *J Clin Microbiol* 1989;27(5):1099–1101.

24 Ward R, Durge NG, Arya en J, Baqai M. Myocardial toxoplasmosis. *Lancet* 1964;2:723–725.

25 Pomeroy C, Miller L, McFarling L, Kennedy C, Filice GA. Phenotypes, proliferative responses, and suppressor function of lung lymphocytes during *Toxoplasma gondii* pneumonia in mice. *J Infect Dis* 1991;164:1227–1232.

26 Jacobs F, Depierreux M, Goldman M, et al. Role of bronchoalveolar lavage in diagnosis of disseminated toxoplasmosis. *Rev Infect Dis* 1991;13:637–641.

27 Cohen SN. Toxoplasmosis in patients receiving immunosuppressive therapy. *JAMA* 1970;211:657–660.

28 Gleason TH, Hamlin WB. Disseminated toxoplasmosis in the compromised host. *Arch Intern Med* 1974;134:1059–1062.

29 Rose MS, Black PJ, Barkhan P. Fatal outcome after combined therapy for myeloblastic leukaemia and toxoplasmosis. *Lancet* 1973;1(803):600.

30 Ryning FW, McLeod R, Maddox JC, Hunt S, Remington JS. Probable transmission of *Toxoplasma gondii* by organ transplantation. *Ann Intern Med* 1979;90(1):47–49.

31 Vietzke WM, Gelderman AH, Grimley PM, Valsamis MP. Toxoplasmosis complicating malignancy. Experience at the National Cancer Institute. *Cancer* 1968;21(5):816–827.

32 Britt RH, Enzmann DR, Remington JS. Intracranial infection in cardiac transplant recipients. *Ann of Neuro* 1981;9:107–119.

33 Froysaker T, Foerster A, Forfang K, et al. Heart transplantation in Norway: one year experience. *Scand J Thor Cardiovasc Surg* 1986;19:193–197.

34 Hall WA, et al. Central nervous system infections in heart and heart-lung transplant recipients. *Arch Neurol* 1989;46:173–177.

35 Hakim M, Esmore D, Wallwork J, English TA. Toxoplasmosis in cardiac transplantation. *Br Med J* 1986;292:1108.

36 McLeod R, Berry PF, Marshall WH, et al. Toxoplasmosis presenting as brain abscesses. *Am J Med* 1979;67:711–714.

37 Montero CG, Martinez AJ. Neuropathology of heart transplantation: 23 cases. *Neurology* 1986;36:1149–1154.

38 Sluiters JF, et al. Indirect enzyme-linked immunosorbent assay for immunoglobulin G and four immunoassays for immunoglobulin M to Toxoplasma gondii in a series of heart transplant recipients. *J Clin Microbiol* 1989;27:529–535.

39 Wreghitt TG, Hakim M, Cory-Pearce R, English TAH, Wallwork J. The impact of donor-transmitted CMV and *Toxoplasma gondii* disease in cardiac transplantation. *Trans Proc* 1986;18(5):1375–1376.

40   Emerson RG, Jardine DS, Milvenan ES, et al. Toxoplasmosis: a treatable neurologic disease in the immunologically compromised patient. *Pediatrics* 1981;67(5):653–655.

41   Fisher MA, Levy J, Helfrich M, Luft BJ, August CS, Starr SE. Detection of *Toxoplasma gondii* in the spinal fluid of a bone marrow transplant recipient. *Ped Infect Dis* 1987;6(1):81–83.

42   Guibeau JC, et al. Aspects temodensitometriques d'un cas de toxoplasmose intra-craniene chez un immuno-deprine. *J Radiol* (Paris) 1983;64:347.

43   Jehn U, Fink M, Gundlach P, et al. Lethal cardiac and cerebral toxoplasmosis in a patient with acute myeloid leukemia after successful allogeneic bone marrow transplantation. *Transplantation* 1984;38(4):430–433.

44   Shepp DH, Hackman RC, Conley FK, Anderson JB, Meyers JD. *Toxoplasma gondii* reactivation identified by detection of parasitemia in tissue culture. *Ann Intern Med* 1985;103(2):218–221.

45   Tang TT, Harb JM, Dunne WJ, et al. Cerebral toxoplasmosis in an immunocompromised host. A precise and rapid diagnosis by electron microscopy. *Am J Epidemiol* 1986;123(1):154–161.

46   Best T, Finlayson M. Two forms of encephalitis in opportunistic toxoplasmosis. *Arch Pathol Lab Med* 1979;103:693.

47   Callaway CS, et al. Electron microscopy studies of *Toxoplasma gondii* in fresh and frozen tissue. *Arch Pathol* 1968;86:484.

48   Flament-Durand J, Coers C, Waelbroeck C, Van Geertruyden J, Toussaint C. Toxoplasmic encephalitis and myositis during treatment with immunodepressive drugs (English translation). *Acta Clinica Belgica* 1967;22(1):44–54.

49   Ghatak NR, Sawyer DR. A morphologic study of opportunistic cerebral toxoplasmosis. *Acta Neuropath* 1978;42(3):217–221.

50   Guerin C, Miguet D, Genin C, et al. Generalized toxoplasmosis in a renal transplant patient (English translation). *La Presse Medicale* 1986;15(21):979.

51   Herb HM, Jontofsohn R, Löffler HD, Heinze V. Toxoplasmosis after renal transplantation. *Clin Nephrol* 1977;8(6):529–553.

52   Hooper DC, Pruitt AA, Rubin RH. Central nervous system infection in the chronically immunosuppressed. *Medicine* 1982;61(3):166–188.

53   Mason JC, Ordelheide KS, et al. Toxoplasmosis in two renal transplant recipients from a single donor. *Transplantation* 1987;44(4):588–591.

54   Mejia G, Leiderman E, Builes M, et al. Transmission of toxoplasmosis by renal transplant. *Am J Kidney Dis* 1983;II(6):615–617.

55   Munda R, Alexander JW, First MR, Gartside PS, Fidler JP. Pulmonary infections in renal transplant recipients. *Ann Surg* 1978;187:126–133.

56   Remington JS. Toxoplasmosis in the adult. *Cancer Res* 1975;50(2):211–227.

57   Reynolds ES, Walls KW, Pfeiffer RI. Generalized toxoplasmosis following renal transplantation. Report of a case. *Arch Intern Med* 1966;118(4):401–405.

58   Rhodes RH, Davis RL, Berne TV, Tatter D. Disseminated toxoplasmosis with brain involvement in a renal allograft recipient. *Bull Los Angeles Neurol Soc* 1977;42(1):16–22.

59   Townsend JJ, Wolinsky JS, Baringer JR, Johnson PC. Acquired toxoplasmosis. a neglected cause of treatable nervous system disease. *Arch Neurol* 1975;32(5):335–343.

60   Tsanaclis AM, de MC. Cerebral toxoplasmosis after renal transplantation. Case report. *Pathol Res Pract* 1986;181(3):339–341.

61   Deleze M, Mintz G, del Carmen, Majia M. *Toxoplasma gondii* encephalitis in systemic lupus erythematosus: a neglected cause of treatable nervous system infection. *J Rheum* 1985;12(5):994–996.

62   Hellman DB, Petri M, Whiting-O'Keefe Q. Fatal infection in systemic lupus erythematosus: the role of opportunistic organisms. *Medicine* 1987;66(5):341–348.

63   Karkouche B, Gremain J, Godeau P, Chomette G. Toxoplasmosis in the immunocompromised host. A report of three anatomiclinical cases (English translation). *Arch Anat Cytol Pathol* 1985;33:281–284.

64   Palmer DG. Systemic lupus erythematosus with cerebral complications [Letter to the Editor]. *N Z Med J* 1988;101(840):91.

65   Nicholson DH, Wolchok EB. Ocular toxoplasmosis in an adult receiving long-term corticosteroid therapy. *Arch Ophthalmol* 1976;94(2):248–254.

66   Pennoit DH, Lameire N, De Tollenaere G. Flare-up of toxoplasmosis caused by corticosteroid therapy of pulmonary sarcoidosis. *Ned Tijdschr Geneeskd* 1970;114:1288–1291.

67   Triki A, Couvreur J. Les manifestations neuromeningees de la toxoplasmose acquise. *Tunis Med* 1971;49:323–329.

68   Chernick NL, Armstrong D, Posner JB, et al. Central nervous system infections in patients with cancer. *Medicine* 1973;52:563–581.

69 Andres TL, et al. Immunohistochemical demonstration of *Toxoplasma gondii*. *Am J Clin Pathol* 1981;75:431–434.

70 Bamford CM. Toxoplasmosis mimicking a brain abscess in an adult with scleroderma. *Neurology* 1975;25:343–345.

71 Bertrand Y, Fegueux N, Rodiere M, Jean R. Toxoplasmose cerebrale fatale chez un enfant leucemique en remission. *Arch Fr Pediatr* 1988;45:347–348.

72 Cheever AW, et al. Necrotizing toxoplasmic encephalitis and herpetic pneumonia complicating treated Hodgkin's disease. *N Eng J Med* 1965;272:26.

73 Fiere, et al. Toxoplasmose intra-cerebrale au cours d'une maladie de Hodgkin d'evolution severe. *Lyon Med* 1970;223:1067–1072.

74 Fortsch D. Toxoplasma encephalitis in adults (English translation). *Deutsche Medizinische Wochenschrift* 1970;95:2362–2366.

75 Kersting G, Neuman J. "Malignant lyphoma" of the brain following renal transplantation. *Acta Neuropathol* 1975;VI(suppl):131.

76 Luft BJ, Billingham M, Remington JS. Endomyocardial biopsy in the diagnosis of toxoplasmic myocarditis. *Transplant Proc* 1986;18:1871–1873.

77 Marty R, Cain ML. Effects of corticosteroid (dexamethasone) administration on the brain scan. *Radiology* 1973;107:117–121.

78 Masson R, Fiere D, Lahneche B, Cordat C, Berger F, Revol L. Toxoplasmose encephalitique pseudotumorale au cours d'une hemopathie. *Nouv Press Med* 1975;4:2499–2502.

79 Meienberg O, Probst A, Schmidlin M, Planta M, Gratwohl A. Cerebrovascular insult and coma in a patient with acute lymphocytic leukemia (English translation). *Schweiz Rundsch Med Prax* 1986;75(45):1351–1355.

80 Narasimhan P, Ahn BH, Levy RN, Glasberg SS. Immunoblastic lymphadenopathy. High serum toxoplasma titer. *N Y State J Med* 1979;79(2):241–244.

81 O'Reilly MJ. Acquired toxoplasmosis: an acute fatal case in a young girl. *Med J Aust* 1954;2:968–969.

82 Prosmanne O, Chalaoui J, Sylvestre J, Lefebvre R. Small nodular pattern in the lungs due to opportunistic toxoplasmosis. *J Can Assoc Radiol* 1984;35(2):186–188.

83 Slavick HE, Lipman IJ. Brain stem toxoplasmosis complicating Hodgkin's disease. *Arch Neurol* 1977;34(10):636–637.

84 Smith GM, Leyland MJ, Crocker J, Geddes AM. Cerebral toxoplasmosis in a patient with Hodgkin's disease. *J Infect* 1987;14(3):243–245.

85 Tang TT, Harb JM, Dunne WM, et al. Reply to Dr. Kean's letter to the editor submitted to *American Journal of Clinical Pathology* 1986.

86 Wolf A, Kaufman MA, Cowen D. Adult toxoplasmosis. *Trans Am Neurol Assoc* 1953;78:284–286.

87 Yeo JH, Jakobiec FA, Iwamoto T, Richard G, Kreissig I. Opportunistic toxoplasmic retinochoroiditis following chemotherapy for systemic lymphoma. A light and electron microscopic study. *Ophthalmology* 1983;98(8):885–898.

88 Michaels MG, Wald ER, Fricker FJ, et al. Toxoplasmosis in pediatric recipients of heart transplants. *Clin Infect Dis* 1992;14:847–851.

89 Barlotta FM, Ochoa M, Neu HC, Ultmann JE. Toxoplasmosis, lymphoma, or both? *Ann Intern Med* 1969;70(3):517–528.

90 Belli AM, Elliott C, Heron CW. Case of the month: an opportunity not to be missed. *Br J Radiol* 1988;61:171–172.

91 Ghatak NR, Zimmerman HM. Fine structure of toxoplasma in the human brain. *Arch Pathol* 1973;95:276–283.

92 Ghatak NR, Poon TP, Zimmerman HM. Toxoplasmosis of the central nervous system in the adult. *Arch Pathol* 1970;89:337–348.

93 Grines C, Plouffe JF, Baird IM, Kandawalla N. Toxoplasma meningoencephalitis with hypoglycorrhachia. *Arch Intern Med* 1981;141:935.

94 Hemsath PA, Pinkerton H. Disseminated cytomegalic inclusion disease and disseminated toxoplasmosis in an adult with myeloid metaplasia. *Am J Clin Pathol* 1956;26:36–41.

95 Kalderon AE, Kikkawa Y, Bernstein J. Chronic toxoplasmosis associated with severe hemolytic anemia. *Arch Int Med* 1964;114:95–102.

96 Keel HJ, von Roth W, Keiser G, Reutter F, Martz G. Uber das Zusammentreffen von Morbus Hodgkin und Toxoplasmose. *Schweiz Med Wochenschr* 1963;93:1465–1469.

97 Knecht H, Rhyner K, Streuli RA. Toxoplasmosis in hairy-cell leukaemia. *Brit J Haematol* 1986;62:65–73.

98 Kusne S, et al. Self-limited toxoplasma parasitemia after liver transplantation. *Transplantation* 1987;44:457–458.

99 Launais B, Laurent G, Benchekroun S, et al. Neuromeningeal and chorioretinal manifestations of toxoplasmosis in a patient with immunodeficiency. *Sem Hop Paris* 1983;59(1):40–42.

100 Lemaire A, Boudin G, Lauras A, Debray J, Lyon G. Toxoplasmose cerebrale decouverte a

l'examen anatomique d'une leucemie mye-loide compliquee de troubles phychiques. *Bull Soc Med Hop, Paris* 1962;13:1102–1107.

101 Lods F. Chorioretinite toxoplasmique acquise au cours d'une leucemie aigue. *Bull Soc Ophthalmol* 1979;79(6–7)539–541.

102 Luna MA, Lichtiger B. Disseminated toxoplasmosis and cytomegalovirus infection complicating Hodgkin's disease. *Am J Clin Pathol* 1971;55(4):499–505.

103 Pilz P, Blinzinger K, Sniesko I. Cerebral toxoplasmosis complicating Hodgkin's disease in the adult. Light and electron-microscopic findings <Original> Cerebrale Erwachsenen-Toxoplasmose bei Morbus Hodgkin. Licht-und elektronenmikroskopische Befunde. *Arch Psychiatr Nervenkr* 1978;225(2):127–134.

104 Powell HC, Gibbs CJ Jr., Lorenzo AM, Lampert PW, Gajdusek DC. Toxoplasmosis of the central nervous system in the adult. Electron microscopic observations. *Acta Neuropathol (Berl)* 1978;41(3):211–216.

105 Strannegard O, Holm SE, Weinfeld A, Westin J. Serologic studies of infections in patients with hematologic malignancy. *Scand J Infect Dis* 1973;5(3):181–186.

106 Theologides A, Lee JC. Concomitant opportunistic infection. *Minn Med* 1970;53:21–23.

107 Budzilowitch GN. Acquired toxoplasmosis: a clinicopathological study of a case. *Am J Clin Pathol* 1961;35:66–76.

108 Renoult E, Chabot F, Aymard B, et al. Generalized toxoplasmosis in two renal transplant recipients who received a kidney from the same donor. *Rev Infect Dis* 1991;13:180–181.

109 Conner E, Menegus M, Cecalupo A, Gigliotti F. Central nervous system toxoplasmosis mimicking a brain abscess in a compromised pediatric patient. *Pediatr Infect Dis* 1984;3(6): 552–555.

110 de Crousaz G, de Tribolet H. Lymphogranulone de Hodgkin stabilise et encephalite necrosante a toxoplasme. *Arch Suiss Neurol Neurochir Psychiatr* 1972;110:1–12.

111 Frenkel JK, Nelson BM, Arias-Stella J. Immunosuppression and toxoplasmic encephalitis: clinical and experimental aspects. *Hum Pathol* 1975;6:97–111.

112 Frenkel JK, Amare M, Larsen W. Immune competence in a patient with Hodgkin's disease and relapsing toxoplasma. *Infection* 1978;6(2):84–91.

113 Green JA, et al. Favorable outcome of central nervous system toxoplasmosis occurring in a patient with untreated Hodgkin's disease. *Cancer* 1980;45(4):808–810.

114 Koeze TH, Klingon GH. Acquired toxoplasmosis. *Arch Neurol* 1964;11:191–197.

115 Leyva WH, Santa Cruz DJ. Cutaneous toxoplasmosis. *J Am Acad Derm* 1986;14(4): 600–605.

116 Mashaly R, Gray F, Poisson M, Rancurel G, Escourolle R, Buge A. Adult acquired cerebral toxoplasmosis. A clinical and neuropathological study (English translation). *Rev Neurol* 1983;139(10):561–568.

117 Mazer S, Araujo JC, Riberiro KC, Kasting G. Unusual computed tomographic presentation of cerebral toxoplasmosis. *Am J Neurosurg* 1983;4:458–460.

118 Toussaint D, Vanderhaeghen J. Ocular toxoplasmosis, trigeminal herpes zoster and pulmonary tuberculosis in a patient with Hodgkin's disease. *Ophthalmol* 1975;171:237–243.

119 Bernard J, Boiron M, Levy JP, et al. Toxoplasmose generalisee associee a une leucemie aigue. *Nouv Rev Fr Heatol* 1962;2:910–914.

120 Dry J, et al. Acute toxoplasmosis with necrotizing vasculitis (English translation). *Ann Med Interne (Paris)* 1979;130(8–9):401–404.

121 Kusne S, Dummer JS, Singh N, et al. Infections after liver transplantation. An analysis of 101 consecutive cases. *Medicine* 1988; 67(2):132–143.

122 Summerfield GP. Demonstration of lesions of cerebral toxoplasmosis by computerized tomography. *Postgrad Med J* 1980;56:112.

123 Tang TT, Dunne WM, Meyer GA, et al. Authors' reply to letter to the editor entitled "Cerebral toxoplasmosis" from L. Cerezo (see also Cerezo, L., pg. 757). *Am J Clin Pathol* 1986.

124 Theologides A, Osterberg K, Kennedy BJ. Cerebral toxoplasmosis in multiple myeloma. *Ann Intern Med* 1966;64(5):1071–1074.

125 Embil JA, Covert AA, Howes WJ, Tanner CE, Staudt M. Visualization of *Toxoplasma gondii* in the cerebrospinal fluid of a child with a malignant astrocytoma. *C M A J* 1985;133:213–214.

126 Gentry LO, Zeluff BJ. Diagnosis and treatment of infection in cardiac transplant patients. *Surg Clin N Am* 1986;66:459–465.

127 Henry JM, Hefner RR, Dillard SH, et al. Primary malignant lymphomas of the CNS. *Cancer* 1974;34:1293–1302.

128 de la Torre FE, Gorraez M. Toxoplasma-induced occlusive hypertrophic arteritis as the cause of discrete coagulative necrosis in the CNS. *Hum Pathol* 1989;20:604–605.

129 Huang TE, Chou SM. Occlusive hypertrophic arteritis as the cause of discrete necrosis in CNS toxoplasmosis in the acquired immu-

nodeficiency syndrome. *Hum Pathol* 1988; 19:1210–1214.

130 Conley FK, Jenkins KA, Remington JS. *Toxoplasma gondii* infection of the central nervous systems. Use of the peroxidase antiperoxidase method to demonstrate toxoplasma in formalin fixed paraffin embedded tissue sections. *Hum Pathol* 1981;12:690–698.

131 Holland GN. Ocular toxoplasmosis in the immunocompromised host. *Intern Ophthal* 1989;13:399–402.

132 Shachor J, Shneyour A, Radnay J, Steiner ZP, Bruderman I. Toxoplasmosis in a patient with common variable immunodeficiency. *Am J Med Sci* 1984;287(3):36–38.

133 Figuier P, Saragoussi JJ, Cavaille-Coll M, LeHoang P, Offret H. Acquired ocular toxoplasmosis and immunosuppression caused by a thymic tumor (English translation). *J Fr Opthalmol* 1984;7(12):813–817.

134 Hoerni B, Vallat M, Durand M, Pesme D. Ocular toxoplasmosis and Hodgkin's disease. *Arch Ophthalmol* 1978;96(1):62–63.

135 Holland GN, O'Connor GR, Diaz RF, Minasi P, Wara WM. Ocular toxoplasmosis in immunosuppressed nonhuman primates. *Invest Ophthalmol Vis Sci* 1988;29:835–841.

136 Newell FW. Toxoplasmosis. In: *Ophthalmology: Principles & Concepts*, 7th Edition. Mosby, 1992:450–451.

137 Derouin F, Gluckman E, Auber P, et al. Toxoplasmosis in bone marrow transplant patients. Evaluation of the risk factors; guidelines for prophylaxis. In: *Proceedings of First International Conference on the Prevention of Infection*, Nice, 1990;#PD2046.

138 Wreghitt TG, et al. Toxoplasmosis in heart and heart and lung transplant recipients. *J Clin Pathol* 1989;42:194–199.

139 Wertlake PT, Winter TS. Fatal toxoplasma myocarditis in an adult patient with acute lymphocytic leukemia. *N Engl J Med* 1965; 273:438–440.

140 Pinkerton J, Henderson RG. Adult toxoplasmosis: previously unrecognized diseases simulating typhus-spotted fever group. *JAMA* 1941:116;807–814.

141 Wreghitt TG, Hakim M, Gray JJ, et al. A detailed study of *Toxoplasma gondii* infections in heart and heart/lung transplant patients at Papworth Hospital, Cambridge. In: *Proceedings of International Symposium on Infections in the Immunocompromised Host*, The Netherlands, 1988.

142 Vinh LT, Barbet JP, Mace B, Rousset S, Huault G. La pneumonie toxoplasmique avec generalisation. *Semaine Des Hopitaux De Paris* 1980:56:744–750.

143 Holliman RE, Johnson J, Burke M, Adams S, Pepper JR. False negative dye-test finding in a case of fatal toxoplasmosis associated with cardiac transplantation. *J Infect* 1990;21: 185–189.

144 Pomeroy C, Filice GA. Pulmonary toxoplasmosis: a review. *Clin Infect Dis* 1992;14: 863–870.

145 Cockerill F, Wilson WR, Carpenter HA, Smith TF, Rosenow EC. Open lung biopsy in immunocompromised patients. *Arch Intern Med* 1985;145:1398–1404.

146 Kennedy BJ, Theologides A. Pulmonary infiltrate. Initial manifestation of toxoplasmosis. *Minn Med* 1971;54:321–325.

147 Maguire GP, Tatz J, Giosa R, Ahmed T. Diagnosis of pulmonary toxoplasmosis by bronchoalveolar lavage. *N Y State J Med* 1986;86(4):204–205.

148 Ludlam GB, Beattie CP. Pulmonary toxoplasmosis. *Lancet* 1963;2:1136–1138.

149 Catteral JR, Hofflin JM, Remington JS. Pulmonary toxoplasmosis. *Am Rev Respir Dis* 1986:133;704–705.

150 Bendelac A, Laporte JP, Marteau M, et al. Detection of a pulmonary localization of *Toxoplasma gondii* in an immunosuppressed patient (letter to the editor). *Presse Med* 1984;13(19):1213–1214.

151 Stinson EB, Bieber CP, Griepp RB, et al. Infectious complications after transplantation in a man. *Ann Intern Med* 1971;74:22–36.

152 Derouin F, Sarfati C, Beauvais B, et al. Laboratory diagnosis of pulmonary toxoplasmosis in patients with acquired immune deficiency syndrome. *J Clin Microbiol* 1989; 27:1661–1663.

153 Mawhorter SD, Effron D, Blinkhorn R, Spagnuolo PJ. Cutaneous manifestations of toxoplasmosis. *Clin Infect Dis* 1991;14: 1084–1088.

154 Justus J. Cutaneous manifestations of toxoplasmosis. *Curr Prob Dermatol* 1972;4:24–47.

155 Binazzi M. Profile of cutaneous toxoplasmosis. *Int J Dermatol* 1986;25:357–363.

156 Topi G, Gandolfo LD, Giacolone B, Griso D, Zardi O, Angiroffo A. Acquired cutaneous toxoplasmosis. *Dermatologica* 1983;167: 24–32.

157 Piringer-Kuchinka A, Martin I, Thalhammer O. Uber die vorzuglich cervico-nuchale Lymphadenitis mit kleinherdiger Epithelioid zellwucherung. *Virchows Arch* [A]1958;351: 535–552.

158 Saxen E, Saxen L. The histological diagnosis of glandular toxoplasmosis. *Lab Invest* 1959; 8:386–394.

159 Stansfeld AF. The histological diagnosis of toxoplasmic lymphadenitis. *J Clin Pathol* 1961;4:565–578.

160 Dorfman RF, Remington JS. Value of lymph node biopsy in the diagnosis of acute acquired toxoplasmosis. *N Eng J Med* 1973; 289:878–881.

161 Weiss LM, Yuan-Yuan C, Berry GJ, Strickler JG, Dorfman RF, Warnke RA. Infrequent detection of toxoplasma gondii genome in toxoplasmic lymphadenitis: A polymerase chain reaction study. *Hum Path* 1992:23:154–158.

162 Gray GF, Kimball AC, Kean BH. The posterior cervical lymph node in toxoplasmosis. *Am J Pathol* 1972;69:349–358.

163 Connolly CS. Hodgkin's disease associated with *Toxoplasma gondii*. *Arch Int Med* 1963; 112:393–396.

164 Bachman F, Keiser G, Martenent AC. Die erworbene Erwachsenen-toxoplasmose. *Hel Med Acta* 1962;29:156–177.

165 Jurges E, Young Y, Eltumi M, et al. Transmission of toxoplasmosis by bone marrow transplant associated with Campath-1G. *Bone Marrow Transplantation* 1992;9:65–66.

166 Karasawa T, Shikata T, Takizawa I, Morita K, Komukai M. Localized hepatic necrosis related to cytomegalovirus and *Toxoplasma gondii*. *Acta Pathol Jpn* 1981;31(3):527–534.

167 Sheagren JN, Lunde MN, Simon HB. Chronic lymphadenopathic toxoplasmosis. A case with marked hyperglobulinemia and impaired delayed hypersensitivity responses during active infection. *Am J Med* 1976;60(2):300–305.

168 Lopez-Ruz MA, Ortego-Centeno N, Herrnandez-Quero J, Miras-Parra F, de la Higuera J. Association of polymyositis and toxoplasmosis (English translation). *Med Clin (Barc)* 1986;87(6):246–248.

169 Hendrickx GFM, Verhage J, Jennekens FGI, van Knapen F. Dermatomyositis and toxoplasmosis. *Ann Neurol* 1978;5:393–395.

170 Hicsonmez G, Kanra G, Gursel T, Yetkin S, Altintas K. Acute lymphoblastic leukemia and toxoplasmosis. *Turk J Pediatr* 1979;21(1): 24–27.

171 Araujo JC. Tumoral forms of toxoplasmosis. In: *Proceedings of the XVIII Latin American Congress of Neurosurgery*, November 1979, p 261.

172 Magnin PH, Casas JG, Korte CG. Cryptococcosis, Hodgkin's disease and toxoplasmosis. Case report with autopsy <Original>

Cryptococcose, Morbus Hodgkin und Toxoplasmose mit Nekropsie. Caso presenta de necropsia. *Mykosen* 1971;14(11):515–523.

173 Vortel V, Peychl L. Two cases of acquired latent focal toxoplasmosis of the brain in a cytostatic & corticosteroid treated neoplastic disease. *Sb Ved Pr Lek Fak Karlovy Univerzity Hradei Kralove* 1970;13:107–111.

174 Mackowiak PA, Demian SE, Sutker WL, et al. Infections in hairy cell leukemia. Clinical evidence of a pronounced defect in cell-mediated immunity. *Am J Med* 1980;68: 718–724.

175 Abell C, Holland P. Acute toxoplasmosis complicating leukemia. *Am J Dis Child* 1969;118:782–787.

176 Green I, Carson PF. A study of skin homografting in patients with lymphoma. *Blood* 1959:14:235.

177 Miller DG, Lizardo JG, Snyderman RK. Homologous and heterologous skin transplantation in patients with lymphomatous disease. *J Natl Cancer Inst* 1969:26:569.

178 Sokol JE, Primikiro M. The delayed skin test response in Hodgkin's disease and lymphosarcoma. *Cancer* 1969;14:597.

179 Eltringham JS, Kaplan HS. Impaired delayed hypersensitivity response in 154 patients with untreated Hodgkin's disease. *Natl Cancer Inst Monogr* 1973;36:127.

180 Aixenberg AC. Studies on delayed hypersensitivity in Hodgkin's disease. *J Clin Invest* 1962;41:1964.

181 King GW, Yanes B, Hurtubise PE, et al. Immune function of successfully treated lymphoma patients. *J Clin Invest* 1976;57:1451.

182 Engleman EG, Benike CJ, Hoppe RT, Kaplan HS. Autologous mixed lymphocyte reaction in patients with Hodgkin's disease: evidence for a T-cell defect. *J Clin Invest* 1980;66:149.

183 Gaines JD, Gilmer A, Remington JS. Deficiency of antigen recognition in Hodgkin's disease. *Natl Cancer Inst Monogr* 1973;36: 117–121.

184 McLeod R, Estes R. Role of lymphocyte blastogenesis to *Toxoplasma gondii* antigens in containment of chronic, latent *Toxoplasma gondii* infections in humans. *Clin Exp Immunol* 1985;62:24–30.

185 Kimball AC, Kean BH, Kellner A. The risk of transmitting toxoplasmosis by transfusion. *Transfusion* 1965;5:447–451.

186 Catterall JR, Black CM, Leventhal JP, Rizk NW, Wachtel JS, Remington JS. Nonoxidative microbicidal activity in normal human

alveolar and peritoneal macrophages. *Infect Immun* 1987;55:1635–1640.

187 **Catterall JR, Sharma SD, Remington JS.** Oxygen-independent killing by alveolar macrophages. *J Exp Med* 1986;163:1113–1131.

188 **Israelski DM, Araujo FG, Wachtel JS, Heinrichs L, Remington JS.** Differences in microbicidal activities of human macrophages against *Toxoplasma gondii* and *Trypanosoma cruzi. Infect Immun* 1990;58(1):263–265.

189 **Stewart DJ, Bodey GP.** Infections in hairy cell leukemia (leukemic reticuloendotheliosis). *Cancer* 1981;47:801–805.

190 **Chrobak L, Bostikova D, Mirova S, Hozak A, Radochova D.** Hairy-cell leukemia and toxoplasmosis. *Neoplasma* 1982;29(4):487–492.

191 **Rose AG, Uys CJ, Novitsky D, Cooper DK, Barnard CN.** Toxoplasmosis of donor and recipient hearts after heterotopic cardiac transplantation. *Arch Pathol Lab Med* 1983; 107(7):368–373.

192 **Volker H, Sigmund M, Kropff M, et al.** Myokarditis durch Toxoplasma gondii und aspergillus fumigatus nach orthoroper herztransplantation. *Z Kardiol* 1991;80:359–362.

193 **Hofflin JM, et al.** Infectious complications in heart transplant recipients receiving cyclosporine and cortiocosteroids. *Ann of Int Med* 1987;106:209–216.

194 **Copeland DJ, Stinson EB.** Human heart transplantation. *Curr Probl Cardiol* 1980;3: 4–51.

195 **Hofflin JM, Postasman I, Baldwin JC, Oyer PE, Stinson EB, Remington JS.** Infectious complications in heart transplant recipients receiving cyclosporine and corticosteroids. *Ann Intern Med* 1987;106:209–216.

196 **Nagington J, Martin AL.** Toxoplasmosis and heart transplantation. *Lancet* 1983;2:679.

197 **Price LA, Bondy PK.** Fatal outcome after combined therapy for myeloblastic leukaemia and toxoplasmosis. *Lancet* 1973;1:727.

198 **Alintas K.** Incidence of toxoplasmosis in cases of Hodgkin's and non-Hodgkin's lymphoma (English translation). *Mikrobiyol Bult* 1983;17(4):251–256.

199 **Derouin F, Debure A, Godeaut E, Lariviere M, Kreis H.** Toxoplasma antibody titers in renal transplant recipients. *Transplantation* 1987;44(4):515–518.

200 **Anthony CW.** Disseminated toxoplasmosis in a liver transplant patient. *J Am Med Wom Assoc* 1972;27:601–603.

201 **Rosner S, Ginzler E, Diamond H, et al.** A multicenter study of outcome in systemic lupus erythematosus: II: Causes of death. *Arthritis Rheum* 1982;25:612–617.

202 **Wilcox MH, et al.** Toxoplasmosis and systemic lupus erythematosus. *Ann Rheum Dis* 1990;49:254–257.

203 **Frenkel JK.** Effects of cortisone, total body irradiation, and nitrogen mustard on chronic, latent toxoplasmosis. *Am J Path* 1957;33(3): 618–619.

204 **Erichsen S, Harboe A.** Toxoplasmosis in chickens. *Acta Path Microbiol Scand* 1953; 33:56–71.

205 **Metzger M, et al.** The influence of zymosan, cortisone and x-rays on the course of experimental toxoplasmosis in white rats. *Arch Immunol Ther Exp (Warsz)* 1963;11:227–233.

206 **O'Connor GR, Frenkel JK.** Dangers of steroid treatment in toxoplasmosis. *Arch Ophthalmol* 1976;94:213.

207 **Sabates R, Pruett RC, Brockhurst RJ.** Fulminant ocular toxoplasmosis. *Am J Ophthalmol* 1981;92:497–503.

208 **Beelen DW, Mahmoud HK, Mlynek ML, et al.** Toxoplasmosis after bone marrow transplantation (English translation). *Hamatol Bluttransfus* 1987;30:574–578.

209 **Pomeroy C, Kline S, Jordan MC, Filice GA.** Reactivation of *Toxoplasma gondii* by cytomegalovirus disease in mice: antimicrobial activities of macrophages. *J Infect Dis* 1989; 160:305–311.

210 **Gelderman AH, Grimley PM, Lunde MN, Rabson AS.** *Toxoplasma gondii* and cytomegalovirus: mixed infection by a parasite and a virus. *Science* 1968;160(3832):1130–1132.

211 **Araujo FG, Barnett EV, Gentry LO, Remington JS.** False-positive anti-toxoplasma fluorescent antibody tests in patients with antinuclear antibodies. *Appl Microbiol* 1971; 22(3):270–275.

212 **Naot Y, Luft BJ, Remington JS.** False positive serological tests in heart transplant recipients. *Lancet* 1981;2:590–591.

213 **Desmonts G.** Central nervous system toxoplasmosis (Letter to the Editor). *Pediat Infect Dis J* 1987;6(9):872–873.

214 **Kijlstra A, et al.** Aqueous humor analysis as a diagnostic tool in toxoplasma uveitis. *Intern Ophthal* 1989;13:383–386.

215 **Derouin F, et al.** Comparative study of tissue culture and mouse inoculation methods for demonstration of *Toxoplasma gondii. J Clin Micro* 1987;25:1597–1600.

216 **Huskinson J, Thulliez P, Remington JS.** Toxoplasma antigens recognized by human

immunoglobulin A antibodies. *J Clin Microbiol* 1990;28(12):2632–2636.

217 Huskinson J, Thulliez P, Remington JS. Toxoplasma antigens recognized by human immunoglobulin A antibodies. *J Clin Microbiol* 1990;28(12):2632–2636.

218 Pinon JM, Toubas D, Marx C, Mougeot G, et al. Detection of specific immunoglobulin E in patients with toxoplasmosis. *J Clin Microbiol* 1990;28:1739–1743.

219 Araujo FG, Remington JS. Antigenemia in recently acquired acute toxoplasmosis. *J Infect Dis* 1980;141:144–150.

220 Burg J, Grover C, Pouletty P, Boothroyd J. Direct and sensitive detection of a pathogenic protozoan, *Toxoplasma gondii*, by polymerase chain reaction. *J Clin Microbiol* 1989;27(8):1787–1792.

221 Weiss LM, Harris C, Berger M, et al: Pyrimethamine concentrations in serum and cerebrospinal fluid during treatment of acute Toxoplasma encephalitis in patients with AIDS. *J Infect Dis* 1988;157:580–583.

222 Leport C, Meulemans A, Dameron, et al: Levels of pyrimethamine in serum of AIDS patients treated for toxoplasmic encephalitis. Presented at the 4th European Congress of Clinical Microbiology (Abstract #843), Nice, April 1989.

223 Hofflin JM, Remington JS. *In vivo* synergism of roxithromycin (RU 965) and interferon against *Toxoplasma gondii*. *Antimicrob Agents Chemother* 1987;31:346–348.

224 Araujo FG, Guptill DR, Remington JS. Azithromycin, a macrolide antibiotic with potent activity against *Toxoplasma gondii*. *Antimicrob Agents Chemother* 1988;32(5):755–757.

225 Araujo FG, Huskinson J, Remington JS. Remarkable *in vitro* and *in vivo* activities of the hydroxynaphthoquinone 566C80 against tachyzoites and tissue cysts of *Toxoplasma gondii*. *Antimicrob Agents Chemother* 1991;35(2):293–299.

226 Huskinson-Mark J, Araujo FG, Remington JS. Evaluation of the effect of drugs on the cyst form of *Toxoplasma gondii*. *J Infect Dis* 1991;164(1):170–177.

227 McCabe RE, Brooks RG, Dorfman RF, Remington JS. Clinical spectrum in 107 cases of toxoplasmic lymphadenopathy. *Rev Infect Dis* 1987;9:754–774.

228 Israelski DM, Remington JS. Activity of gamma interferon in combination with pyrimethamine or clindamycin in treatment of murine toxoplasmosis. *Eur J Clin Microbiol Infect Dis* 1990;9(5):358–360.

229 Chang HR, Grau GE, Pechere JC. Role of TNF and IL-1 in infections with *Toxoplasma gondii*. *Immunology* 1990;69(1):33–37.

230 Sharma SD, Hofflin JM, Remington JS. In vivo recombinant interleukin 2 administration enhances survival against a lethal challenge with *Toxoplasma gondii*. *J Immunol* 1985;135:4160–4163.

231 Orellana MA, Suzuki Y, Araujo FG, Remington JS. Role of beta interferon in resistance to *Toxoplasma gondii* infection. *Infect Immun* 1991;59(9):3287–3290.

232 Karasawa T, Takizawa I, Morita K, et al. Polymyosites and toxoplasmosis. *Acta Pathol Jpn* 1981;31(4):675–680.

Index